50 Landmark Papers

every

Vascular and Endovascular Surgeon Should Know

50 Landmark Papers

every

Vascular and Endovascular Surgeon Should Know

EDITED BY

Juan Carlos Jimenez, MD, MBA
Professor of Surgery
Gonda (Goldschmied) Vascular Center
David Geffen School of Medicine at UCLA
Los Angeles, California

Samuel Eric Wilson, MD
Distinguished Professor of Surgery and Chair Emeritus
University of California Irvine
Irvine, California

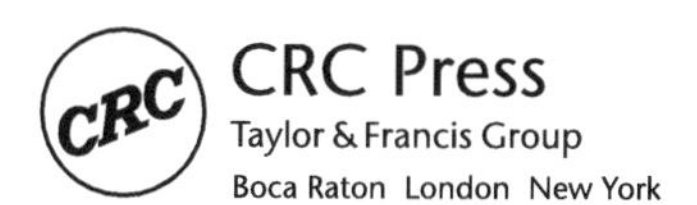
CRC Press
Taylor & Francis Group
Boca Raton London New York

CRC Press is an imprint of the
Taylor & Francis Group, an **informa** business

First edition published 2021
by CRC Press
6000 Broken Sound Parkway NW, Suite 300, Boca Raton, FL 33487-2742

and by CRC Press
2 Park Square, Milton Park, Abingdon, Oxon, OX14 4RN

CRC Press is an imprint of Taylor & Francis Group, LLC

ISBN: 9781138335356 (hbk)
ISBN: 9781138334380 (pbk)
ISBN: 9780429434020 (ebk)

Typeset in Times LT Std
by Nova Techset Private Limited, Bengaluru & Chennai, India

Contents

Section One Cerebrovascular

Section Two Infrarenal Aortic Aneurysm

Section Three Aortic Dissection

Section Six Visceral Occlusive Disease

Section Seven Peripheral Artery Aneurysms

Section Eight Venous

Section Nine Vascular Medicine

Section Ten Miscellaneous Topics

Preface

The evolution of vascular surgery over the past decade has brought profound and rapid changes to our practice. Endovascular techniques are now our predominant intervention. Certainly, no field of modern surgery has experienced so many changes in such a brief period of time. Accordingly, we thought it would be worthwhile to capture those key articles establishing these changes in practice, bearing in mind that vascular surgery measures its success by the scientific method. We should proudly acknowledge that vascular surgeons have responded by changing training paradigms and mastering evolving technological advances.

We have assembled this volume of expert reviews remembering Henry Ford's assertion that:

> *"I invented nothing new. I simply assembled the discoveries of other men behind whom were centuries of work ... Progress happens when all the factors that make for it are ready and then it is inevitable. To teach that a comparatively few men are responsible for the greatest forward steps of mankind is the worst sort of nonsense."*

Our aim is to provide the research that supports our current standards of practice. As there are many more than 50 studies which have impacted our specialty, we acknowledge this collection is neither exclusive nor definitive. In our opinion, however, the selected studies contain essential knowledge for all 21st-century vascular and endovascular surgeons.

Abstracts for the manuscripts and an author or expert review are provided. Our reviewers have assessed the impact of the paper on current practice. We thank our reviewers who have contributed their expertise selflessly.

Juan Carlos Jimenez, MD, MBA
Samuel Eric Wilson, MD

Contributors

Mark Ajalat
Division of Vascular Surgery
David Geffen School of Medicine at UCLA
Los Angeles, California

Mark Archie
Division of Vascular and Endovascular Surgery
Harbor–UCLA Medical Center
Los Angeles, California

Meena Archie
Division of Vascular Surgery
David Geffen School of Medicine at UCLA
Los Angeles, California

Samuel P. Arnot
Pitzer College
Claremont, California

Enrico Ascher
Division of Vascular Surgery
New York University
New York, New York

Ali Azizzadeh
Division of Vascular and Endovascular Surgery
Cedars-Sinai Medical Center
Los Angeles, California

Donald Baril
Division of Vascular Surgery
David Geffen School of Medicine at UCLA
Los Angeles, California

Adam W. Beck
Division of Vascular Surgery and Endovascular Therapy
University of Alabama at Birmingham
Birmingham, Alabama

Michael Belkin
Division of Vascular and Endovascular Surgery
Brigham and Women's Heart and Vascular Center
Boston, Massachusetts

Thakshyanee Bhuvanakrishna
University Hospitals Southampton
Southampton, United Kingdom

Nina Bowens
Division of Vascular and Endovascular Surgery
Harbor–UCLA Medical Center
Los Angeles, California

Neal S. Cayne
Division of Vascular Surgery
New York University
New York, New York

Rabih Chaer
Division of Vascular Surgery
University of Pittsburgh Medical Center
Pittsburgh, Pennsylvania

Benjamin B. Chang
Division of Vascular Surgery
Albany Medical College
Albany Medical Center Hospital
Albany, New York

K.M. Charlton-Ouw
Department of Cardiothoracic and Vascular Surgery
McGovern Medical School
University of Texas
Houston, Texas

Tristen T. Chun
Division of Vascular Surgery
David Geffen School of Medicine at UCLA
Los Angeles, California

Jayer Chung
Division of Vascular and Endovascular Therapy
Baylor College of Medicine
Houston, Texas

Dawn Marie Coleman
Division of Vascular and Endovascular Surgery
University of Michigan
Ann Arbor, Michigan

Anthony Comerota
Inova Heart and Vascular Institute
Inova Alexandria Hospital
Alexandria, Virginia

Michael Conte
Division of Vascular and Endovascular Surgery
University of California, San Francisco
San Francisco, California

R. Clement Darling III
Division of Vascular Surgery
Albany Medical Center Hospital
Albany, New York

Brian DeRubertis
Division of Vascular Surgery
David Geffen School of Medicine at UCLA
Los Angeles, California

C.A. Durham
Houston Methodist Hospital
Houston, Texas

Matthew Eagleton
Division of Vascular and Endovascular Surgery
Massachusetts General Hospital
Boston, Massachusetts

Anthony L. Estrera
Department of Cardiothoracic and Vascular Surgery
McGovern Medical School
University of Texas
Houston, Texas

Steven M. Farley
Division of Vascular Surgery
David Geffen School of Medicine at UCLA
Los Angeles, California

Julie Freischlag
Wake Forest Baptist Medical Center
Winston-Salem, North Carolina

Justin Galovich
Division of Vascular Surgery
David Geffen School of Medicine at UCLA
Los Angeles, California

Hugh Gelabert
Division of Vascular Surgery
David Geffen School of Medicine at UCLA
Los Angeles, California

Peter Gloviczki
Gonda Vascular Center
Mayo Clinic
Rochester, Minnesota

Jerry Goldstone
Division of Vascular Surgery
Stanford University School of Medicine
Palo Alto, California

Roger Greenhalgh
Vascular Surgical Research Group
Imperial College
London, United Kingdom

Juan Carlos Jimenez
Gonda (Goldschmied) Vascular Center
David Geffen School of Medicine at UCLA
Los Angeles, California

William D. Jordan
Division of Vascular and Endovascular Surgery
Emory University
Atlanta, Georgia

Nii-Kabu Kabutey
Division of Vascular and Endovascular Surgery
University of California, Irvine
Irvine, California

Vikram S. Kashyap
Division of Vascular Surgery
University Hospitals
Case Western Reserve University
Cleveland, Ohio

Alexander H. King
University Hospitals Cleveland Medical Center
Cleveland, Ohio

Paul B. Kreienberg
Division of Vascular Surgery
Albany Medical College
Albany Medical Center Hospital
Albany, New York

Peter F. Lawrence
Division of Vascular Surgery
David Geffen School of Medicine at UCLA
Los Angeles, California

Gregory A. Magee
Division of Vascular Surgery and Endovascular Therapy
Keck Medical Center of USC
Los Angeles, California

Hazel Marecki
Division of Vascular Surgery
University of Massachusetts Medical School
Worcester, Massachusetts

Charles C. Miller III
Division of Cardiothoracic and Vascular Surgery
McGovern Medical School
University of Texas
Houston, Texas

Joseph L. Mills
Division of Vascular and Endovascular Therapy
Baylor College of Medicine
Houston, Texas

Wesley S. Moore
Division of Vascular Surgery
David Geffen School of Medicine at UCLA
Los Angeles, California

Rameen Moridzadeh
Division of Vascular Surgery
David Geffen School of Medicine at UCLA
Los Angeles, California

Ian Nordon
Vascular and Endovascular Surgery
University Hospitals Southampton
Southampton, United Kingdom

D. Ocazionez
Department of Diagnostic and Interventional Imaging
University of Texas Medical School at Houston
Memorial Hermann Hospital
Houston, Texas

Jessica Beth O'Connell
Division of Vascular Surgery
David Geffen School of Medicine at UCLA
Los Angeles, California

Gustavo S. Oderich
Aortic Center
Mayo Clinic
Rochester, Minnesota

Zoë Öhman
BIBA Medical
London, United Kingdom

Joe Pantoja
Division of Vascular Surgery
David Geffen School of Medicine at UCLA
Los Angeles, California

Woosup M. Park
Vascular Surgery
Cleveland Clinic Abu Dhabi
Abu Dhabi, United Arab Emirates

Gaurav M. Parmar
Division of Vascular Surgery and Endovascular Therapy
University of Alabama at Birmingham
Birmingham, Alabama

Rhusheet Patel
Division of Vascular Surgery
David Geffen School of Medicine at UCLA
Los Angeles, California

William J. Quinones-Baldrich
Division of Vascular Surgery
David Geffen School of Medicine at UCLA
Los Angeles, California

H.M. Ray
Department of Cardiothoracic and Vascular Surgery
McGovern Medical School
University of Texas
Houston, Texas

David Rigberg
Division of Vascular Surgery
David Geffen School of Medicine at UCLA
Los Angeles, California

Fiona Rohlffs
Vascular Surgical Research Group
Imperial College
London, United Kingdom

Hazim J. Safi
Division of Cardiothoracic and Vascular Surgery
McGovern Medical School
University of Texas at Houston
Houston, Texas

Harleen K. Sandhu
Division of Cardiothoracic and Vascular Surgery
McGovern Medical School
University of Texas
Houston, Texas

Andres Schanzer
Division of Vascular and Endovascular Surgery
University of Massachusetts Medical School
Worcester, Massachusetts

Gaurav Sharma
Division of Vascular and Endovascular Surgery
Brigham and Women's Heart and Vascular Center
Boston, Massachusetts

Cynthia K. Shortell
Division of Vascular and Endovascular Surgery
Department of Surgery
Duke University School of Medicine
Durham, North Carolina

Emanuel Ramos Tenorio
Aortic Center
Mayo Clinic
Rochester, Minnesota

Steven Tohmasi
University of California, Irvine School of Medicine
Irvine, California

Jesus G. Ulloa
Division of Vascular Surgery
David Geffen School of Medicine at UCLA
Los Angeles, California

Frank J. Veith
Division of Vascular and Endovascular Surgery
New York University Medical School
New York, New York

and

Division of Vascular and Endovascular Surgery
Cleveland Clinic Lerner College of Medicine
Case Western Reserve University
Cleveland, Ohio

Gabriela Velázquez
Division of Vascular and Endovascular Surgery
Wake Forest Baptist Medical Center
Winston-Salem, North Carolina

Fred Weaver
Division of Vascular Surgery and Endovascular Therapy
Keck Medical Center of USC
Los Angeles, California

E. Hope Weissler
Division of Vascular and Endovascular Surgery
Duke University
Durham, North Carolina

Samuel Eric Wilson
University of California Irvine
Irvine, California

Karen Woo
Division of Vascular Surgery
David Geffen School of Medicine at UCLA
Los Angeles, California

Chapter 1

Beneficial Effect of Carotid Endarterectomy in Symptomatic Patients with High-Grade Carotid Stenosis

North American Symptomatic Carotid Endarterectomy Trial Collaborators, Barnett HJM, Taylor DW, Haynes RB et al. N Engl J Med. 1991 Aug 15;325(7):445–53

ABSTRACT

Background Without strong evidence of benefit, the use of carotid endarterectomy for prophylaxis against stroke rose dramatically until the mid-1980s, then declined. Our investigation sought to determine whether carotid endarterectomy reduces the risk of stroke among patients with a recent adverse cerebrovascular event and ipsilateral carotid stenosis.

Methods We conducted a randomized trial at 50 clinical centers throughout the United States and Canada, in patients in two predetermined strata based on the severity of carotid stenosis—30%–69% and 70%–99%. We report here the results in the 659 patients in the latter stratum, who had had a hemispheric or retinal transient ischemic attack or a nondisabling stroke within the 120 days before entry and had stenosis of 70%–99% in the symptomatic carotid artery. All patients received optimal medical care, including antiplatelet therapy. Those assigned to surgical treatment underwent carotid endarterectomy performed by neurosurgeons or vascular surgeons. All patients were examined by neurologists 1, 3, 6, 9, and 12 months after entry and then every 4 months. Endpoints were assessed by blinded, independent case review. No patient was lost to follow-up.

Results Life-table estimates of the cumulative risk of any ipsilateral stroke at 2 years were 26% in the 331 medical patients and 9% in the 328 surgical patients—an absolute risk reduction (+/– SE) 17% +/– 3.5% (P less than 0.001). For a major or fatal ipsilateral stroke, the corresponding estimates were 13.1% and 2.5%—an absolute risk reduction of 10.6% +/– 2.6% (P less than 0.001). Carotid endarterectomy was still found to be beneficial when all strokes and deaths were included in the analysis (P less than 0.001).

Conclusions Carotid endarterectomy is highly beneficial to patients with recent hemispheric and retinal transient ischemic attacks or nondisabling strokes and ipsilateral high-grade stenosis (70%–99%) of the internal carotid artery.

EXPERT COMMENTARY BY SAMUEL ERIC WILSON

We decided to include this article because it describes the clinical research that saved carotid endarterectomy (CEA) as the most effective treatment over the last 30 years for moderate to severe symptomatic carotid stenosis. In the 1980s, neurologists and internists became concerned about the results of CEA, particularly the varying indications for operation and reports of high levels of postoperative complications. One example of this skepticism is seen in the 1984 journal article in *Stroke* in which the author asks, "Carotid Endarterectomy: Does It work?"[2] Recognizing the steep decline in CEA operations, vascular surgeons decided to demonstrate efficacy by defining clear cut indications for CEA[3] and proceeding with three cooperative trials: an NIH-sponsored trial (NASCET),[1] the VA Cooperative Study 309,[4] and a European trial.[5] All three trials showed such an unexpected, impressive reduction in ipsilateral stroke after CEA in moderate to severe symptomatic patients that a clinical alert was published in *Stroke* before the formal publication of NASCET results.[6]

As described in the abstract, the 659 patients who had a hemispheric transient attack, nondisabling stroke or retinal transient ischemic attack within 120 days of entry, and had 70%–99% stenosis were randomized to best medical treatment versus medical treatment and CEA. The cumulative risk for ipsilateral stroke at 2 years follow-up was 26% in the 331 medical patients and was decreased to 9% in the 328 surgical patients ($p < 0.001$). The VA Cooperative Trial found that after one year there was a reduction in stroke or crescendo transient ischemic attacks in men from 19.4% in medically treated patients to 7.7% in CEA patients. ($p = 0.011$).[2] These studies, and others, established irrefutably the role of carotid endarterectomy in preventing stroke. A 2015 international systematic review found that 31 of 33 (94%) published guidelines for CEA in patients who had 50%–99% symptomatic stenosis recommended CEA.[7]

The benefit of CEA may be greater if an operation is performed soon after the transient ischemic event. A retrospective review of clinical outcome at the Mayo Clinic showed that CEA can be done with "acceptable risk in properly selected symptomatic patients within 2 weeks" of the transient ischemic attack.[8]

The appropriate use of CEA still has room for improvement. In the records of 3,167 CEAs done in four Canadian provinces, Kennedy et al. found adherence to strict criteria for appropriateness to vary from 78% to 46% and inappropriate use to be 10% overall.[9]

The precise role and methods of carotid stenting are currently under clinical investigation. The lesson of how comparative, randomized clinical trials established the value of CEA, if followed, will provide reliable future guidelines.

REFERENCES

1. North American Symptomatic Carotid Endarterectomy Trial Collaborators. Beneficial effect of carotid endarterectomy in symptomatic patients with high grade stenosis. *N Eng J Med*. 1991:325:445–53.
2. Warlow C. Carotid endarterectomy: Does it work? *Stroke*. 1984;15(6): 068–76.
3. Wilson SE, Mayberg MR, and Yatsu FM. Defining the indications for carotid endarterectomy. *Surgery*. 1988;104:923–3.
4. Mayberg MR, Wilson SE, Yatsu F et al. Carotid endarterectomy and prevention of cerebral ischemia in symptomatic carotid stenosis. Veterans Affairs Cooperative Studies Program 309 Trialist Group. *JAMA*. 1991;266:3289–94.
5. Randomized trial of endarterectomy for recently symptomatic carotid stenosis: Final results of the MRC European Carotid Surgery Trial (ECST). *Lancet*. 1998;351:1379–87.
6. NASCET Investigators. Clinical Alert: Benefit of carotid endarterectomy for patients with high-grade stenosis of internal carotid artery. *Stroke*. 1991;22:816–7.
7. Abbott AL, Paraskevas KI, Kakkos SK et al. Systematic review of guidelines for the management of asymptomatic and symptomatic carotid stenosis. *Stroke*. 2015;46:3288–3301.
8. Brinjikji W, Rabinstein AA, Meyer FB et al. Risk of early carotid enterectomy for symptomatic carotid stenosis. *Stroke*. 2010;41:2186–2190.
9. Kennedy J, Quan H, Ghali WA, and Feasby TE. Variations in rates of appropriate carotid endarterectomy for stroke prevention in 4 Canadian provinces. *CMAJ*. 2004;171:455–459.

CHAPTER 2

Stenting versus Endarterectomy for Treatment of Carotid-Artery Stenosis

Brott TG, Hobson RW 2nd, Howard G, Roubin GS, Clark WM, Brooks W, Mackey A, Hill MD, Leimgruber PP, Sheffet AJ et al.
CREST Investigators. N Engl J Med. 2010 Jul 1;363(1):11–23

ABSTRACT

Background Carotid-artery stenting and carotid endarterectomy are both options for treating carotid-artery stenosis, an important cause of stroke.

Methods We randomly assigned patients with symptomatic or asymptomatic carotid stenosis to undergo carotid-artery stenting or carotid endarterectomy. The primary composite endpoint was stroke, myocardial infarction, or death from any cause during the periprocedural period or any ipsilateral stroke within 4 years after randomization.

Results For 2,502 patients over a median follow-up period of 2.5 years, there was no significant difference in the estimated 4-year rates of the primary endpoint between the stenting group and the endarterectomy group (7.2% and 6.8%, respectively; hazard ratio with stenting, 1.11; 95% confidence interval, 0.81 to 1.51; P = 0.51). There was no differential treatment effect with regard to the primary endpoint according to symptomatic status (P = 0.84) or sex (P = 0.34). The 4-year rate of stroke or death was 6.4% with stenting and 4.7% with endarterectomy (hazard ratio, 1.50; P = 0.03); the rates among symptomatic patients were 8.0% and 6.4% (hazard ratio, 1.37; P = 0.14), and the rates among asymptomatic patients were 4.5% and 2.7% (hazard ratio, 1.86; P = 0.07), respectively. Periprocedural rates of individual components of the endpoints differed between the stenting group and the endarterectomy group: for death (0.7% vs. 0.3%, P = 0.18), for stroke (4.1% vs. 2.3%, P = 0.01), and for myocardial infarction (1.1% vs. 2.3%, P = 0.03). After this period, the incidences of ipsilateral stroke with stenting and with endarterectomy were similarly low (2.0% and 2.4%, respectively; P = 0.85).

Conclusions Among patients with symptomatic or asymptomatic carotid stenosis, the risk of the composite primary outcome of stroke, myocardial infarction, or death did not differ significantly in the group undergoing carotid-artery stenting and the group undergoing carotid endarterectomy. During the periprocedural period, there was a higher risk of stroke with stenting and a higher risk of myocardial infarction with endarterectomy. (ClinicalTrials.gov number, NCT00004732.)

AUTHOR COMMENTARY BY WESLEY S. MOORE

Research Question/Objective The primary objective of the CREST trial was to compare the outcomes of carotid artery stenting (CAS) with those of carotid endarterectomy (CEA) among symptomatic and asymptomatic patients with extracranial carotid stenosis. The primary endpoint, for comparison, was a composite of stroke, myocardial infarction or death from any cause during the periprocedural period or any ipsilateral stroke within 4 years of randomization.

Study Design Prospective, multicentered randomized trial in which patients with symptomatic or asymptomatic carotid stenoses were allocated to either CEA or transfemoral CAS.

Sample Size 2,502 patients.

Follow-Up This initial report was published after the last patient entered had completed 1 year of follow-up. The median follow-up for the entire group, at time of this initial publication, was 2.5 years.

Inclusion/Exclusion Criteria Patients were included if they were considered average risk for either CEA or CAS. Patients were considered symptomatic if they had a territorial TIA or nondisabling stroke within 180 days of randomization. They had to have a 50% stenosis, or greater, of the study artery by angiography, or 70% or greater by duplex ultrasound, MRA, or CTA. Patients were considered asymptomatic if they never had symptoms in the distribution of the study artery or if prior symptoms, such as TIA, were absent for at least 180 days prior to randomization. Patients were excluded if they had confounding variables such as prior disabling stroke, atrial fibrillation, myocardial infarction within 30 days of randomization, or unstable angina.

Intervention or Treatment Received CEA was performed as per an approved surgeon's practice. 90% of CEA was performed under general anesthesia, 62.4% had patch closure, and 56.7% had a shunt employed during clamping for CEA. CEA patients received 325 mgm of aspirin (ASA) within 48 hours of operation in 92.1% of cases and 91.1% continued ASA following operation. All patients received standard medical therapy, as needed, to treat hypertension, diabetes, and hyperlipidemia. CAS was performed as per published guidelines using the transfemoral approach. The protocol required the use of the Acculink stent and, where possible, the Accunet filter distal protection device. At least 48 hours prior to stenting, patients received ASA 325 mgm twice daily and clopidogrel 75 mgm twice daily. After stenting, patients received one or two doses of ASA 325 mgm daily and either clopidogrel 75 mgm daily or ticlopidine 250 mgm twice daily for 4 weeks. Continuation of antiplatelet drugs after 4 weeks was recommended for all patients. Standard medical therapy for hypertension, diabetes, and hyperlipidemia was at discretion of the treating physician.

Results The 4-year primary endpoint, which was a composite of periprocedural death, any stroke, myocardial infarction, and ipsilateral stroke within 4 years of randomization, was 7.2% for CAS and 6.8% for CEA. This difference was not statistically different. However, 61/1,262 (4.8%) patients randomized to CAS died or had a stroke in the periprocedural interval. This is compared to 33/1,240 (2.7%) patients randomized to CEA in the same time interval. That difference is statistically significant in favor of CEA. Fourteen patients randomized to CAS had a nonfatal myocardial infarction (MI) compared to 28 patients randomized to CEA. That difference is statistically significant in favor of CAS.[1]

Study Limitations The major limitation of this study was the decision to formulate a composite endpoint for primary analysis. By adding death, any stroke, myocardial infarction, and any ipsilateral stroke within 4 years of the study into a single endpoint, it is implied that each of those complications are of equal importance, when they clearly are not. It is only when the individual complications are broken out that it is possible to discern that CAS carried nearly twice the periprocedural death/stroke rate when compared to CEA.

Relevant Studies There have been several prospective randomized trials comparing transfemoral carotid stenting to carotid endarterectomy. The EVA-3S trial was a prospective randomized trial carried out in France. 525 patients, who had recently become symptomatic and had at least a 60% carotid stenosis, were randomly allocated to either CAS or CEA. The study was stopped early by the safety monitoring committee because the complications of stroke and death were clearly and significantly higher in CAS. The patients continued to be followed, and by the end of 4 years, 11.1% of CAS patients had suffered death or stroke compared with 6.2% of CEA patients. This difference was entirely accounted for by the higher periprocedural event rate with CAS.[2] The large ICSS (International Carotid Stenting Study) trial reported similar results. Between May 2001 and October 2008, 1,713 symptomatic patients from 50 academic centers in Europe, Australia, New Zealand, and Canada were enrolled and randomized to either CAS or CEA. The risk of stroke, death, or procedural myocardial infarction 120 days after randomization was significantly higher in CAS patients compared to CEA (8.5% vs. 5.2%).[3]

Study Impact The CREST trial results have been used by interventionists to claim that CAS results are equivalent to CEA. Unfortunately, this is not an accurate assessment. The design error of lumping death, stroke, and MI into a single primary endpoint has led to this misinterpretation. Since all carotid artery interventions have, as their primary objective, the prevention of stroke and stroke-related death, then those two adverse outcomes must be the primary basis of comparison. Nonfatal myocardial infarction is an important adverse outcome, but that event alone cannot compare with death and stroke. In CREST, there were nine deaths in the CAS group compared to four in the CEA group. There were 52 strokes in the CAS group compared to 29 in the CEA group. The only outcome measure that favored CAS

Table 2.1 Adverse Primary Events and Cumulative Penalty Point Value

	CAS #	CAS Points	CEA #	CEA Points	P Value
Death	9	90	4	40	
Major Stroke	11	88	8	64	
Minor Stroke	41	287	21	147	
MI	14	70	28	140	
Total		535		391	<0.0001

over CEA was nonfatal MI where there were 28 in the CEA group compared to 14 in the CAS group. In retrospect, it might have been better to assign a weighting to each of the three major adverse events. In order to assign a penalty point score for each adverse event, we can look at this from the patient's perspective. In the CREST trial, SF-36 questionnaires were performed in living patients comparing the physical and mental impact of a complication to patients without the complication. Obviously, death speaks for itself. From the patient's perspective, the complication that had the greatest impact on their lives was a major stroke. This was followed closely by minor stroke. Interestingly, at the end of one year, MI, from the patient's perspective, had no effect on their physical or mental well-being. With this observation, from the patient's perspective, I would like to offer a possible scoring system to measure adverse events. I would assign 10 penalty points to death, 8 penalty points to major stroke, 7 penalty points to minor stroke, and 5 penalty points to MI. The results of this analysis are summarized in Table 2.1. In summary, CAS earned 535 penalty points compared to 391 penalty points for CEA. That difference was statistically significant with $P < 0.0001$.

REFERENCES

1. Brott TG, Hobson RW II, Howard G et al. Stenting versus endarterectomy for treatment of carotid-artery stenosis. *N Engl J Med*. 2010;363:11–23.
2. Mas JL, Trinquart L, Leys D et al., for the EVA-3S Investigators. Endarterectomy versus angioplasty in patients with symptomatic severe carotid stenosis (EVA-3S trial). Results up 4 years from a randomized, multicenter trial. *Lancet Neurol*. 2008;7:895–92.
3. International Study Investigators. Carotid artery stenting compared with endarterectomy in patients with symptomatic carotid stenosis (International Carotid Stenting Study): An interim analysis of a randomized controlled trial. *Lancet*. 2010;375:985–97.

Chapter 3

Endarterectomy for Asymptomatic Carotid Artery Stenosis

Walker MD, Marler JR, Goldstein M et al. JAMA. 1995;273(18):1421–8. doi: 10.1001/jama.1995.03520420037035

EXPERT COMMENTARY BY WESLEY S. MOORE

Research Question/Objective To determine whether the addition of carotid endarterectomy to aggressive medical management can reduce the incidence of cerebral infarction in patients with asymptomatic carotid artery stenosis.

Study Design Prospective, randomized, multicenter trial.

Sample Size 1,662 patients.

Follow-Up Patients were entered between December 1987 and December 1993. Publication of results occurred in 1995.[1] After randomization the patients were seen at 1 month and then at 3-month intervals alternating between telephone and clinic visits. At conclusion of the study, the median follow-up interval was 2.7 years with 4,657 patient years of observation.

Inclusion/Exclusion Criteria Inclusion criteria consisted of documentation of at least a 60% diameter reducing stenosis as documented by intra-arterial contrast angiography and duplex doppler ultrasound. Patients had to be between ages 40 and 79 years. Exclusion criteria included prior cerebrovascular events in the distribution of the study artery or vertebral-basilar symptoms within 45 days of randomization. Also excluded were patients who were intolerant of aspirin or had a medical condition that would likely lead to death or disability within 5 years of randomization.

Intervention or Treatment Received Patients in both the surgical and medical randomized groups received what was considered optimal medical management at that time. This included 325 mgm of aspirin daily. Patients were counseled regarding risk factor modification including blood pressure management, diabetes control, tobacco cessation, alcohol moderation, and a healthy diet. Patients randomized to surgical care had to undergo carotid endarterectomy within 2 weeks of randomization. No effort was made to specify details of the surgical procedure or choice of anesthesia. However, surgeons who wished to participate in the study were required to submit their prior surgical experience and results to a surgical management committee for review and approval. Criteria were established to identify those surgeons, whose experience and results were deemed to be well qualified for participation.[2]

Results The event rate of ipsilateral stroke or death in those randomized to surgery within 30 days of randomization was 2.3%. However, it should be noted that complications of preoperative angiography were counted against the surgery arm since it was argued that an angiogram would not have been performed if surgery had not been contemplated. The complications of preoperative angiography of stroke and death, in the surgery group, was 1.2%.

The study achieved significance after a median follow-up of 2.7 years. The incidence of ipsilateral periprocedural stroke/death or a subsequent stroke in any distribution for the surgical group was 5.1% compared to 11% for the medical group. This difference was statistically significant with $P = 0.004$.

Study Limitations At the time when this study was performed and published in 1995, it was regarded as a model of clinical science with no limitations identified. However, with the passage of time and medical progress, several limitations can now be identified in light of today's practice. By today's standards, patients did not receive optimal medical management. Statins had yet to be invented, no specific criteria for blood pressure control had been mandated, HbA1c was not used to monitor diabetic patients, exercise programs were not included, and abstinence of tobacco products, while recommend, was not mandated or monitored. From the surgical management perspective, intra-arterial contrast angiography, the single largest cause of post-randomization stroke and stroke related death in the study, is now seldom if ever performed.[3]

Relevant Studies Prior to publication of this study (ACAS), a prospective randomized study, performed in the Veterans Affairs Hospital system, was published. It, too, documented the benefit of adding carotid endarterectomy to medical management over medical management alone.[4] However, following publication, the trial was criticized in that transient ischemic attacks (TIAs) were included as endpoints together with stroke and death. While the study also showed a trend in favor of surgery in reducing stroke and death, the study was not sufficiently powered to use stroke and death alone for endpoints.

During the conduct of the ACAS trial, a similar study was initiated in the United Kingdom (UK). The UK trial, entitled the Asymptomatic Carotid Surgery Trial (ACST), continued after publication of ACAS and was subsequently published. It included the largest number of patients of any similar trial to date (larger than ACAS) and came to the identical conclusion, thus validating the ACAS results.[5]

Study Impact With the publication of ACAS, the prior VA study, and subsequent ACST trial, the relatively common practice of offering carotid endarterectomy (CEA) to patients with "high-grade" asymptomatic carotid stenosis now had level 1 evidence to support that practice. The number of CEAs performed in the United States rapidly exceeded 100,000/year with more than 90% being performed in asymptomatic patients. With development of duplex scanning, more and more patients were being offered CEA using that diagnostic parameter alone. With the development of magnetic resonance angiography (MRA) and computed tomographic angiography (CTA), the list of noninvasive imaging options has widened. Unfortunately, this has led to CEA being overused beyond what was justified based upon ACAS. The threshold carotid stenosis in ACAS was a 60% diameter reducing lesion as documented by contrast angiography. Using duplex scanning, that usually meant that it would need to fall into the category 80%–99% stenosis or a peak systolic velocity of at least 230 cm/sec and an ICA/CC ratio of at least 4. The average clinician who sees a duplex scan report stating that there is a 60%–79% lesion present assumes that this also corresponds to a similar percent stenosis as measured by contrast angiography, when it clearly does not. Likewise, MRA also tends to overread percent stenosis as does CTA.

Finally, medical management, as a form of primary prevention, has clearly improved over the years. The introduction of statin therapy to reduce LDL levels has had a remarkable impact upon atherosclerotic plaque stabilization and now figures prominently in primary prevention. This has led to a re-examination of the role of CEA in patients with asymptomatic carotid stenosis with the advent of the CREST 2 study. CREST 2 is a two-track, prospective, randomized, controlled trial that is designed to compare the benefit of either carotid stent/angioplasty (CAS) plus intensive medical management or CEA plus intensive medical management versus intensive medical management alone. Intensive medical management includes 325 mgm aspirin daily, the use of a statin drug to keep LDL cholesterol below 70 mgm/dcL, and medical management to keep systolic blood pressure below 130 mmHg. For diabetic patients it means careful control to maintain their HbA1c below 7%. Intensive medical management also includes an exercise program supervised to accommodate a patient's tolerance, as well as a program to help those still using tobacco products, to quit. At this time, the study enrollment is at about the halfway mark. Once enrollment is complete and the last patient has had 2 years of follow-up, we will know whether or not ACAS is still relevant.[6,7]

REFERENCES

1. Endarterectomy for asymptomatic carotid artery stenosis. Executive Committee for the Asymptomatic Carotid Atherosclerosis Study. *JAMA* 1995;273:1421–8.
2. Moore WS, Vescera CL, Robertson JT, Baker WH, Howard, VJ, and Toole JF. Selection process for surgeons in the Asymptomatic Carotid, Atherosclerosis Study. *Stroke.* 1991;22:1353–7
3. Chervu A and Moore WS. Carotid endarterectomy without arteriography. *Ann Vasc Surg.* 1994;8:296–302.
4. Hobson RW II, Weiss DG, and Fields WS, for the Veterans Affairs Cooperative Study Group. Efficacy of carotid endarterectomy for asymptomatic carotid stenosis. *N Engl J Med.* 1993;328:221–7.

5. Haliday A, Mansfield A, Marro J et al. MRC Asymptomatic Carotid Surgery Trial (ACST). Collaborative Group. Prevention of disabling and fatal strokes by successful carotid endarterectomy in patients without neurological symptoms: Randomized controlled trial. *Lancet*. 2004;363(9420):1491–502.
6. Moore, WS. Issues to be addressed and hopefully resolved in the carotid revascularization endarterectomy versus stenting trial 2. *Angiology*. 2015;1–3
7. Howard, VJ, Meschia JF, Lal BK et al., on behalf of the CREST-2 investigators. Carotid revascularization and medical management for asymptomatic carotid stenosis: Protocol of the CREST-2 trials. *Int J Stroke*. 2017;12:770–8.

CHAPTER 4

A Multi-Institutional Analysis of Transcarotid Artery Revascularization Compared to Carotid Endarterectomy

Kashyap VS, King AH, Foteh MI, Janko M, Jim J, Motaganahalli RL, Apple JM, Bose S, Kumins NH. J Vasc Surg. 2019 Jul;70(1):123–9. doi: 10.1016/j.jvs.2018.09.060. Epub 2019 Jan 6

ABSTRACT

Objective Transcarotid artery revascularization (TCAR) is a novel approach to carotid intervention that uses a direct carotid cut-down approach coupled with cerebral blood flow reversal to minimize embolic potential. The initial positive data with TCAR indicates that it may be an attractive alternative to transfemoral carotid artery stenting and possibly carotid endarterectomy (CEA) for high-risk patients. The purpose of this study was to present 30-day and 1-year outcomes after treatment by TCAR and to compare these outcomes against a matched control group undergoing CEA at the same institutions.

Methods A retrospective review of all patients who underwent TCAR at four institutions between 2013 and 2017 was performed to evaluate the use of the ENROUTE Transcarotid Neuroprotection System (Silk Road Medical, Inc, Sunnyvale, Calif). TCAR patients had high-risk factors and were either enrolled in prospective trials or treated with a commercially available TCAR device after U.S. Food and Drug Administration approval. Contemporaneous patients undergoing CEA at each institution were also reviewed. Patients were propensity matched in a 1:1 (CEA:TCAR) fashion with respect to preoperative comorbidities. Data were analyzed using statistical models with a P value of less than 0.05 considered significant. Individual and composite stroke, myocardial infarction, and death at 30 days and 1 year postoperatively were assessed.

Results Consecutive patients undergoing TCAR or CEA were identified (n = 663) and compared. Patients undergoing the TCAR procedure (n = 292) had higher rates of diabetes (P = 0.01), hyperlipidemia (P = 0.02), coronary artery disease (P < 0.01), and renal insufficiency (P < 0.01) compared with unmatched CEA patients (n = 371). Stroke rates were similar at 30 days (1.0% TCAR vs. 1.1% CEA) and 1 year

(2.8% TCAR vs. 3.0% CEA) in the unmatched groups. After propensity matching by baseline characteristics including gender, age, symptom status (36.3%, 35.3%) and diabetes, 292 TCAR patients were compared with 292 CEA patients. TCAR patients were more likely to be treated preoperatively and postoperatively with clopidogrel (preoperatively, 82.2% vs. 39.4% [P < 0.01]; postoperatively, 98.3% vs. 36.0% [P < 0.01]) and statins (preoperatively, 88.0% vs. 75.0% [P < 0.01]; postoperatively, 97.8% vs. 78.8% [P < 0.01]). Stroke (1.0% TCAR vs. 0.3% CEA; P = 0.62) and death (0.3% TCAR vs. 0.7% CEA; P = NS) rates were similar at 30 days and comparable at 1 year (stroke, 2.8% vs. 2.2% [P = 0.79]; death 1.8% vs. 4.5% [P = 0.09]). The composite endpoint of stroke/death/myocardial infarction at 1 month postoperatively was 2.1% vs. 1.7% (P = NS). TCAR was associated with a decreased rate of cranial nerve injury (0.3% vs. 3.8%; P = 0.01).

Conclusions These early data suggest that patients undergoing TCAR, even those with high-risk comorbidities, achieve broadly similar outcomes compared with patients undergoing CEA while mitigating cranial nerve injury. Further comparative studies are warranted.

AUTHOR COMMENTARY BY VIKRAM S. KASHYAP AND ALEXANDER H. KING

As with any new technology, there can be some initial skepticism. We were early participants of trials studying transcarotid artery revascularization (TCAR). As our experience grew, we were heartened by the good results even in the most challenging patients. Thus, we collaborated with other early adopters of TCAR to understand the outcomes from this procedure. In this propensity-matched study of transcarotid artery revascularization (TCAR) to carotid endarterectomy (CEA), we aimed to directly compare postoperative outcomes of patients with atherosclerotic carotid bifurcation disease after undergoing TCAR or CEA. This was a multicenter retrospective review of prospectively collected data from 663 patients at four institutions. Patients were matched on the basis of baseline characteristics so that the best matched 292 TCAR and CEA patients were compared with respect to individual and composite stroke, death, and myocardial infarction at 30 days and 1 year postoperatively. We found similar results of stroke, death, and myocardial infarction at both 30 days and 1 year, but a markedly increased risk of cranial nerve injury in the CEA group (3.1% vs. 0.3%, P = 0.01), with only half resolving by 6 months.

Despite advances in technology and stent design, transfemoral carotid artery stenting (TFCAS) has failed to gain popularity, largely due to the nearly doubled risk of perioperative stroke rate compared to CEA. This may be due to unprotected catheterization of the aortic arch and crossing the carotid lesion in order to place an embolic filter. In addition, a transfemoral approach relies on a porous, floating filter with unknown apposition to the vessel wall to capture all embolic material. Hence, there was an unmet need for a minimally invasive option to treat carotid artery disease in patients with high-risk factors precluding CEA.

The results of our study demonstrated promising initial data for the potential widespread use of TCAR, particularly in patients at high risk for surgery. The obligate reversal of cerebral blood flow with TCAR is a compelling feature when treating a carotid plaque with risk of embolization. The limited common carotid artery exposure required for TCAR led to only one patient suffering a transient vagus nerve injury, manifested by hoarseness. The short working length makes the procedure easy to perform and quick to master. We have published data on the learning curve associated with TCAR and found only 10 to 15 cases required to gain technical proficiency.[1] More importantly, patients in the early phase of the learning curve are not at increased risk for postoperative complications.

TCAR with carotid blood flow reversal as neuroprotection is a relatively new procedure in the treatment of carotid bifurcation disease and appears to be a promising treatment alternative to transfemoral stenting and carotid endarterectomy in high surgical risk patients. The short learning curve and relative simplicity of the procedure are hallmarks of this minimally invasive procedure to treat carotid artery disease. We hope that these data will lead to further prospective comparative studies of TCAR in high-risk and standard-risk patients with carotid disease.

REFERENCE

1. King AH, Kumins NH, Foteh MI, Jim J, Apple JM, and Kashyap VS. The learning curve of transcarotid artery revascularization. *J Vasc Surg*. 2019;70(2):516–521.

CHAPTER 5

Immediate Repair Compared with Surveillance of Small Abdominal Aortic Aneurysm

Aneurysm Detection and Management, Veterans Affairs Cooperative Study Group, Lederle FA, Wilson SE, Johnson GR et al. Immediate repair compared with surveillance of small abdominal aortic aneurysms. N Engl J Med. 2002 May 9;346(19):1437–44

ABSTRACT

Background Whether elective surgical repair of small abdominal aortic aneurysms improves survival remains controversial.

Methods We randomly assigned patients 50 to 79 years old with abdominal aortic aneurysms of 4.0 to 5.4 cm in diameter who did not have high surgical risk to undergo immediate open surgical repair of the aneurysm or to undergo surveillance by means of ultrasonography or computed tomography every 6 months with repair reserved for aneurysms that became symptomatic or enlarged to 5.5 cm. Follow-up ranged from 3.5 to 8.0 years (mean, 4.9).

Results A total of 569 patients were randomly assigned to immediate repair and 567 to surveillance. By the end of the study, aneurysm repair had been performed in 92.6% of the patients in the immediate-repair group and 61.6% of those in the surveillance group. The rate of death from any cause, the primary outcome, was not significantly different in the two groups (relative risk in the immediate-repair group as compared with the surveillance group, 1.21; 95% confidence interval, 0.95 to 1.54). Trends in survival did not favor immediate repair in any of the prespecified subgroups defined by age or diameter of aneurysm at entry. These findings were obtained despite a low total operative mortality of 2.7% in the immediate-repair group. There was also no reduction in the rate of death related to abdominal aortic aneurysm in the immediate-repair group (3.0%) as compared with the surveillance group (2.6%). Eleven patients in the surveillance group had rupture of abdominal aortic aneurysms (0.6% per year), resulting in seven deaths. The rate of hospitalization related to abdominal aortic aneurysm was 39% lower in the surveillance group.

Conclusions Survival is not improved by elective repair of abdominal aortic aneurysms smaller than 5.5 cm, even when operative mortality is low.

EXPERT COMMENTARY BY SAMUEL ERIC WILSON, SAMUEL P. ARNOT, AND JUAN CARLOS JIMENEZ

When the Aneurysm Detection and Management (ADAM) Trial[1] began, patient accrual in 1992 endovascular repair was still undergoing laboratory investigation. Publications by Volodos in 1986 from Russia, and Parodi, Argentina, in 1991 showed the promise and clinical feasibility of the minimally invasive technique. Some surgeons, however, worried that if endovascular aneurysm repair (EVAR) proved safer than open repair, as it did, there would be relaxation of the size limits for repair, i.e., small aneurysms would be repaired without evidence of benefit. Others thought that delay in repair, as would occur in an observation group, could lead to a higher postoperative morbidity and mortality as the patients aged or that ruptures were likely to occur even in small aneurysms. Guidelines from societies were indefinite. Given this clinical equipoise, the RAND Corporation along with the Society for Vascular Surgery advocated for clinical trial.

The principal goal of the ADAM trial was to determine if early repair of small abdominal aortic aneurysms (AAAs), soon after discovery, resulted in better life expectancy than observation with serial ultrasound until expansion or symptoms mandated repair.

Study Design This was a prospective, randomized, clinical trial of "immediate" open surgery (within 6 weeks of diagnosis) versus serial observations by ultrasound every 6 months for AAAs 4.0–5.5 cms in diameter. If symptoms occurred, size reached 5.5 cms, or diameter grew 1 cm in 1 year or 0.7 cms in 6 months patients under observation were referred for open surgery.

Sample Size 569 patients were randomized to immediate repair and 567 to surveillance.

Follow-Up Until threshold size for intervention was reached (5.5 cms), rapid expansion or symptoms occurred.

Inclusion/Exclusion Criteria Included were AAAs between 4 and 5.5 cms. The major exclusion criteria were previous aortic surgery, chronic obstructive pulmonary disease, recent myocardial infarct, and chronic renal failure.

Treatment Patients were randomized to early, open AAA repair or follow-up with ultrasound measurement of AAA diameter.

Results Early survival benefit in the surveillance group, primarily due to the higher 30-day postoperative mortality in the surgical group, but no difference in survival at 5 years and 10 years. Rupture rate in those patients under surveillance was less than 1%/year. A Cochrane Database analysis of the ADAM and UKSAT pooled data also found that there was no outcome difference according to age or diameter.[2]

Study Limitations Patients selected were good risk unlike the majority of patients likely to be encountered in practice. Some AAAs expanded rapidly with 30% reaching threshold size in 3 years and 40% by 4 years. Few women were study participants.

Relevant Studies The contemporaneous UK Small Aneurysm Trial (Greenhalgh) found essentially the same outcome.[3]

Study Impact There were two major findings: first, an accurate description of the natural history of small AAAs, showing a less than 1% rupture rate per year, justifying close observation; and second, the realization that significant numbers of small aneurysms expand during follow-up requiring repair. The low rupture rate for small aneurysms was now known, accurately providing useful information to patients in deciding on intervention. The mean linear expansion rate of AAAs was calculated to be 0.26 cm/year over a mean follow-up period of 3.7 years.[4] One must bear in mind that individual patient expansion may have a staccato growth pattern.

Another important result was that even after introduction of a method of repair (EVAR) with a one-third 30-day mortality at 30 days versus that of open surgery (approximately 1% vs. 4%), the new technique did not accelerate the overall number of procedures.[5] It is interesting to compare this with prostatectomy where introduction of robotic surgery, along with PSA testing, almost doubled the rate without conclusive evidence of improved cancer cures or decrease in serious morbidity.

Secondary outcomes included recognition of the high incidence of AAAs in men between ages 50 and 79 who were screened with ultrasound. An AAA of 4 cm or greater was discovered in 1,031 of 73,451 (1.4%). This finding supported the approval of screening for AAA in this age group.

Risk factors for aneurysm disease were clearly identified to be predominately tobacco use, hypertension, and atherosclerosis. A family history was noted in 5.1%. Negative risk factors included female sex and diabetes mellitus.[6]

Lest the risk of rupture in larger AAAs be underestimated, it is well to reflect that screening for the ADAM trial detected 198 patients who had AAAs of at least 5.5 cms but were not fit for elective open repair. The 1-year incidence of rupture was 9.4% for AAAs of 5.5 to 5.9 cms and 10.2% for AAAs between 6.0 and 6.9 cms.[7]

The ADAM trial established guidelines on intervention for aortic aneurysms which have stood the test of time into the EVAR era.

REFERENCES

1. Lederle FA, Wilson SE, Johnson GR et al. Immediate repair compared with surveillance of small abdominal aortic aneurysms. *N Engl J Med*. 2002 May 9;346(19):1437–44.
2. Filardo G, Powell JT, Martinez MA et al. Surgery for small asymptomatic abdominal aortic aneurysms. *Cochrane Database Syst Rev*. 2015 Feb 8;(2), CD001835. doi: 10.1002/14651858.pub4.
3. The UK Small Aneurysm Trial Participants. Mortality results for randomized controlled trial of early elective surgery or ultrasonographic surveillance for small abdominal aortic aneurysms. *Lancet*. 1998;352:1649–55.
4. Bhak RH, Wininger M, Johnson GR et al. Factors associated with small abdominal aortic aneurysm expansion rate. *JAMA Surg*. 2015 Jan;150(1):44–50.
5. Chang DC, Easterlin MC, Montesa C et al. Adoption of endovascular repair of abdominal aortic aneurysm in California: Lessons for future dissemination of surgical technology. *Ann Vasc Surg*. 2012 May;26(4):468–75.
6. Lederle FA, Johnson GR, Wilson SE et al. Prevalence and associations of abdominal aortic aneurysm detected through screening. Aneurysm Detection and Management (ADAM) Veterans Affairs Cooperative Study Group. *Anals Intern. Med*. 1997 March;126(6):441–9.
7. Lederle FA, Johnson GR, Wilson SE et al. Rupture rate of large abdominal aortic aneurysms in patients refusing or unfit elective repair. *JAMA*. 2002 Jun 12;287(22):2968–72.

Chapter 6

Experience with 1509 Patients Undergoing Thoracoabdominal Aortic Operations

Svensson LG, Crawford ES, Hess KR, Coselli JS, Safi HJ.
J Vasc Surg. 1993 Feb;17(2):357–68; discussion 368–70

EXPERT COMMENTARY BY HARLEEN K. SANDHU, CHARLES C. MILLER III, ANTHONY L. ESTRERA, AND HAZIM J. SAFI

Research Question The purpose of this study was to retrospectively identify variables associated with early death and postoperative complications in patients undergoing thoracoabdominal aortic operations.

Study Design Retrospective cohort study.

Sample Size 1,509 patients (first operation in each).

Follow-Up 10 years for mortality.

Inclusion/Exclusion Presence of thoracoabdominal aortic aneurysm amenable to surgical repair. Consecutive series of open surgical repairs for 30 years, from 1960–1991.

Intervention or Treatment Received In the majority, open surgical repair utilizing clamp-and-sew technique; two randomized trials were imbedded in the cohort—one using cerebrospinal fluid drainage compared to clamp-and-sew and one using distal aortic perfusion compared to clamp-and-sew.

Results Aortic cross-clamp time and visceral ischemic time had strong correlations with risk of spinal cord ischemia. Multiple risk factors for early mortality were identified, including increasing age, poor renal function (Figure 6.1), chronic obstructive pulmonary disease, coronary artery disease, concurrent proximal aneurysm, and cross-clamp time. The addition of postoperative events retained all of the above variables and showed that postoperative events, including stroke, cardiac, renal, and gastrointestinal complications were also important predictors. Variables associated with spinal cord ischemia were clamp time, rupture, age, renal dysfunction, and concurrent proximal aneurysm.

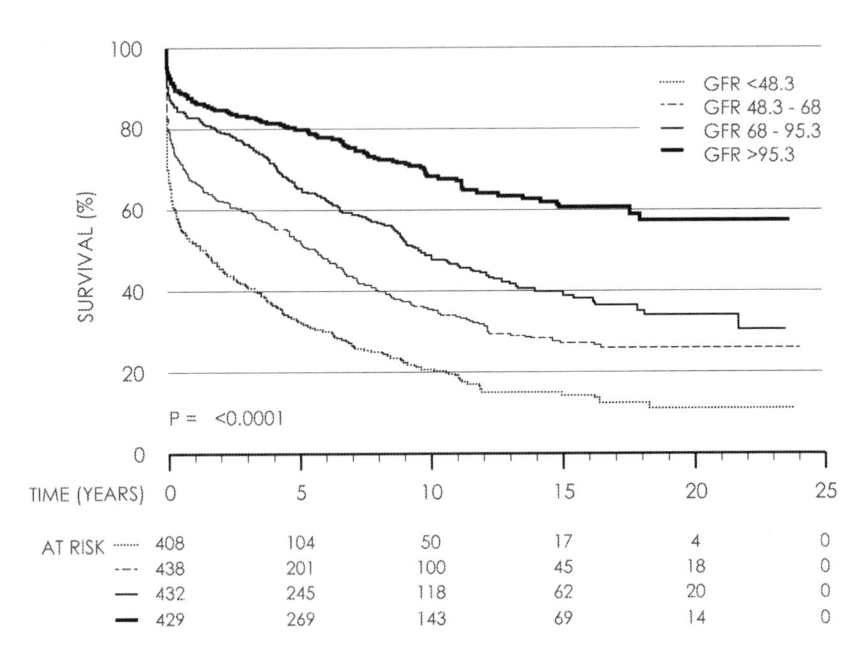

Figure 6.1 25-year patient survival after thoracoabdominal aortic repair by baseline renal function as measured by calculated glomerular filtration rate. (Adapted from Estrera AL et al. *Ann Surg*. 2015 Oct;262(4):660–8.)

Study Limitations This was a retrospective series with an observational cohort. Treatment subgroups from imbedded trials were not clearly identified and reported on separately.

Relevant Studies This 1993 paper remains a landmark for thoracoabdominal aortic aneurysm (TAAA) open surgical repair in the first well-characterized generation of this procedure, mostly using a single modality, the clamp-and-sew technique. The observations come primarily from the vast experiences of Dr. E. Stanley Crawford, a true master surgeon, and his protégées. The paper was brilliantly analyzed by Dr. Lars G. Svensson and emphasizes the challenges surgeons face when repairing TAAA—the most difficult aneurysms in the body. TAAA repair places multiple organ systems at risk and demands multiorgan system preservation. The paper is among the first to systematically address the pattern and interplay of pre-operative risk factors for mortality (immediate, 30-day, and long term) in a large sample using sophisticated statistical techniques, as well as pre-operative and intra-operative factors contributing to spinal cord ischemia.

Intra-operatively, the paper addresses the issue of the correlation between the extent of the aneurysm and the clamp time, where it evaluates the effects of total aortic clamp/ischemic time and also stratifies these effects according to extent of the aortic repair. During the Crawford era, where minimal countermeasures other than surgical speed and sequential clamping were used, extents II and I were high risk for spinal cord ischemia. Extents III and IV were called low-risk. Subsequently, with our group's identification and publication of extent V—which includes anything below the sixth intercostal space above the renal vessels—when we removed it from the admixed extent III, extent III became a risk factor for paraplegia, as important as in extent II.

Figure 6.2, located on page 364 of the paper, shows the Kaplan-Meier long-term survival. What is striking in these four panels is that the association between renal impairment and survival is much stronger than the previously described association between spinal cord ischemia (paralysis and paraparesis) and death. The authors further found that dissection was not associated with long-term survival.

The paper also analyzed renal complications and the correlations between pre-operative renal function, atherosclerotic disease, renal arterial occlusive disease, pre-operative creatinine, and visceral ischemic time. These all correlate with postoperative renal failure, as defined by the increase of 1 mg creatinine postoperatively times two above the pre-operative baseline or the institution of hemodialysis.

We believe this is a landmark article, that all vascular surgeons should know, because it includes a summative report of a large number of patients that were, for the most part, treated with a single technique, clamp-and-sew, and is based on the work of an incredibly technically skilled surgeon in Dr. Crawford. It can be thought of as the benchmark for this technique, as practiced at its highest level, and the base case against which to compare future improvements in the field. It is true that, embedded in this experience are a small number of patients that received some form of alternative treatment strategy, for example, profound hypothermic circulatory arrest, which resulted in a high incidence of mortality and did not protect against spinal cord

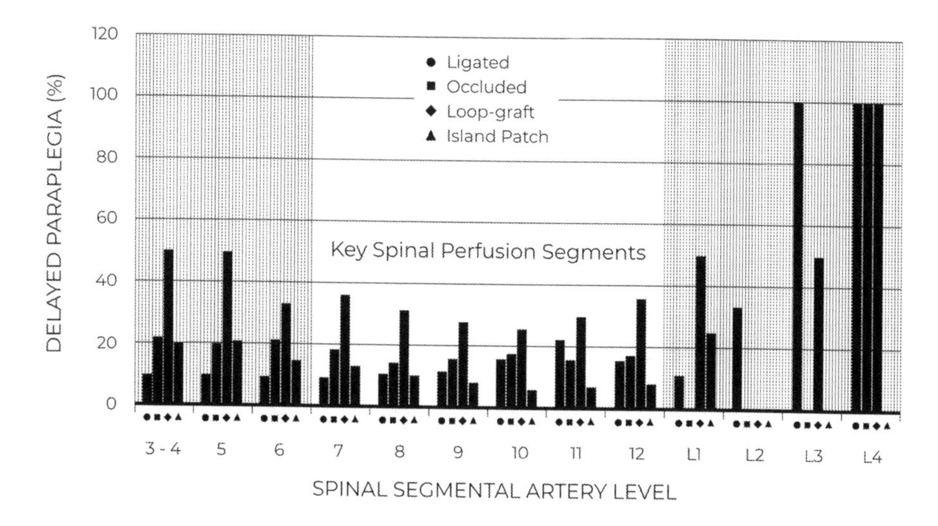

Figure 6.2 Risk of spinal cord ischemia by intercostal artery status/management. (Adapted from Afifi RO et al. *J Thorac Cardiovasc Surg*. 2018 Apr;155(4):1372–8.)

ischemia any more effectively than clamp-and-sew. In addition, two small randomized trials, one involving use of distal aortic perfusion, which we used prospectively in extents I-IV, and a separate trial of cerebrospinal fluid (CSF) drainage in extents II and I, only intra-operatively, were included in this series. Both of these trials were negative at the time and, therefore, were considered to be a part of this global experience.

Despite its prominence and importance as a landmark study in the field, this paper should be read carefully and considered in the context of its time. It provided the impetus to Dr. Crawford and his protégées to venture into ways to prevent the most dreaded complication with the spinal cord ischemia, which limits the lifespan of patients—both in immediate and delayed fashion. Some subsequent investigators ventured into the use of profound hypothermia circulatory arrest. It has been reported to be most effective in cases involving the upper half of the descending thoracic aorta but, in fact, this is where it is not really needed—and it carries a high risk of death in extent II TAAA, with the dreaded complication of bleeding to the left lung. The group from Boston, headed by Richard Cambria, adapted principles of hypothermic organ protection to use in regional CSF drainage, meaning cooling the spinal cord by using catheter in the proximal spinal compartment and then draining distally. However, the shortcoming of this procedure is it doesn't cool the spinal cord uniformly—with the upper portion getting cold and the lower portion remaining less cold. A further problem is that the CSF pressure is increased by perfusion into the rigid spinal column, which correlates with complications and some clinical work, especially that from Ramon Berguer and his associates, which showed paralysis in the upper extremities—in addition to lack of adequate protection to the spinal cord.

With regard to the pulmonary complications, as was shown in the past, it is correlated with underlying pulmonary disease, measured pulmonary function and the surgical management of the central portion of the diaphragm, cutting straight or radially. In our subsequent work on preserving the tendinous portion of the diaphragm and protecting the left phrenic nerve, diaphragm management was shown to have a major impact on pulmonary morbidity and ventilation time.[1] Dr. Crawford's paper also addresses the grave complications of gastrointestinal ischemia, which could be related to either lack of blood supply or embolism.

Having trained with Dr. Crawford and having seen the best possible outcomes of clamp-and-sew, our group decided to combine CSF drainage, which was done by Miyamoto,[2] Blaisdell and Cooley,[3] and Bower,[4] as well as distal aortic perfusion, with the work of Connolly,[5] in order to lower the CSF pressure, and augment distal aortic pressure, in order to give the surgeon ample time to do the operation without haste[6] during the repair of proximal anastomosis, reattachment of lower intercostal arteries, as well as the visceral perfusion. In the past, perfusion to the celiac trunk negated all of the ischemic effect of the clamp on the liver and the bowel and cooling the kidneys.[7] That has been our mainstay, corroborated by colleagues Drs. Joseph Coselli and Lars Svensson,[8] who worked on using vasodilators in the spinal cord both on animals and the human model.

Dr. Crawford's work was a major landmark in the history of vascular surgery and represents the pinnacle of what was achievable in its historic context. His protégées have considered this work to be the standard against which any future innovations should be judged, and incremental improvements that have since become widely adopted, such as cerebrospinal fluid drainage, distal aortic perfusion, and aggressive intercostal artery salvage, have been made possible because of Dr. Crawford's courageous pioneering work.

REFERENCES

1. Engle J, Safi HJ, Miller CC III, Campbell MP, Harlin SA, Letsou GV, Lloyd MD KS, and Root DB. The impact of diaphragm management on prolonged ventilator support after thoracoabdominal aortic repair. *J Vasc Surg.* 1999 Jan;29(1): 150–6.
2. Miyamoto K, Ueno A, Wada T, and Kimoto S. A new and simple method of preventing spinal cord damage following temporary occlusion of the thoracic aorta by draining the cerebrospinal fluid. *J Cardiovasc Surg (Torino).* 1960 Sep;1:188–97.
3. Blaisdell FW, and Cooley DA. The mechanism of paraplegia after temporary thoracic aortic occlusion and its relationship to spinal fluid pressure. *Surgery.* 1962 Mar;51:351–5.
4. Bower TC, Murray MJ, Gloviczki P, Yaksh TL, Hollier LH, and Pairolero PC. Effects of thoracic aortic occlusion and cerebrospinal fluid drainage on regional spinal cord blood flow in dogs: Correlation with neurologic outcome. *J Vasc Surg.* 1989 Jan;9(1):135–44.
5. Connolly JE, Wakabayashi A, German JC, Stemmer EA, and Serres EJ. Clinical experience with pulsatile left heart bypass without anticoagulation for thoracic aneurysms. *J Thorac Cardiovasc Surg.* 1971 Oct;62(4):568–76.
6. Estrera AL, Sandhu HK, Charlton-Ouw KM, Afifi RO, Azizzadeh A, Miller CC 3rd, and Safi HJ. A quarter century of organ protection in open thoracoabdominal repair. *Ann Surg.* 2015 Oct;262(4):660–8.
7. Afifi RO, Sandhu HK, Zaidi ST, Trinh E, Tanaka A, Miller CC 3rd, Safi HJ, and Estrera AL. Intercostal artery management in thoracoabdominal aortic surgery: To reattach or not to reattach? *J Thorac Cardiovasc Surg.* 2018 Apr;155(4):1372–8.
8. Lima B, Nowicki ER, Blackstone EH, Williams SJ, Roselli EE, Sabik JF 3rd, Lytle BW, and Svensson LG. Spinal cord protective strategies during descending and thoracoabdominal aortic aneurysm repair in the modern era: The role of intrathecal papaverine. *J Thorac Cardiovasc Surg.* 2012 Apr;143(4):945–52.

CHAPTER 7

Results of the United States Multicenter Prospective Study Evaluating the Zenith Fenestrated Endovascular Graft for Treatment of Juxtarenal Abdominal Aortic Aneurysms

Fenestrated Study Investigators, Oderich GS, Greenberg RK, Farber M, Lyden S, Sanchez L, Fairman R, Jia F, Bharadwaj P. J Vasc Surg. 2014 Dec; 60(6):1420–8.e1–5. doi: 10.1016/j.jvs.2014.08.061. Epub 2014 Sep 5

EXPERT COMMENTARY BY GUSTAVO S. ODERICH AND EMANUEL RAMOS TENORIO

Research Question/Objective This study reports the results of a prospective, multicenter trial designed to evaluate the safety and effectiveness of the Zenith fenestrated endovascular graft (Cook Medical, Bloomington, IN) for treatment of juxtarenal abdominal aortic aneurysms (AAAs, Figure 7.1).

Methods 67 patients with juxtarenal AAAs (neck >4 and <15 mm) were prospectively enrolled in 14 centers in the United States from 2005 to 2012. Custom-made fenestrated stent grafts were designed with one to three fenestrations on the basis of analysis of computed tomography data sets. Follow-up included clinical examination, laboratory studies, mesenteric-renal duplex ultrasound, abdominal radiography, and computed tomography imaging at hospital discharge and at 1 month, 6 months, and 12 months and yearly thereafter up to 5 years.

Results There were 54 male and 13 female patients with a mean age of 74 ± 8 years enrolled. Mean aneurysm diameter was 60 ± 10 mm. A total of 178 visceral arteries required incorporation with small fenestrations in 118, scallops in 51, and large fenestrations in nine. Of these, all 118 small fenestrations (100%), eight of the scallops (16%) and one of the large fenestrations (11%) were aligned by stents. Technical success was 100%. There was one postoperative death within 30 days (1.5%). Mean length of hospital stay was 3.3 ± 2.1 days. No aneurysm ruptures or conversions were noted during a mean follow-up of 37 ± 17 months (range, 3–65 months). Two patients (3%) had migration ≥10 mm with no endoleak, both due to cranial progression of aortic disease. Of

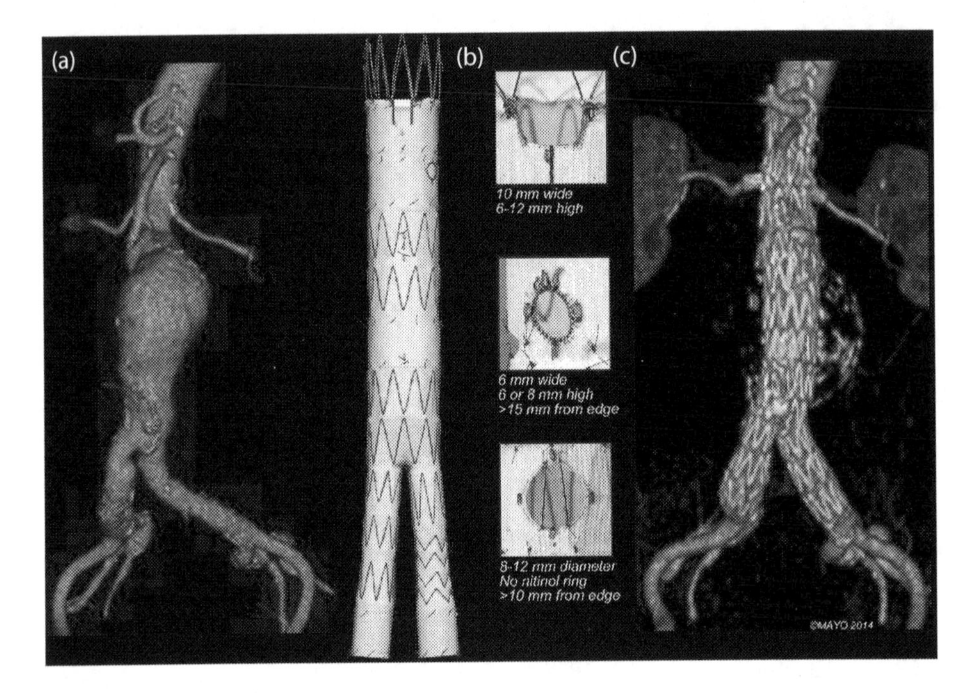

Figure 7.1 (a) Preoperative computed tomography angiography (CTA) of a patient with juxtarenal abdominal aortic aneurysm (AAA) treated by Zenith fenestrated stent graft (b). (c) Follow-up CTA with patent stent graft and no endoleak. (Reproduced with permission of Mayo Foundation for Medical Education and Research. All rights reserved.)

a total of 129 renal arteries targeted by a fenestration, there were four (3%) renal artery occlusions and 12 (9%) stenoses. Fifteen patients (22%) required secondary interventions for renal artery stenosis/occlusion in 11 patients, type II endoleak in three patients, and type I endoleak in one patient. At 5 years, patient survival was 91% ± 4%, and freedom from major adverse events was 79% ± 6%; primary and secondary patency of targeted renal arteries was 81% ± 5% and 97% ± 2%, freedom from renal function deterioration was 91% ± 5%, and freedom from secondary interventions was 63% ± 9%.

Study Limitations The primary limitations of this study relate to the nonrandomized design and lack of surgical control group, which preclude any definitive comparison with open surgical repair or alternative endovascular techniques beyond a discussion of historical results. Despite the study's mean follow-up of >3 years, many patients have not reached their 5-year endpoint, thereby restricting the power of our statistical analysis. Finally, the stringent anatomic requirements used in this study should be taken into consideration in comparing results with alternative techniques, such as parallel grafts or open repair.

Conclusions This prospective study demonstrates that endovascular repair of juxtarenal AAAs with the Zenith fenestrated AAA stent graft is safe and effective.

Mortality and morbidity are low in properly selected patients treated in centers with experience in these procedures.

Fenestrated endovascular aortic repair (FEVAR) has evolved over the past 20 years from an experimental and investigational treatment for complex AAA to an acceptable alternative to open surgical repair, especially in high-risk patients. Gradually this technique has been utilized to treat a broader range of patients and is now considered first-line therapy for complex AAA at some experienced centers.[1] Published series dating back to 2004 have demonstrated the safety and efficacy of the technique, with favorable perioperative morbidity and mortality rates.[2] Previous reviews of the reported literature and meta-analyses have reported impressive early and midterm results, with overall mortality ranging from 0% to 4.1% (Table 7.1).[1,3–10] Technical success in these series has been reported as >95%, with comparably low type I (2.5%–6%) and type III (1.0%–4.3%) endoleak rates and low rates of postoperative new-onset dialysis (0%–3%). Collective data regarding outcomes following FEVAR can be challenging to interpret and generalize, however, because there exists an inherent variability in the inclusion criteria for patient groups analyzed, indications for repair, techniques utilized, and respective outcome parameters among published reports. In the manuscript under discussion, the observation of high technical success (100%), low mortality (1.5%), rare incidence of type I or type III endoleaks (1.5%), high target vessel patency (97%), and lack of conversion to open repair or aneurysm rupture relate to the integrity of the device, support the safety, effectiveness, and durability of the Zenith fenestrated stent graft, and serve as a benchmark for comparison with other devices or alternative endovascular techniques to treat similar anatomy. However, generalizability of successful outcomes following FEVAR to less experienced centers remains unproven in the literature, and re-intervention rates, even among the most experienced centers and especially in the mid- to long term, remain a concern.

The ongoing evolution of endovascular techniques has resulted in a steady decline of open aortic repair since 2000 and has been discussed in several papers.[11] Concerns have been raised regarding training of young vascular surgeons and the need for additional methods to provide that training. At this moment, sufficient aortic surgery training with open infrarenal aneurysm surgery can still be offered in younger patients or aorto-bifemoral bypasses in arteriosclerotic patients, but the number of open complex abdominal and thoracoabdominal surgery cases has reduced to 10–15 cases per year. Further centralization of complex aortic surgery will certainly be needed to maintain high quality and education of trainees. As the more complex endovascular techniques also deserve centralization, it seems clear that a further centralization toward aortic centers, preferably offering both open and endovascular surgery, is a must.

The United States Zenith fenestrated stent graft trial is the first pivotal pre-marked approval study to evaluate use of fenestrated stent grafts for short neck and juxtarenal aortic aneurysms. The study has shown that fenestrated endovascular repair can be performed with high technical success, low mortality, and low morbidity in selected patients with minimum infrarenal seal zone of 4–15 mm by experienced operators.

Table 7.1 Contemporary Reports of Fenestrated Stent Grafts for Complex Abdominal Aortic Aneurysms

Author	Year	Aneurysm Type	n	Vessels	Technical Success	30-Day Mortality	Dialysis	Endoleaks	Branch Patency	Re-Intervention	Follow-Up (Months)
Quiñones-Baldrich et al.[3]	2013	JRA	31	124	97%	0.0%	3.2%	3.2%	94%	13%	23
Kristmundsson et al.[4]	2014	JRA	54	134	98%	3.7%	0.0%	31%	96%	37%	67
Oderich et al.[5]	2014	JRA	67	178	100%	1.5%	0.0%	1.5%	97%	22%	37
Mastracci et al.[6]	2015	JRA, Extent IV	610	1463	98%	NR	NR	9.6%	93%	26%	96
Patel et al.[7]	2015	JRA	150	313	92%	8.0%	NR	1.3%	89%	6.7%	32
Verhoeven et al.[1]	2016	JRA, SRA	281	896	97%	0.7%	0.7%	11%	98%	5.3%	21
Katsargyris et al.[8]	2017	JRA, SRA	384	983	97%	0.5%	0.2%	NR	99%	2.1%	20
Roy et al.[9]	2017	JRA	173	572	95%	5.2%	0.0%	10%	90%	20%	34
Colgan et al.[10]	2018	JRA	101	255	97%	3.0%	0.9%	15%	98%	9.0%	12

Advantages are the low rate of cardiac and pulmonary complications and a remarkably low rate of new onset dialysis, all relatively common problems with open surgical repair.[5] As compared to the alternative endovascular techniques of parallel stent grafts or short neck EVAR with endo-anchors, fenestrated stent grafts allow for a longer proximal seal zone and more reliable exclusion of the aneurysm no early type IA endoleak. Despite these advantages, the study has shown a relatively high rate of renal artery re-interventions for in-stent restenosis or occlusion. It is important to highlight that the clinical trial utilized primarily bare metal balloon-expandable stents, instead of covered stent grafts, which have been shown to lower the rates of neointimal hyperplasia leading to re-interventions.

Some aspects of the trial should be carefully analyzed prior to making generalizations. All patients met a rigid clinical and anatomical criterion and had their devices carefully planned and approved by the National Principal Investigator (Dr. Roy Greenberg), in addition to an experienced sizing team.[2] Operators had extensive experience with endovascular aortic repair and techniques of renal and mesenteric artery stenting. The frequent imaging surveillance protocol allowed early recognition of stent-related problems and endoleaks, which otherwise would have gone undetected.

The Zenith fenestrated stent graft has design limitations imposed by the original trial design. Although outside the United States these devices can be manufactured with almost no design constraint with respect to the number of fenestrations and the delivery system, in the United States the stent is approved with a maximum of three fenestrations, of which only two are reinforced by nitinol ring. Therefore, the design is applicable to approximately two-thirds of the overall patient population of complex abdominal aortic aneurysms. Patients with pararenal or paravisceral aneurysms, and those with extent IV thoracoabdominal aortic aneurysms are not ideally suited for the current version of the Zenith fenestrated stent graft. In these cases, devices designed with four fenestrations and a supra-celiac seal zone provide a more durable alternative and reliable seal. To overcome these anatomical constraints, ongoing and future design trials, such as the Gore thoracoabdominal multibranched endoprosthesis (TAMBE) and the Cook Zenith fenestrated plus trials, will investigate the more extensive designs.

REFERENCES

1. Verhoeven E, Katsargyris A, Oikonomou K, Kouvelos G, Renner H, and Ritter W. Fenestrated endovascular aortic aneurysm repair as a first line treatment option to treat short necked, juxtarenal, and suprarenal aneurysms. *European Journal of Vascular and Endovascular Surgery*. 2016;51(6):775–81.
2. Greenberg R, Haulon S, O'neill S, Lyden S, and Ouriel K. Primary endovascular repair of juxtarenal aneurysms with fenestrated endovascular grafting. *European Journal of Vascular and Endovascular Surgery*. 2004;27(5):484–91.
3. Quiñones-Baldrich WJ, Holden A, Mertens R et al. Prospective, multicenter experience with the Ventana Fenestrated System for juxtarenal and pararenal aortic aneurysm endovascular repair. *Journal of Vascular Surgery*. 2013;58(1):1–9.

4. Kristmundsson T, Sonesson B, Dias N, Törnqvist P, Malina M, and Resch T. Outcomes of fenestrated endovascular repair of juxtarenal aortic aneurysm. *Journal of Vascular Surgery*. 2014;59(1):115–20.
5. Oderich GS, Greenberg RK, Farber M et al. Results of the United States multicenter prospective study evaluating the Zenith fenestrated endovascular graft for treatment of juxtarenal abdominal aortic aneurysms. *Journal of Vascular Surgery*. 2014;60(6):1420–8. e5.
6. Mastracci TM, Eagleton MJ, Kuramochi Y, Bathurst S, and Wolski K. Twelve-year results of fenestrated endografts for juxtarenal and group IV thoracoabdominal aneurysms. *Journal of Vascular Surgery*. 2015;61(2):355–64.
7. Patel SD, Constantinou J, Simring D et al. Results of complex aortic stent grafting of abdominal aortic aneurysms stratified according to the proximal landing zone using the Society for Vascular Surgery classification. *Journal of Vascular Surgery*. 2015;62(2): 319–25. e2.
8. Katsargyris A, Oikonomou K, Kouvelos G, Mufty H, Ritter W, and Verhoeven EL. Comparison of outcomes for double fenestrated endovascular aneurysm repair versus triple or quadruple fenestrated endovascular aneurysm repair in the treatment of complex abdominal aortic aneurysms. *Journal of Vascular Surgery*. 2017;66(1):29–36.
9. Roy I, Millen A, Jones S et al. Long-term follow-up of fenestrated endovascular repair for juxtarenal aortic aneurysm. *British Journal of Surgery*. 2017;104(8):1020–7.
10. Colgan FE, Bungay PM, Burfitt N et al. Operative and 1-Year Outcomes of the Custom-Made Fenestrated Anaconda Aortic Stent Graft—A UK Multicenter Study. *Annals of Vascular Surgery*. 2018;46:257–64.
11. Sachs T, Schermerhorn M, Pomposelli F, Cotterill P, O'malley J, and Landon B. Resident and fellow experiences after the introduction of endovascular aneurysm repair for abdominal aortic aneurysm. *Journal of Vascular Surgery*. 2011;54(3):881–8.

CHAPTER 8

Outcomes Following Endovascular vs Open Repair of Abdominal Aortic Aneurysm: A Randomized Trial

Open Versus Endovascular Repair (OVER) Veterans Affairs Cooperative Study Group, Lederle FA, Freischlag JA, Kyriakides TC et al. JAMA. 2009 Oct 14;302(14):1535–42. doi: 10.1001/jama.2009.1426

ABSTRACT

Context Limited data are available to assess whether endovascular repair of abdominal aortic aneurysm (AAA) improves short-term outcomes compared with traditional open repair.

Objective To compare postoperative outcomes up to 2 years after endovascular or open repair of AAA in a planned interim report of a 9-year trial.

Design, Setting, and Patients A randomized, multicenter clinical trial of 881 veterans (aged > or = 49 years) from 42 Veterans Affairs Medical Centers with eligible AAA who were candidates for both elective endovascular repair and open repair of AAA. The trial is ongoing and this report describes the period between October 15, 2002, and October 15, 2008.

Intervention Elective endovascular (n = 444) or open (n = 437) repair of AAA.

Main Outcome Measures Procedure failure, secondary therapeutic procedures, length of stay, quality of life, erectile dysfunction, major morbidity, and mortality.

Results Mean follow-up was 1.8 years. Perioperative mortality (30 days or inpatient) was lower for endovascular repair (0.5% vs. 3.0%; P = .004), but there was no significant difference in mortality at 2 years (7.0% vs. 9.8%, P = .13). Patients in the endovascular repair group had reduced median procedure time (2.9 vs. 3.7 hours), blood loss (200 vs. 1000 mL), transfusion requirement (0 vs. 1.0 units), duration of mechanical ventilation (3.6 vs. 5.0 hours), hospital stay (3 vs. 7 days), and intensive care unit stay (1 vs. 4 days), but required substantial exposure to fluoroscopy and contrast. There were no differences between the 2 groups in major morbidity, procedure failure, secondary therapeutic procedures, aneurysm-related hospitalizations, health-related quality of life, or erectile function.

Conclusions In this report of short-term outcomes after elective AAA repair, perioperative mortality was low for both procedures and lower for endovascular than open repair. The early advantage of endovascular repair was not offset by increased morbidity or mortality in the first 2 years after repair. Longer-term outcome data are needed to fully assess the relative merits of the 2 procedures.

Trial Registration clinicaltrials.gov Identifier: NCT00094575.

EXPERT COMMENTARY BY JULIE FREISCHLAG AND GABRIELA VELÁZQUEZ

Research Question/Objective Several studies have addressed early and long-term outcomes comparing endovascular versus open repair for abdominal aortic aneurysms. When endovascular repair became widely available, the thought was that its minimally invasive nature would result in better overall outcomes. This was true for reduced perioperative mortality, hospital stay, and intensive care unit stay; however, there were more frequent re-interventions. Most importantly several reports showed the survival advantage was lost within 2 years.[2,3] Some of these large randomized studies were conducted in Europe which led us to question if these results would be applicable to U.S. practice. The goal of this study was to compare postoperative outcomes up to 2 years after endovascular or open repair.

Study Design Randomized multicenter clinical trial from 42 Veterans Affairs Medical Centers. Primary outcome long-term all-cause mortality.

Sample Size 881 patients.

Follow-Up 2 years.

Inclusion/Exclusion Criteria

Inclusion Criteria Abdominal aortic aneurysm at least 5 cm, associated iliac aneurysm with maximum diameter of at least 3 cm or maximum diameter of at least 4.5 cm plus either rapid enlargement (at least 0.7 cm in 6 months or 1 cm in 12 months), or saccular morphology. Patient had to meet the manufacturer's indications for the endovascular system that would be used if so assigned.

Exclusion Criteria Abdominal aortic aneurysm <5 cm, not candidates for both procedures and/or failed to complete evaluation, prior abdominal aortic surgery, need for urgent repair.

Intervention or Treatment Received Pending randomization, patients would undergo open repair involving sutured anastomoses of an anatomically placed vascular graft through an abdominal or retroperitoneal incision. Endovascular repair involved the transluminal introduction of an expandable grafts system through the femoral arteries. Only endovascular systems approved the U.S. Food and Drug Administration could be used in the study.

Results The two randomized groups had similar demographic characteristics. Forty-one patients had an AAA less than 5 cm, and these patients underwent intervention for co-existing iliac aneurysm, rapid enlargement, or saccular morphology. All 109 physicians who participated in the study were vascular surgeons. Endovascular repair resulted in significantly reduced procedure time, duration of mechanical ventilation, hospital and ICU stays, blood loss, and transfusion requirement, but required substantial exposure to fluoroscopy and contrast.

Perioperative mortality was significantly higher for open repair at 30 days and during hospitalization. There was no significant difference in all-cause mortality at 2 years. Mortality after perioperative period was similar in the two groups. No differences were observed between the two groups in procedure failures, secondary therapeutic procedures, aneurysm-related hospitalizations, or 1-year major morbidity. See Tables 8.1 and 8.2.

Study Limitations N/A

Relevant Studies In commentary.

Study Impact This paper followed a series of early reports showing the benefit of endovascular repair reducing perioperative morbidity and mortality compared to open repair. Prospective randomized trials like the UK EVAR trial, DREAM, and the European multicenter registry EUROSTAR showed decreased mortality within 30 days in the groups undergoing endovascular repair for AAA.[2–4] The OVER trial

Table 8.1 Details of Aneurysm Repair by Randomly Assigned Group

	Median (Interquartile Range)	
	Endovascular Repair (n = 439)	**Open Repair (n = 429)**
Patients with aorta as distal attachment site (vs. iliac/femoral), No. (%)	23 (5.2)	190 (44.3)
Time from randomization to repair, d	18.0 (10.0–28.0)	17.0 (9.0–26.0)
Duration of procedure, h	2.9 (2.3–3.7)	2.7 (2.9–4.7)
Duration of mechanical ventilation, h	3.6 (3.0–4.5)	5.0 (4.0–9.1)
Duration of fluoroscopy, min	23.0 (17.0–31.0)	0
Volume of contrast used, mL	132.5 (96.5–176.0)	0
Estimated blood loss, mL	200 (150–400)	1000 (650–2000)
Banked red cell transfusion within 24 h, unit	0	1.0 (0–3.0)
Duration of hospital stay for initial repair, d	3.0 (2.0–5.0)	7.0 (6.0–10.0)
Time in intensive care unit, d	1.0 (1.0–2.0)	4.0 (3.0–6.0)

Note: Patients who had no repair (refused, aborted, and never completed, or died before repair) are not included. $P < 0.001$ for all comparisons of means, except time from randomization to repair ($P = 0.36$).

Table 8.2 All Outcome Measures

Outcomes	No. (%) of Patients Endovascular Repair (n = 444)	Open Repair (n = 437)	*P* Value
All-cause mortality	31 (7.0)	43 (9.8)	0.13
Before AAA repair	2 (0.5)	1 (0.2)	>0.99
Within 30 d after repair	1 (0.2)	10 (2.3)	0.006
Within 30 d after repair or during hospitalization	2 (0.5)	13 (3.0)	0.004
AAA diameter <5.5 cm	1 (0.5)	5 (2.6)	0.10
AAA diameter ≥5.5 cm	1 (0.4)	8 (3.2)	0.02
After 30 d or hospitalization	27 (6.1)	29 (6.6)	0.74
Cause of death	**(n = 31)**	**(n = 43)**	
AAA-related[a]	6 (1.4)	13. (3.0)	0.10
Cardiovascular	9 (2.0)	4 (0.9)	0.26
Cancer	10 (2.3)	15 (3.4)	>0.99
Other[b]	5 (1.1)	7 (1.6)	0.54
Unknown	1 (0.2)	4 (0.9)	0.21
Patients with procedure failure	58 (13.1)	51 (11.7)	0.53
Patients with no repair attempted	4 (0.9)	5 (1.1)	0.75
Patients with aborted initial procedure	8 (1.8)	6 (1.4)	0.61
Patients having second therapeutic procedures	46 (10.4)	40 (9.2)	0.73
All secondary therapeutic procedures, no. of events	61	55	
Patients with any 1-year major morbidity	18 (4.1)	20 (4.6)	0.70
Myocardial infarction	6 (1.4)	12 (2.7)	0.14
Stroke	7 (1.6)	4 (0.9)	0.38
Amputation	1 (0.2)	3 (0.7)	0.37
Renal failure requiring dialysis	5 (1.1)	3 (0.7)	0.73
Patients with new or worsened claudication	37 (8.3)	20 (4.6)	0.02
All postrepair, aneurysm-related hospitalizations, no. of events	108	86	

Abbreviation: AAA, abdominal aortic aneurysm.

[a] Includes all deaths within 30 days after repair or during hospitalization.

[b] Includes cerebrovascular disease, injury, pneumonia, other infections, and unexplained sudden deaths not considered AAA related.

would be the first large prospective randomized trial to do this comparison in the United States. At the time of this original article, 45,000 patients were undergoing elective AAA repair resulting in 1,400 deaths. The increasing use of aortic stent grafts to repair aneurysms was expected to decrease the number of periprocedural deaths, which in most studies was the case. However, long-term survival proved to be no different compared to open. When the OVER trial was conducted, both groups had low perioperative mortality, but it was even lower for the endovascular group, which was similar to other European results. This early advantage was not offset by increased morbidity or mortality in the endovascular group in the first 2 years after repair. The authors of this trial were convinced that with the years, evolving technology and improvement in the endovascular systems used would definitely impact long-term outcomes. However, 3 years later, the OVER trial investigators published their long-term data comparing endovascular and open repair for abdominal aortic aneurysms which resulted in similar long-term survival. Perioperative survival advantage of endovascular repair was sustained for several years but rupture after endovascular repair remained a concern. Endovascular repair led to better long-term survival in younger patients, but not in the older patients for whom benefit was most expected.[5]

It appeared long-term results would be similar to early reports which prompted the authors to evaluate the cost-effectiveness of open versus endovascular repair for AAA as a follow up of this trial. Lower costs due to shorter hospitalization for initial repair with endovascular approach were offset by increased costs from AAA-related secondary procedures and imaging studies. After follow-up to 9 years, survival, quality of life, costs, and cost-effectiveness did not differ between open or endovascular repair.[6]

A significant concern was the number of late ruptures associated with EVAR that did not occur in the open repair group. It is well known now that endoleaks are quite common, presenting in 20%–50% of patients with EVAR. A sub-analysis was performed to identify risk factors and long-term outcomes of endoleaks with emphasis on aneurysm sac diameter, rupture, and mortality. Presence of endoleaks resulted in increased aneurysm diameter over time and this was statistically significant. Delayed type II endoleaks (>1 year following EVAR) were associated with aneurysm enlargement compared to early ones. Of patients with endoleaks, 31.9% received secondary intervention. The initial size of the aneurysm sac predicted the need for secondary intervention. There was no difference in aneurysm size or length of survival between type II and other types of endoleaks.[7]

In the most recent extended follow-up report, patients in the OVER trial were followed for 14 years. No difference was observed between endovascular and open repair in the primary outcome of all-cause mortality. Younger patients had a somewhat higher long-term overall survival undergoing endovascular repair, but among older patients, endovascular repair resulted in lower long-term survival. Another difference in this extended follow-up is the number of patients who underwent secondary therapeutic procedures in both groups. They were significantly higher in the endovascular group. It is of note that postoperative mortality was lower in this trial than in the European trials.[8]

All these findings, throughout years of follow-up, have helped treating physicians with their decision-making and patient counseling when treating abdominal aortic aneurysms. Despite evolving technology in endograft design and delivery systems, long-term survival remains similar in open versus endovascular repair. Patients prefer the endovascular repair due to its noninvasive nature with them having less pain following the procedure, shorter hospital stays, lower perioperative mortality, and earlier return to work and other activities. However, we are pushing the envelope to treat more and more infra-renal aneurysms with challenging anatomy. Future outcomes regarding cost effectiveness and secondary interventions may be affected by these advances. We have to remember that rupture after EVAR remains a concern, and we have to be diligent in following these patients who may potentially develop aneurysmal enlargement requiring intervention years after their repair. The OVER trial original article and related reports have been the largest prospective randomized trial with extended long-term follow-up conducted in the United States.

REFERENCES

1. Lederle FA, Freischlag JA, Kyriakides TC et al. Outcomes following endovascular vs open repair of abdominal aortic aneurysm: A randomized trial Open Versus Endovascular Repair (OVER) Veterans Affairs Cooperative Study Group. *JAMA*. 2009 Oct 14;302(14):1535–42.
2. The United Kingdom EVAR Trial Investigators. Endovascular versus open repair of abdominal aortic aneurysm. *N Engl J Med*. 2010;362:1863–71.
3. De Bruin JL, Baas AF, Buth J, Prinssen M, Verhoeven EL, Cuypers PW, Van Sambeek MR, Balm R, Grobbee DE, and Blankensteijn JD. Long term outcome of open or endovascular repair of abdominal aortic aneurysm. *N Engl J Med*. 2010;362(20):1881–9.
4. Lurs LJ, Buth J, and Lehiji RJ, for the EUROSTAR Collaborators. Long term results of endovascular abdominal aortic aneurysm treatment with the first generation of commercially available stent grafts. *Arch Surg*. 2007;142:33–41.
5. Lederle FA, Freischlag JA, Kyriakides TC, Padberg FT Jr, Matsumura JS, Kohler TR, Kougias P, Jean-Claude J, Cikrit DF, and Swanson KM. For the OVER Veterans Affairs Cooperative Study Group. Long term comparison of endovascular and open repair of abdominal aortic aneurysm. *NEJM*;367(21):1988–97.
6. Stroupe KT, Lederle FA, Matsumara JS, Kyriakides TC, Jonk YC, Ge L, and Freischlag JA. Open Versus Endovascular Repair OVER, Veterans Affairs Cooperative Study Group. Cost Effectiveness of open versus endovascular repair of abdominal aortic aneurysm in the OVER trial. *J Vasc Surg*. 2012;56(4):901–9.
7. Lal BK, Zhou W, Li Z, Kyriakides T, Matsumura J, Lederle FA, and Freischlag J; OVER Veterans Affairs Cooperative Study Group. *J Vasc Surg*. 2015;62(6):1394–404.
8. Lederle FA, Kyriakides TC, Stroupe KT, Freischlag JA, Padberg FT Jr, Matsumura JS, Huo Z, and Johnson GR. OVER Veterans Affairs Cooperative Study Group. *NEJM*;380(22):2126–35.

CHAPTER 9

Collected World and Single Center Experience with Endovascular Treatment of Ruptured Abdominal Aortic Aneurysms

RAAA Investigators, Veith FJ, Lachat M, Mayer D, Malina M, Holst J, Mehta M, Verhoeven EL, Larzon T, Gennai S, Coppi G, Lipsitz EC et al. *Ann Surg. 2009 Nov;250(5):818–24*

ABSTRACT

Background Case and single center reports have documented the feasibility and suggested the effectiveness of endovascular aneurysm repair (EVAR) of ruptured abdominal aortic aneurysms (RAAAs), but the role and value of such treatment remain controversial.

Objective To clarify these we examined a collected experience with use of EVAR for RAAA treatment from 49 centers.

Methods Data were obtained by questionnaires from these centers, updated from 13 centers committed to EVAR treatment whenever possible, and treatment details were included from a single center and information on 1,037 patients treated by EVAR and 763 patients treated by open repair (OR).

Results Overall 30-day mortality after EVAR in 1,037 patients was 21.2%. Centers performing EVAR for RAAAs whenever possible did so in 28% to 79% (mean 49.1%) of their patients, had a 30-day mortality of 19.7% (range: 0%–32%) for 680 EVAR patients and 36.3% (range: 8%–53%) for 763 OR patients ($P < 0.0001$). Supraceliac aortic balloon control was obtained in 19.1% ± 12.0% (SD) of 680 EVAR patients. Abdominal compartment syndrome was treated by some form of decompression in 12.2% ± 8.3% (±SD) of these EVAR patients.

Conclusion These results indicate that EVAR has a lower procedural mortality at 30 days than OR in at least some patients and that EVAR is better than OR for treating RAAA patients provided they have favorable anatomy; adequate skills, facilities, and protocols are available; and optimal strategies, techniques, and adjuncts are employed.

AUTHOR COMMENTARY BY FRANK J. VEITH

On November 23, 1992, I led the group that performed the first endovascular graft repair of an aortic aneurysm (EVAR) in North America.[1,2] The patient had a large (7.5 cm) symptomatic infrarenal abdominal aortic aneurysm (AAA), but such severe cardiac and pulmonary disease that an open repair would not be possible. The team performing the procedure was comprised of three vascular surgeons (Juan Parodi, Michael Marin, Frank Veith) and two interventional radiologists (Claudio Schonholz, Jacob Cynamon). The endograft used was a Dacron graft to which was sewn a large Palmaz balloon expandable stent. The patient did well and became asymptomatic. His AAA was excluded.[1,2]

Encouraged by this first case, our vascular group at Montefiore Medical Center in New York then embarked on a program of surgeon-made endovascular graft treatment for a variety of occlusive, aneurysmal, and traumatic vascular lesions in patients who were mainly too high a risk for standard open surgical treatment.[3,4]

It soon became apparent that these endovascular graft treatments worked, often in otherwise hopeless situations.[3] Since some of these early patients had large symptomatic AAAs, we had the idea of using this technology to treat ruptured AAAs. This concept was feasible because our AAA endograft system was comprised of a large tulip-shaped PTFE graft to which was sewn a large Palmaz stent.[3,5] This stent secured the proximal end of the endograft to the AAA neck, and the distal end of the endograft was brought out through the delivery system's femoral insertion site. Then the excess endograft was cut off and its remaining end was secured to the inside of the femoral artery by an endovascular anastomosis. The procedure was completed by occluding the opposite common iliac artery and performing a femoro-femoral bypass.[5]

This endograft system was particularly suited to treating ruptured AAAs because it was a one-size-fits-most and because it could be fabricated, sterilized, and available for treating an urgent or emergent condition without delay. Because of this availability, we were able on April 24, 1994 to perform the first EVAR to treat a ruptured AAA anywhere.[5]* The patient was inoperable for open repair because of both local and systemic risk factors. Nevertheless, his ruptured AAA was excluded, and he lived 3 years longer before dying of his comorbidities.[5]

This experience prompted us to employ EVAR to treat 11 other ruptured AAA patients who were for various reasons unsuitable for treatment by an open repair.[6,7] In all of these patients, the ruptured AAA was excluded. Only two patients died after their procedure, a low 17% mortality for these first 12 high-risk patients.[6,7]

This prompted us in 1995 to advocate treating all ruptured AAAs by EVAR if the AAA anatomy was suitable and the facilities, grafts, and skills to perform the

* Another case was performed after ours by Yusuf, Hopkinson et al. However, this case was published before ours because of rapid publication in *Lancet* (1994;344:1645).

procedure were available.[7] At first, this recommendation was greeted with skepticism and even disdain. Those who opposed our suggestion believed that patients would not survive the time delay required to complete the endovascular procedure and thereby gain aortic control. To counteract this possibility we advocated what we called "hypotensive hemostasis." This was a policy of totally restricting fluid resuscitation, even if the patient was hypotensive, and permitting any hypotension that occurred to persist. With this technique most (~80%) of ruptured AAA patients could be successfully treated by EVAR. If the few (~20%) remaining patients developed total cardio-vascular collapse despite hypotensive hemostasis, we also innovated techniques for obtaining balloon control of the supraceliac aorta to facilitate successful EVAR treatment.[6–8]

Because most authorities in the late 1990s and early 2000s did not accept our recommendation that EVAR and endovascular techniques were the best way to treat ruptured AAAs, we collected the world experience with the procedure and reported it in the article abstracted previously.[7] This article showed many things. Most importantly it showed that in institutions like ours that favored EVAR over open repair whenever possible, the ruptured AAA mortality was much lower (see abstract).[7] It also detailed strategies and technical adjuncts to facilitate EVAR in this setting.[7] However, many felt our favorable results were based on patient selection and that randomized controlled trials were necessary to determine the best treatment for ruptured AAAs.

As a result, three RCTs were carried out, one each in the Netherlands, France, and the United Kingdom. All three of these RCTs showed no early mortality benefit to EVAR over open repair. However, we believed that all of these RCTs were performed with major methodological flaws which we detailed in a 2015 article.[9] So despite the results of these three RCTs, we still believe EVAR is the best way to treat ruptured AAAs if the skills, grafts, and facilities are available and the anatomy is suitable. This opinion has also been vindicated by the now generally accepted superiority of EVAR for the treatment of ruptured AAAs if it can be performed.

Interestingly, the later results of the largest of these RCTs (the IMPROVE trial) show the superiority of EVAR in terms of better late survival and lower costs in the treatment of ruptured AAAs.[10] Thus it appears that in 2019 most experts and practicing vascular surgeons accept the concept that EVAR is the best way to treat ruptured AAAs, if one can do so—a concept that, when we presented it in years past, was greeted with much negativity and even some derision.

REFERENCES

1. Parodi JC, Marin ML, and Veith FJ. Transfemoral endovascular stented graft repair of an abdominal aortic aneurysm. *Arch Surg*. 1995;130:549–52.
2. Veith FJ, Marin ML, Cynamon J, Schonholz C, and Parodi JC. 1992: Parodi, montefiore, and the first abdominal aortic aneurysm stent graft in the United States. *Ann Vasc Surg*. 2005;19:749–51.

3. Veith FJ. Presidential address: Transluminally placed endovascular stented grafts and their impact on vascular surgery. *J Vasc Surg*. 1994;20:855–60.
4. Veith FJ, Cynamon J, Schonholz CJ, and Parodi JC. Early endovascular grafts at Montefiore Hospital and their effect on vascular surgery. *J Vasc Surg*. 2014;59:547–50.
5. Marin ML, Veith FJ, Cynamon J et al. Initial experience with transluminally placed endovascular grafts for the treatment of complex vascular lesions. *Ann Surg*. 1995;222:449–69.
6. Ohki T, and Veith FJ. Endovascular grafts and other image-guided catheter-based adjuncts to improve the treatment of ruptured aortoiliac aneurysms. *Ann Surg*. 2000;4:466–79.
7. Veith FJ, Lachat M, Mayer D et al. Collected world and single center experience with endovascular treatment of ruptured abdominal aortic aneurysms. *Ann Surg*. 2009;250:818–24.
8. Berland T, Veith FJ, Cayne NS, Mehta M, Mayer D, and Lachat M. Technique of supraceliac balloon control of the aorta during endovascular repair of ruptured abdominal aortic aneurysms. *J Vasc Surg*. 2013;57:272–5.
9. Veith FJ, and Rockman CB. The recent randomized trials of EVAR versus open repair for ruptured abdominal aortic aneurysms are misleading. *Vascular*. 2015;23:217–9.
10. Ulug P, Sweeting MJ, Gomes M et al. for the IMPROVE Trial Investigators: Comparative clinical effectiveness and cost effectiveness of endovascular strategy v open repair for ruptured abdominal aortic aneurysm: Three year results of the IMPROVE randomised trial. *BMJ*. 14 Nov 2017;359:j4859.

CHAPTER 10

Repair of Extensive Aortic Aneurysms: A Single-Center Experience Using the Elephant Trunk Technique over 20 Years

Estrera AL, Sandhu HK, Miller CC 3rd, Charlton-Ouw KM, Nguyen TC, Afifi RO, Azizzadeh A, Safi HJ. *Ann Surg. 2014 Sep;260(3):510–6; discussion 517–8*

ABSTRACT

Objectives We report the early and late outcomes after repair of extensive aortic aneurysms using the 2-stage elephant trunk (ET) technique.

Background Management of aneurysm involving the entire aorta is a significant challenge. Given the anatomical complexity, the staged ET procedure was devised. A paucity of long-term data of outcomes of this approach exists.

Methods A single-center retrospective analysis of a prospectively collected database of all patients undergoing repair for extensive aortic aneurysm was performed.

Results Between 1991 and 2013, we repaired 3,012 aneurysms of the ascending or thoracoabdominal aorta. Of these, we performed 503 operations in 348 patients using the ET technique. Mean age was 62.4 ± 14.3 years, and 156/346 (45.1%) operations were in women; 288 patients underwent first-stage ET with 157 receiving a complete second-stage repair. Index repair early mortality was 29/317 (9.1%). Completion stage early mortality was 17/186 (9.1%). Stroke after first-stage ET repair was 10/297 (3.4%), and immediate neurologic deficit after the second-stage ET repair was 6/206 (2.9%). In the 131 patients who did not receive a second-stage repair, 17.8% died in the interval between 31 and 45 days.

Conclusions Extensive aortic aneurysm is a complex problem, but it can be managed safely with a 2-stage open procedure. Those patients who could not complete the completion repair fared poorly. Better predictors for early outcome need to be determined. The use of ET technique remains a valuable approach for repair of extensive aortic aneurysm.

AUTHOR COMMENTARY BY ALI AZIZZADEH AND ANTHONY L. ESTRERA

Extensive aortic aneurysms involving most of, or in some cases, the entire aorta, are particularly challenging clinical problems. Untreated, these extensive aneurysms pose a high risk of rupture and death. From a surgical management perspective, the proximal and distal thoracic aorta require differing access leading to the staged approach for repair. Although the single "clam shell" incision has been applied to extensive aneurysms confined to the thoracic cavity, the staged approach has become more widely accepted. The technical challenge in performing the open second stage repair was controlling the proximal descending thoracic aorta for the anastomosis. At risk during this maneuver was injury to the left main pulmonary artery and bleeding.

In 1983, Hans Borst[1] and colleagues described the "elephant trunk" technique. This is a staged procedure in which the ascending aorta and aortic arch are repaired through a sternotomy and a portion of aortic graft is left extending unanchored into the proximal descending aorta, to be retrieved via a subsequent thoracotomy/thoracoabdominal incision and sutured end-to-end to a second graft used to repair the remaining distal aortic segment. The staged nature of this procedure allows for a period of recovery between the operative encounters that reduces the burden on the patient and improves the tractability of the procedure for the care team. When feasible, performing the sternotomy first can result in a shorter time interval between the proximal and distal operations, since recovery time following sternotomy is generally shorter and less painful than recovery for thoracotomy. A downside of staging the procedure—especially for large-diameter aneurysms or those in high-risk patients, such as those with Marfan syndrome—is that risk of rupture in the untreated segment remains until the entirety of the disease has been addressed.

We started looking into our experience with management of extensive aortic aneurysms in the late 1990s and have since reported our short, mid, and long-term outcomes periodically.[2–5] In a recent review from our group, we provide an in-depth commentary on the changes in the techniques and evolution of the elephant trunk strategy in current times, along with the present-day indications for it with tips from our surgical technique and management during the staged repair of extensive aortic aneurysms using elephant trunk.[6] Our 2014 paper[5] presented at the 134th American Surgical Association Annual Meeting and published in the *Annals of Surgery*, extended Borst's pioneering work to assess the risk factors and outcomes of each stage of the procedure and also to review the experience of the patient cohort in the interval between the stages. This paper described the results of 503 operations in 348 patients using the elephant trunk technique. These patients were identified from a total cohort of 3,012 repairs of the aortic root, ascending, arch, descending thoracic, or thoracoabdominal aorta, performed between 1991 and 2013. Results for stage 1 were reported as 30-day outcomes following stage 1, interval outcomes were reported as outcomes occurring between 30 and 45 days post-stage 1, and stage 2 outcomes were reported as those occurring within 30 days following stage 2.

Mortality following stage 1 was 8.4% and after stage 2 10.2%. In all, 2.2% died during the prescribed recovery interval of 30 to 45 days while 30% of patients intended for second-stage surgery did not recover sufficiently to undergo second-stage repair within a median interval of 2.3 months. Of those, 17.8% died. Also, 57% of stage 1 procedures were performed prophylactically, meaning that an elephant trunk was left in the descending aorta that was considered to be at risk for future expansion but was not dilated enough to warrant repair at the time of the first stage. Long-term survival in the prophylactic cohort was 75% at 5 years—similar to that of patients undergoing complete two-stage repair.

Results of elephant trunk repair in our center are comparable to the results of each type or repair performed conventionally for limited extent disease in our usual patient cohort. Interval repair mortality was low at 2.2% during the waiting period—and may well accumulate to less than the incremental mortality that would be accrued if one-shot, single-stage repair was attempted. Although the "interval mortality" was low, there was mortality related to rupture while waiting for the second stage to be completed. It was the concern of the "interval mortality" that led to the single-staged repair using the "frozen elephant trunk" (also devised by the Hannover group).[7] In this procedure, a stent graft attached to a standard impregnated polyester graft is deployed into the descending thoracic aorta. Using the polyester graft, a standard ascending and arch replacement is then completed.

Observations related to the "intention to treat" the second stage procedure were notable. Early in our experience using this approach for extensive aortic aneurysms, we observed that those who did not complete the second-stage procedure had a late mortality similar to those who did not undergo a procedure at all. This suggested that if a patient was not willing to undergo both stages of the elephant trunk procedure, then no intervention should be offered. Our subsequent analysis in our work analyzed the second-stage groups in more detail. In the group that did not return for the second stage, three groups were identified: "prophylactic;" "nonreturners;" and "too frail." The prophylactic group—patients in whom the second stage was not indicated (aortic diameter <5 cm)—did well with surveillance with a 5-year survival of 73%. The nonreturners were patients who had indications for the second stage but refused to return—the intention was to treat this group. This group's 5-year survival was 43%. Finally, the too frail group witnessed no survivors beyond 2 years, suggesting these patients should not have undergone any procedure.

In conclusion, these results establish two things: (1) a standard against which endovascular procedures should be judged as new technologies are developed; (2) a rational guide to management for those who cannot be repaired by endovascular technique. As the commercially produced frozen elephant trunk devices become more available, it is likely that the traditional elephant trunk procedure will be replaced by this hybrid approach. In the United States, current endovascular options to address the ascending aorta and aortic arch are limited—and a significant proportion of these aneurysms may not be suitable for endovascular repair with any existing technology. Therefore, surgical options remain an essential element of the procedural armamentarium, and best practices for these complex problems need to be developed, refined, and disseminated.

REFERENCES

1. Borst HG, Walterbusch G, and Schaps D. Extensive aortic replacement using "elephant trunk" prosthesis. *Thorac Cardiovasc Surg*. 1983;31(1):37–40.
2. Safi HJ, Miller CC, Estrera AL et al. Staged repair of extensive aortic aneurysms: Morbidity and mortality in the elephant trunk technique. *Circulation*. 2001;104(24):2938–42.
3. Estrera AL, Miller CC, Porat EE et al. Staged repair of extensive aortic aneurysms. *Ann Thorac Surg*. 2002;74(5):S1803–5; discussion S1825–32.
4. Safi HJ, Miller CC, Estrera AL et al. Staged repair of extensive aortic aneurysms: Long-term experience with the elephant trunk technique. *Ann Surg*. 2004;240:677–85.
5. Estrera AL, Sandhu HK, Miller CC et al. Repair of extensive aortic aneurysms. *Ann Surg*. 2014;260(3):510–8.
6. Tanaka A and Estrera AL. Elephant trunk: Argument for all arches. *Semin Cardiothorac Vasc Anesth*. 2016;20(4):322–6.
7. Karck M, Chavan A, Hagl C, Friedrich H, Galanski M, and Haverich A. The frozen elephant trunk technique: A new treatment for thoracic aortic aneurysms. *J Thorac Cardiovasc Surg*. 2003 Jun;125(6):1550–3.

CHAPTER 11

Endovascular versus Open Repair of Abdominal Aortic Aneurysm in 15-Years' Follow-Up of the UK Endovascular Aneurysm Repair Trial 1 (EVAR Trial 1): A Randomized Controlled Trial

Patel R, Sweeting MJ, Powell JT, Greenhalgh RM, EVAR Trial Investigators.

ABSTRACT

Background Short-term survival benefits of endovascular aneurysm repair (EVAR) versus open repair of intact abdominal aortic aneurysms have been shown in randomised trials, but this early survival benefit is lost after a few years. We investigated whether EVAR had a long-term survival benefit compared with open repair.

Methods We used data from the EVAR randomised controlled trial (EVAR trial 1), which enrolled 1,252 patients from 37 centers in the UK between September 1, 1999, and August 31, 2004. Patients had to be aged 60 years or older, have aneurysms of at least 5.5 cm in diameter, and deemed suitable and fit for either EVAR or open repair. Eligible patients were randomly assigned (1:1) using computer-generated sequences of randomly permuted blocks stratified by center to receive either EVAR (n = 626) or open repair (n = 626). Patients and treating clinicians were aware of group assignments; no masking was used. The primary analysis compared total and aneurysm-related deaths in groups until mid-2015 in the intention-to-treat population. This trial is registered at ISRCTN (ISRCTN55703451).

Results We recruited 1,252 patients between September 1, 1999, and August 31, 2004. 25 patients (four for mortality outcome) were lost to follow-up by June 30, 2015. Over a mean of 12.7 years (SD 1.5; maximum 15.8 years) of follow-up, we recorded 9.3 deaths per 100 person-years in the EVAR group and 8.9 deaths per 100 person-years in the open-repair group (adjusted hazard ratio [HR] 1.11, 95% CI 0.97–1.27, p = 0.14). At 0–6 months after randomisation, patients in the EVAR group had a lower mortality (adjusted HR 0.61, 95% CI 0.37–1.02 for total mortality; and 0.47, 0.23–0.93 for aneurysm-related mortality, p = 0.031), but beyond 8 years of follow-up open-repair had a significantly lower mortality (adjusted HR 1.25, 95% CI 1.00–1.56, p = 0.048 for total mortality; and 5.82, 1.64–20.65, p = 0.0064 for aneurysm-related mortality). The increased aneurysm-related mortality in the EVAR group after 8 years was mainly attributable to secondary aneurysm sac rupture (13 deaths [7%] in EVAR vs. two [1%] in open repair), with increased cancer mortality also observed in the EVAR group.

Conclusion EVAR has an early survival benefit but an inferior late survival compared with open repair, which needs to be addressed by lifelong surveillance of EVAR and re-intervention if necessary.

EXPERT COMMENTARY BY FIONA ROHLFFS, ZOË ÖHMAN, AND ROGER GREENHALGH

The EndoVascular Aneurysm Repair (EVAR) trial (EVAR trial 1) is the world's first randomized controlled trial comparing the new endovascular aneurysm repair with open repair as gold standard. The 30-day operative mortality for EVAR was 1.7% versus 4.7% for open repair.[1] Four years after randomization all-cause mortality was similar in the two groups, although there was a persistent reduction in aneurysm-related deaths in the EVAR group of 3%.[2] There was now continuing need for ongoing diligent surveillance. At 10 years, no difference was seen in all-cause mortality nor aneurysm-related mortality and already EVAR was associated with increased rates of graft-related complications and re-interventions and was becoming more costly.[3]

Also at this stage, it was noticed that there were no ruptures from open repair and a low rate of rupture following EVAR but mortality after secondary rupture was high though very few seemed to be spontaneous.[4] Secondary aortic sac rupture was seen mainly in a "cluster" of patients associated almost always with annual sac growth with underlying type I, III, II with sac growth, kinking, and graft migration with a 67% mortality. All of the EVAR trial centers were warned to look out for this "cluster" which seemed to predict the increased risk of secondary sac rupture and death.

In this 15-year follow-up report, loss to follow-up was enormous and by the end, only 10% of the group were still followed by annual consultation and CT scan. The patients simply gave up attending! At the same time, the early survival benefit of EVAR was lost with an inferior late survival compared with open repair. The authors realized that this should be addressed by lifelong surveillance of EVAR and re-interventions if required.[5] Therefore, sac expansion and secondary sac rupture could occur unheralded and patients could die of secondary sac rupture never diagnosed.

This approach was pursued[6] with observations on the trajectories of sac growth seeking to develop a dynamic prognostic model to enable stratification of risk for secondary rupture or need for rupture preventing re-intervention (RPR). Ultimately, the aim is to use discreet event simulation (DES) to determine optimal follow-up protocol as 40% of endovascular repair patients with little sign of sac expansion and potentially at low risk of rupture compared with those who did have sac expansion where there was an 85% risk of secondary sac rupture and death within 2 years. Thus high-level predictability of rupture and timely planned endovascular re-intervention is potentially achievable from annual sac growth monitoring.

This 15-year follow-up report has been used by the National Institute of Clinical Excellence (NICE) as the basis of finding that endovascular aneurysm repair is not cost-effective. NICE are basing their decision to challenge funding of endovascular repair upon the findings and this manuscript in particular, with its sub-optimal world first poor follow-up system rather than to learn from the trial and seek to keep patients safe by affordable and effective follow-up.

In the meantime, a probe connected to a mobile phone can be used to measure sac diameter annually in the community and whereas original follow-up protocol for the EVAR world's first randomized controlled trial was clearly sub-optimal, the use of a mobile phone handheld Doppler in the community to establish sac diameter annually could provide encouragement that endovascular repair will be cost effective in the future.

It is thought that this empowers the patient to check the annual sac diameter themselves or with the help of a family member or at the local doctor's practice. This avoids annual visits to the vascular center and CT scan.

In the final NICE aortic guidelines, funding for EVAR is limited but not withdrawn. NICE is aware of the ongoing observational study on EVAR follow up "Detection of EVAR sac expansion using ultrasound surveillance" the "DETECT" study coordinated from Imperial College, London and involving all London University vascular centers and two centers in Helsinki and Tampere, Finland. On modeling, EVAR is expected to be cost effective using this approach.

REFERENCES

1. Greenhalgh RM, Brown LC, Kwong GP et al. Comparison of endovascular aneurysm repair with open repair in patients with abdominal aortic aneurysms (EVAR trial 1), 30–day operative mortality results: Randomised controlled trial. *Lancet*. Sept 2004;364:843–848.
2. Greenhalgh RM, Brown LC, Epstein D et al. Endovascular aneurysm repair versus open repair in patients with abdominal aortic aneurysm (EVAR trial 1) randomised controlled trial. *Lancet*. Jun 2005;365:2179–86.
3. Greenhalgh RM, Brown LC, Powell JT et al. Endovascular versus open repair of abdominal aortic aneurysm. *New Engl J Med*. 2010;362(20):1863–71.
4. Wyss TR, Brown LC, Powell JT et al. Rate and predictability of graft rupture after endovascular and open abdominal aortic aneurysm repair: Data from the EVAR Trials. *Ann Surg*. 2010;252(5): 805–12.
5. EVAR trial investigators, Patel R, Sweeting MJ et al. Endovascular versus open repair of abdominal aortic aneurysm in 15-years' follow-up of the UK endovascular aneurysm repair trial 1 (EVAR trial 1): A randomised controlled trial. *Lancet*. 2016;388(10058):2366–74.
6. Grootes I, Barrett JK, Ulug P et al. Predicting risk of rupture and rupture-preventing reinterventions utilising repeated measures on aneurysm sac diameter following endovascular abdominal aortic aneurysm repair. *Br J Surg*. Sept 2018;105(10):1294–1304.

CHAPTER 12

Long-Term Survival and Secondary Procedures after Open or Endovascular Repair of Abdominal Aortic Aneurysms

van Schaik TG, Yeung KK, Verhagen HJ, de Bruin JL, van Sambeek MRHM, Balm R, Zeebregts CJ, van Herwaarden JA, Blankensteijn JD.
DREAM Trial Participants. J Vasc Surg. 2017 Nov;66(5):1379–89

ABSTRACT

Objective Randomized trials have shown an initial survival benefit of endovascular over conventional open abdominal aortic aneurysm repair but no long-term difference up to 6 years after repair. Longer follow-up may be required to demonstrate the cumulative negative impact on survival of higher re-intervention rates associated with endovascular repair.

Methods We updated the results of the Dutch Randomized Endovascular Aneurysm Management (DREAM) trial, a multicenter, randomized controlled trial comparing open with endovascular aneurysm repair, up to 15 years of follow-up. Survival and re-interventions were analyzed on an intention-to-treat basis. Causes of death and secondary interventions were compared by use of an events-per-person year analysis.

Results There were 178 patients randomized to open and 173 to endovascular repair. Twelve years after randomization, the cumulative overall survival rates were 42.2% for open and 38.5% for endovascular repair, for a difference of 3.7 percentage points (95% confidence interval, −6.7 to 14.1; $P = .48$). The cumulative rates of freedom from re-intervention were 78.9% for open repair and 62.2% for endovascular repair, for a difference of 16.7 percentage points (95% confidence interval, 5.8–27.6; $P = .01$). No differences were observed in causes of death. Cardiovascular and malignant disease account for the majority of deaths after prolonged follow-up.

Conclusions During 12 years of follow-up, there was no survival difference between patients who underwent open or endovascular abdominal aortic aneurysm repair, despite a continuously increasing number of re-interventions in the endovascular repair group. Endograft durability and the need for continued endograft surveillance remain key issues.

EXPERT COMMENTARY BY KAREN WOO

Hypothesis The hypothesis being tested in the study was that longer-term follow-up may demonstrate a cumulative negative impact on survival of higher re-intervention rates associated with endovascular abdominal aortic aneurysm (AAA) repair compared to open AAA repair.

Study Design The original Dutch Randomized Endovascular Aneurysm Management (DREAM)[1] study was a prospective randomized clinical trial of endovascular versus open AAA repair, beginning in November 2000. Data acquisition for the original DREAM study ended on February 1, 2009. In this long-term follow-up study, the data was collected retrospectively from February 1, 2009 on by reviewing medical records, death records, and contacting involved physicians, patients, and relatives.

Sample Size In the original DREAM study, 351 patients were randomly assigned: 178 to endovascular AAA repair and 173 to open AAA repair. Six patients did not undergo repair after randomization. Of the remaining 345 patients, 174 were assigned to open repair and 171 to endovascular repair. There were six crossovers: five who were initially assigned to open repair underwent endovascular repair and one who was assigned to endovascular underwent open repair. There were three conversions from endovascular to open repair and one aborted endovascular repair. Ultimately, open repair was completed in 173 and endovascular repair was completed in 171. At the time data acquisition ended for the original DREAM study on February 1, 2009, 229 patients were reported to be alive.

Follow-Up The primary informed consent for the original DREAM study included 2 years of follow-up. With the additional retrospective long-term follow-up, the median total follow-up was 10.2 years (IQR 5.0–12.5 years).

INCLUSION/EXCLUSION CRITERIA FOR THE ORIGINAL DREAM STUDY:[2]

Inclusion

- Asymptomatic AAA measuring ≥5 cm in diameter
- Considered suitable candidates for either open or endovascular AAA repair
- Adequate infrarenal neck
- Aorto-iliac anatomical configuration suitable for EVAR according to the criteria of the device used
- Patient having a life expectancy of at least 2 years and cleared for transabdominal intervention

Exclusion

- Ruptured AAA or symptomatic AAA, which requires emergency surgery
- Maximum aneurysm diameter <5.0 cm

- Juxtarenal or suprarenal AAA I
- Inflammatory AAA (more than wall thickening)
- Infrarenal neck unsuitable for endovascular fixation or aorto-iliac configuration otherwise unsuitable for EVAR
- Bilateral retroperitoneal incision required for EVAR
- Sacrifice of both hypogastric arteries required
- Anatomical variations, i.e., horseshoe kidney, arteries requiring reimplantation (accessory renal arteries or indispensable IMA)
- Patient unsuitable for laparotomy (i.e., multiple abdominal surgical interventions)
- Administration of contrast agent not possible: proved, severe systemic reaction to contrast agent
- Active infection present
- Transplantation patients
- Limited life expectation due to other illness (<2 years)
- Non-iatrogenic bleeding diathesis
- Connective tissue disease

Intervention or Treatment Received In the original DREAM study, patients were randomized to open versus endovascular AAA repair. In this long-term follow-up study, no additional intervention or treatment was rendered. The data were analyzed on an intent-to-treat basis from the original study.

Results The mean age of the original cohort was 70 years with 92% male and 44% with coronary artery disease. Demographics and comorbidities were equally distributed between the open and endovascular groups. The completeness of follow-up (calculated as the ratio of the total observed person-time of follow-up to the potential time of follow-up) in the study was 98.4% (37.177/37.775 months) for all patients. Eight patients were lost to follow-up: three (1.7%) after open and five (2.9%) after endovascular repair. At 12 years, there was no significant difference in cumulative overall survival rates for open versus endovascular repair (42.2% vs. 38.5%, $P = 0.48$). There was also no significant difference in aneurysm-related mortality for open versus endovascular repair (7.7% vs. 3.1%, $P = 0.33$). At 12 years, the cumulative rate of freedom from secondary procedure was higher for open versus endovascular repair (78.9% vs. 62.2%, $P = 0.01$). The rate of secondary procedures was significantly lower in the open versus endovascular repair groups (2.8 events per 100 person-years vs. 6.6 events per 100 person-years, $P<0.001$). This was predominantly driven by a higher rate of interventions for incomplete aneurysm exclusion in the endovascular repair group (event rate ratio 0.04, $P<0.001$). However, there was no significant difference in re-intervention-free survival for open versus endovascular repair (34.9% vs. 26.5%, $p = 0.13$).

Study Limitations The long-term follow-up of this study is both its strength and the source of its most significant limitations. Since the DREAM study was initiated in 2000, the management of type II endoleaks has evolved significantly. In the early part of the trial, aggressive management of type II endoleak may have led to more interventions than they would with current management of type II endoleak. This may have resulted in an inflated rate of secondary interventions after endovascular repair. Furthermore, the majority of the endovascular repair devices used in this trial are not available today. This limits the generalizability of the results to current practices. The retrospective nature of the long-term follow-up data collection presents several potential risks for the data. There is a risk of inaccurate recording of data in the medical record and a greater risk of inaccurate recollection of secondary interventions and/or health status by patients and families. In addition, four times the number of patients in the endovascular repair group continued with active surveillance following the initial DREAM study completion compared with the open repair group. This could lead to ascertainment bias resulting in a higher rate of complications being detected in the endovascular group due to closer surveillance.

Relevant Studies Three other randomized studies of open versus endovascular AAA repair have been performed: (1) Comparison of endovascular aneurysm repair with open repair in patients with abdominal aortic aneurysm (EVAR-1),[3] (2) Open Versus Endovascular Repair (OVER),[4] and (3) Anevrysme de l'aorte abdominale: Chirurgie versus Endoprothese (ACE).[5]

Study Impact Numerous studies, both prospective and retrospective, have demonstrated the improved mortality for endovascular AAA repair compared to open in the short term (approximately 2 years after index repair) with no difference in mortality following the initial period. With respect to long-term follow-up, there is also a large body of work that demonstrates similar findings to the DREAM long-term follow-up. The 15-year follow-up results of the EVAR-1 trial demonstrated significantly higher rates of re-intervention in the EVAR group (adjusted hazard ratio 2.42, $p<0.0001$).[6] EVAR-1 also showed an increased aneurysm-related mortality in the EVAR group after 8 years, mainly attributable to secondary aneurysm sac rupture. There were 13 (7%) deaths in the EVAR group compared to two (1%) in the open repair group. The 9-year follow-up results of the OVER study demonstrated no difference in the probability of all-cause mortality beginning at 3 years after the index operation.[7] There were six aneurysm ruptures confirmed in the endovascular group compared to none in the open repair group ($P=0.03$).

A number of large-scale retrospective analyses have demonstrated similar findings with no survival advantage of endovascular repair over open repair after the initial 1.5–3 year postoperative period.[8,9] In a propensity score matched analysis of Medicare patients with 8 years of follow-up, the rate of aneurysm rupture was 5.4% in the endovascular repair group compared to 1.4% in the open repair group ($P<0.0001$).[8]

Endovascular AAA repair has rapidly become the preferred approach for AAA repair with high demand by patients for a minimally invasive approach and willingness of physicians to accommodate. However, the long-term follow-up results of the DREAM study, along with the related body of data, underscore the fact that endovascular AAA repair is not a "cure" in the same way that an open AAA repair is. Patients who undergo endovascular repair must understand this point and the importance of lifelong follow-up after endovascular AAA repair. This is an important discussion that surgeons should have as part of the informed consent for AAA repair. Some physicians have even incorporated a contract into the consent process which the patient signs that confirms understanding and agreement to comply with regular lifelong follow-up.

The results of this study also call into question the appropriateness of performing endovascular AAA on young, relatively healthy patients, who are good candidates for open AAA repair and may have a life expectancy of more than 10 years. Open AAA repair requires increased investment in the initial perioperative period but is associated with the long-term benefit of requiring less surveillance and fewer re-interventions. Conversely, endovascular AAA repair requires considerably less investment in the perioperative period with a concordant lifelong investment in surveillance and a higher incidence of re-interventions. This trade-off should be taken into consideration along with the unique circumstances surrounding each patient and discussed in detail with patients and their families.

REFERENCES

1. Prinssen M, Verhoeven EL, Buth J et al. A randomized trial comparing conventional and endovascular repair of abdominal aortic aneurysms. *N Engl J Med.* 2004;351(16):1607–18.
2. Prinssen M, Buskens E, and Blankensteijn JD. The Dutch Randomised Endovascular Aneurysm Management (DREAM) trial. Background, design and methods. *J Cardiovasc Surg.* 2002;43(3):379–84.
3. Greenhalgh RM, Brown LC, Kwong GP, Powell JT, and Thompson SG. Comparison of endovascular aneurysm repair with open repair in patients with abdominal aortic aneurysm (EVAR trial 1), 30–day operative mortality results: Randomised controlled trial. *Lancet (London, England).* 2004;364(9437):843–8.
4. Lederle FA, Freischlag JA, Kyriakides TC et al. Outcomes following endovascular vs open repair of abdominal aortic aneurysm: A randomized trial. *JAMA.* 2009;302(14):1535–42.
5. Becquemin JP, Pillet JC, Lescalie F et al. A randomized controlled trial of endovascular aneurysm repair versus open surgery for abdominal aortic aneurysms in low- to moderate-risk patients. *J Vasc Surg.* 2011;53(5):1167–73.e1161.
6. Patel R, Sweeting MJ, Powell JT, and Greenhalgh RM. Endovascular versus open repair of abdominal aortic aneurysm in 15-years' follow-up of the UK endovascular aneurysm repair trial 1 (EVAR trial 1): A randomised controlled trial. *Lancet (London, England).* 2016;388(10058):2366–74.
7. Lederle FA, Freischlag JA, Kyriakides TC et al. Long-term comparison of endovascular and open repair of abdominal aortic aneurysm. *N Engl J Med.* 2012;367(21):1988–97.
8. Schermerhorn ML, Buck DB, O'Malley AJ et al. Long-term outcomes of abdominal aortic aneurysm in the Medicare population. *N Engl J Med.* 2015;373(4):328–38.
9. Behrendt C-A, Sedrakyan A, Rieß HC et al. Short-term and long-term results of endovascular and open repair of abdominal aortic aneurysms in Germany. *J Vasc Surg.* 2017;66(6):1704–11.e1703.

CHAPTER 13

Twelve-Year Results of Fenestrated Endografts for Juxtarenal and Group IV Thoracoabdominal Aneurysms

Mastracci TM, Eagleton MJ, Kuramochi Y, Bathurst S, Wolski K. J Vasc Surg. 2015 Feb;61(2):355–64

ABSTRACT

Objective The practice of using fenestrated endografts to treat juxtarenal and group IV thoracoabdominal aortic aneurysms (TAAA) has become more accepted, but long-term outcomes are still unknown. We report long-term survival, complications, and branch-related outcomes from a single-center experience.

Methods The study included consecutive patients enrolled prospectively into a physician-sponsored investigational device exemption classified as undergoing group IV TAAA or juxtarenal aneurysm repair by the treating surgeon using fenestrated endografts. Device morphology was used to subclassify this group of patients. Long-term survival and composite outcomes of secondary intervention, branch occlusion, stent migration, endoleak, aneurysm growth, or spinal cord injury were calculated. Descriptive analysis of branch-related outcomes and need for any re-intervention was performed. Univariate and multivariate analysis of mortality and the composite outcome was performed to determine associative risks.

Results Long-term survival for patients with juxtarenal and group IV TAAA treated with fenestrated stent grafts was 20% at 8 years. Multivariate analysis showed long-term survival for this patient population was negatively associated with increasing age, congestive heart failure, cancer, and previous aneurysm repair. The risk of spinal cord ischemia (SCI) in this group was 1.2% and the risk of aortic-related mortality was 2%. The risk of a spinal event increased with coverage above the celiac artery (52 mm of coverage above the celiac artery in patients with SCI vs. 33 mm without SCI; $P = 099$). More complex device configurations were more likely to require an increased rate of re-interventions, and patients with celiac fenestrations were more likely to experience celiac occlusions over time (3.5% vs. 0.5%; $P = 019$). However, less complex designs were complicated by an increased risk of type I endoleak over time (10.4% for renal fenestrations only vs. 1.9% for others; $P < 0.01$). As experience evolved, there was a trend to increase the number of fenestrations in devices treating the same anatomy.

Conclusions The use of fenestrated devise to treat juxtarenal and group IV TAAA is safe and effective in long-term follow-up. Mortality in this population is largely not aortic related. Devices designed for fenestrated repair of juxtarenal and group IV thoracoabdominal aneurysms within a physician sponsored investigational device exemption have changed over time. Further research is needed to determine the best configuration to treat aneurysms requiring coverage proximal to the celiac artery.

AUTHOR COMMENTARY BY MATTHEW EAGLETON

This study represents the culmination of data collected as part of a physician-sponsored investigational device exemption (PS-IDE) trial initiated by the late Dr. Roy Greenberg in 2001. Patient enrollment occurred only 2 years after the use of fenestrated endografts was initially reported and 4 years prior to the initiation of the United States multicenter prospective study evaluating the Cook Zenith fenestrated endovascular graft for treatment of juxtarenal abdominal aortic aneurysms (AAA).[1,2] Dr. Greenberg's PS-IDE data represent the outcomes from the first large-scale use of this technology to treat patients. The investigational program allowed for enrollment of patients who were considered high risk for conventional surgery—either on a physiologic or anatomic basis. The data collected, which was done in a prospective fashion, included both imaging (computed tomography, duplex ultrasound, and plain film radiography) and clinical follow-up information. The technology was in its infancy at the initiation of the study, with first outcomes reported in 2004.[3] Outcomes from these procedures contributed vastly to improvements in all aspects of fenestrated aortic endografting including patient selection, procedural details, imaging requirements, follow-up paradigms, and the technology utilized. The patients and complexity of disease treated also changed over time—with more challenging and extensive anatomy being incorporated into the enrollment criteria. Patients began being treated with branched endograft technology, and the treatment options were expanded to those with thoracoabdominal aortic aneurysms (TAAA). The data also represent physician learning curves. During the 12 years of the study evaluated in this manuscript, three physicians were involved in the performance of the procedures, including Drs. Greenberg, Mastracci, and Eagleton. This PS-IDE ultimately ceased enrollment of patients in early 2018.

Technology evolution heavily weighted outcomes in this series. One of the changes in technology that occurred over time was the transition from an un-supported fenestration to the use of primary nitinol-reinforced fenestrations. The alteration in this stent graft morphology provided a secure link with the bridging stents and the aortic component that allowed for more extensive aneurysms to be treated. This is linked to the transition away from the use of bare metal bridging stents, utilized only to keep the fenestrations aligned, to balloon-expandable stent graft systems such as the Jomed (Abbott Vascular, Santa Clara, CA) and iCAST stents (Atrium Medical, Hudson, NH). This program was able to demonstrate, during this time, that there was improved renal artery patency if covered stent grafts were used as opposed to bare metal stents.[4] In addition, in that same analysis, duplex criteria for assessing renal artery stenosis was shown to be altered, thus adjusting follow-up assessment paradigms. In addition to improved patency, the use of reinforced fenestrations and balloon-expandable stent grafts aneurysms of the aorta could be treated in which the fenestrations on the stent graft did not abut the aortic wall—the exclusion of the aneurysms became dependent upon obtaining a seal between the bridging stent and the fenestrations. And while this interaction seemed tenuous at first glance, it resulted in relatively low rates of stenosis, occlusion, component separation, or endoleak development.[5]

One of the key findings of this study is that, with experience, as the treatment plans become more complicated with the incorporation of more target vessels, this can be accomplished with minimal increase in patient morbidity. Initial application of this technology involved a thought process similar to EVAR. Attempts were made to achieve a 15 mm seal zone with an attempt to incorporate as few of the visceral vessels as possible. One of the early concerns was branch patency and durability, in particular as graft designs became more complicated. Branch durability in these sets of aneurysms, as well as more complicated ones, has proven to be outstanding.[4] Unfortunately, with shorter aortic coverage, there was a high rate of type Ia endoleak development approaching 10%. Given this, the authors opted to treat patients more aggressively and provide more aortic coverage in the visceral segment, even if it meant incorporating more visceral vessels in the fenestrated repair. This significantly reduced the incidence of type Ia endoleaks (1%–3%). The trade-off, however, was an increase in the rate of type 3 endoleaks, also approaching 10%. These endoleaks, however, were significantly easier to manage with either balloon angioplasty or the placement of an additional bridging stent as compared to treating a type Ia endoleak after FEVAR. This led to trends toward higher rates of branch re-intervention in those patients treated with trans-celiac coverage, but this outweighed the detrimental effect of a type Ia endoleak.[6]

One of the risks with extending coverage of the aorta is the potential for inducing spinal cord ischemia. This is a greater problem for patients undergoing repair of more extensive aneurysms, such as type II and III thoracoabdominal aortic aneurysms. There are adjunctive measures that can be employed to help ameliorate this risk, such as the use of spinal drains. One of the knowledge gaps at the time, however, was when these ancillary maneuvers should be necessary and when (from an anatomic perspective) the risk of spinal ischemia increased. In this analysis, we were able to demonstrate that coverage of approximately 5 cm above the celiac artery is associated with a potentially greater risk of developing symptoms related to spinal cord ischemia. The study was limited for this analysis, though, as spinal cord injury only occurred in 7 patients making it likely underpowered for adequate statistical conclusions. It may be that this is the threshold at which time adjuncts, such as the use of subarachnoid drains, may be helpful. Certainly, more information and understanding of this complication is necessary before more firm recommendations can be made.

Technical success was 97%, which given the evolution of devices, procedures, and surgeons during that time is spectacular. In addition, freedom-from-aneurysm related mortality was nearly 98% at 8 years. Long-term survival, however, was poor with survival at 8-years of only 20%. Multivariate analysis demonstrated that long-term survival was negatively influenced by increasing age, congestive heart failure, cancer, and prior aneurysm repair. These results are not surprising, and the long-term poor survival is likely representative of the high-risk patient population that were enrolled in this trial. Given the outstanding technical success of these procedures, and the excellent long-term durability of these procedures, the use of fenestrated and branched technology could safely be used outside of the limitations of the enrollment criteria of this PS-IDE and be used in "normal-risk" and "low-risk" patients. Outcomes assessment of long-term data in these populations may help us to better understand the true long-term durability of these procedures. As has been demonstrated with most endovascular procedures, we will likely continue to observe higher rates of re-intervention with fenestrated endografts compared to open surgery. Given the low perioperative mortality, great long-term freedom from aneurysm-related mortality, and excellent branch vessel patency, these types of procedures will replace conventional surgery in all anatomically suitable patients.

REFERENCES

1. Browne TF, Hartley D, Purchase S et al. A fenestrated covered suprarenal aortic stent. *Eur J Vasc Endovasc Surg*. 1999;18:445–9.
2. Oderich GS, Greenberg RK, Farber M et al. Results of the United States multicenter prospective study evaluating the Zenith fenestrated endovascular graft for treatment of juxtarenal abdominal aortic aneurysms. *J Vasc Surg*. 2014;60:1420–8.
3. Greenberg RK, Haulon S, Lyden SP et al. Endovascular management of juxtarenal aneurysms with fenestrated endovascular grafting. *J Vasc Surg*. 2004;39:279–87.
4. Mohabbat W, Greenberg RK, Mastracci TM et al. Revised duplex criteria and outcomes for renal stents and stent grafts following endovascular repair of juxtarenal and thoracoabdominal aortic aneurysms. *J Vasc Surg*. 2009;39: 827–37.
5. Mastracci TM, Greenberg RK, Eagleton MJ et al. Durability of branches in branched and fenestrated endografts. *J Vasc Surg*. 2013; 57: 926–33.
6. O'Callaghan A, Greenberg RK, Eagleton MJ et al. Type Ia endoleaks after fenestrated and branched endografts may lead to component instability and increased aortic mortality. *J Vasc Surg*. 2015; 61: 908–14.

CHAPTER 14

Predictors of Failure of Medical Management in Uncomplicated Type B Aortic Dissection

Lou X, Duwayri YM, Chen EP, Jordan WD Jr, Forcillo J, Zehner CA, Leshnower BG. Ann Thorac Surg. 2019 Feb;107(2):493–8

ABSTRACT

Background Optimal medical therapy (OMT) for uncomplicated type B aortic dissection (uTBAD) provides excellent short-term outcomes but is associated with a high incidence of failure. This study identified predictors of aortic intervention and mortality in uTBAD patients undergoing OMT.

Methods A retrospective review of the Emory University School of Medicine aortic database identified 314 uTBAD patients undergoing OMT from 2000 to 2016. Two hundred sixty-three (84%) patients had imaging at presentation analyzed for maximum aortic diameters (ADs), false lumen (FL) status, and visceral vessel perfusion. Cox proportional hazards models were constructed to estimate hazard ratios (HRs) and identify predictors of OMT failure.

Results The mean age of patients was 58 ± 12 years, and 67% were men. FL status was patent in 59.4%, partially thrombosed in 39.8%, and completely thrombosed in 0.8% of patients. Over a median follow-up of 5.6 (interquartile range, 1.4 to 8.5) years, 44.9% of patients failed OMT and underwent intervention (n = 58 open, n = 83 endovascular). The estimated incidence of OMT failure was 46%. Multivariate analysis identified the presence of diabetes, renal failure, DeBakey 3B dissection, and a descending thoracic AD of 4.5 cm or greater (HR, 1.39; 95% confidence interval, 1.24 to 1.56; $p < 0.001$) to be independent predictors of failure of OMT. FL status or the distribution of visceral vessels arising from the FL did not predict OMT failure.

Conclusions There is a significant incidence of OMT failure in uTBAD patients. A descending thoracic AD of 4.5 cm or greater at the time of diagnosis is an independent predictor of failure of OMT.

AUTHOR COMMENTARY BY WILLIAM D. JORDAN

Research Question/Objective To determine the factors associated with failure of medical management when treating uncomplicated type B aortic dissection.

Study Design Retrospective analysis of institutional database from patients treated from 2000–2016.

Sample Size 314 patients.

Follow-Up 5.6 years mean follow-up.

Inclusion/Exclusion Criteria Patients who required hospitalization for acute uncomplicated aortic dissection but were managed medically on initial presentation. Prior type A dissection or prior aortic intervention patients were excluded.

Intervention or Treatment Received All patients started with medical therapy to include blood pressure control until pain had resolved and systolic pressure was documented as less than 140 mmHg. Patients were considered to have failed medical management if they required aortic intervention or died from aortic related causes.

Results Sixteen patients (5.1%) died during the initial hospitalization and 84 patients (26.8%) died during the course of the study. 146 patients (46%) failed this initial medical treatment due to mortality or need for aortic repair. Factors that predicted failure of medical therapy included aortic diameter >4.5 cm at presentation, dissection involving the visceral arteries, partial thrombosis of the false lumen, diabetes, end-stage renal disease, and recent tobacco use. With multivariate analysis, tobacco use was no longer significant. The false lumen patency was only marginally significant in the univariate analysis and no longer important when evaluated with multivariate processing.

Study Limitations The cause of late mortality in the 35 patients could be identified in only 8 patients—four aortic related and four non-aortic related. The remaining 27 patients died of unclear causes and may represent an even higher rate of aortic failure. Also, there was not an established protocol for medical treatment of these dissection patients, and we do not have details of the antihypertensive regimen.

Relevant Studies The ADSORB study showed no clear survival benefit for treating aortic dissection early, but there was an improvement in aortic remodeling, potentially related to false lumen thrombosis.[1] While INSTEAD focused primarily on complicated dissection patients, those investigators also identified improved aortic remodeling in the patients treated with an endograft.[2]

Study Impact Much of our established treatment paradigm for uncomplicated type B aortic dissection is related to historical studies that showed a high mortality rate from open surgical repair. Our subsequent collective surgical bias has focused on medical therapy to avoid the surgical pitfalls of sewing to a fragile aortic wall. In 2005, thoracic aortic endografts became commercially available and were used, outside of their intended instruction for use, for aortic stabilization due to the surgical interest in seeking an alternative to open repair. In 2012, the endografts became "approved" by the FDA to include aortic dissection, and the medical community has generally accepted this treatment paradigm. Currently, we are plagued with determining which patients should be repaired acutely and which should maintain a treatment with a medical regimen. The motivation for early treatment includes improved aortic remodeling as seen on surveillance imaging. After early aortic endografting, the false lumen often thrombosis completely, the distal aortic segment remodels nicely, and both patient and doctor are relieved of the long-term failure mode. The prevailing opinion suggests that earlier treatment promotes better aortic remodeling[3] due to the elasticity of the aortic septum. That is, we can return to a normal aorta and make the septum "stick" to the main aortic wall if we treat sooner in the pathologic process. This concept of earlier treatment seems to align with our general medical concept that early detection and treatment leads to better results. However, our skepticism creates some concern. We may cause more harm if we act too soon as some aortic dissections remodel quite well with medical management including control of blood pressure. This study reinforces some of the existing factors for known late failure after aortic dissection—large aortic diameter. However, there is less concern about the false lumen status as some studies have suggested.[4] The study further analyzes the number of outflow vessels from the false lumen under the pretense that more outflow reduces the pressure of the false lumen and minimizes the late failure of expansion.[5] However, this study did not support that hypothesis.

While the current efforts seek to identify factors for late aortic failure after acute type B aortic dissection (aTBAD), our understanding seems rudimentary. We have recently changed classification to include acute, sub-acute, and chronic based upon time interval from the onset of symptoms[6] but we ultimately are hoping to identify an aortic "flap" that will remodel well and respond positively to the endograft. Currently, baseline aortic diameter seems to be our best predictor of success, but we have enormous opportunity to identify more precise markers that could characterize the aortic septum as one that remodels well in establishing a normal aortic outcome.

Ultimately, this study reflects some of the shifting interest to treat uTBAD earlier than previously suggested. A large aortic diameter (4.0 cm in some studies, 4.5 cm in this study) seems to be the most reliable predictor for late failure and thus may be considered a good current predictor. In our own practice, we tend to be more aggressive toward treating these patients earlier, sometimes during the same admission. However, we still need to follow these patients carefully to understand that our treatment is successful in promoting aortic stability—no further degeneration, dissection, malperfusion, or expansion. Our clinical markers remain crude and we have yet to understand which patients' aortic tissue is most responsive when we treat early and with an endograft.

REFERENCES

1. Brunkwall J, Lammer J, Verhoeven E, Taylor P. ADSORB: A Study on the efficacy of endovascular grafting in uncomplicated acute dissection of the descending aorta. *Eur J Vasc Endovasc Surg*. 2012;44(1):31–6.
2. Nienaber CA, Kische S, Rousseau H et al. Endovascular repair of type B aortic dissection: Long-term results of the randomized investigation of stent grafts in aortic dissection trial. *Circ Cardiovasc Interv*. 2013;6:407–16.
3. Leshnower BG, Duwayri YM, Chen EP et al. Aortic remodeling after endovascular repair of complicated acute type B aortic dissection. *Ann Thorac Surg*. 2017;103:1878–85.
4. Tsai TT, Evangelista A, Nienaber CA et al. Partial thrombosis of the false lumen in patients with acute type B aortic dissection. *NEJM*. 2007;357:349–59.
5. Kamman AV, Brunkwall J, Verhoeven EL, Heijmen RH, Trimarchi S. ADSORB trialists. Predictors of aortic growth in uncomplicated type B aortic dissection from the Acute Dissection Stent Grafting or Best Medical Treatment (ADSORB) database. *J Vasc Sur*. 2017;65(4):964–971.e3.
6. Lombardi J. *Reporting Standards Update (with STS): Type B Aortic Dissections*. Vascular Annual Meeting, National Harbor, MD. June 14, 2019.

CHAPTER 15

Predictors of Intervention and Mortality in Patients with Uncomplicated Acute Type B Aortic Dissection

Ray HM, Durham CA, Ocazionez D, Charlton-Ouw KM, Estrera AL, Miller CC 3rd, Safi HJ, Azizzadeh A. J Vasc Surg. 2016 Dec;64(6):1560–8

ABSTRACT

Background Patients with uncomplicated acute type B aortic dissection (uATBAD) have historically been managed with medical therapy. Recent studies suggest that high-risk patients with uATBAD may benefit from thoracic endovascular aortic repair. This study aims to determine the predictors of intervention and mortality in patients with uATBAD.

Methods All patients admitted with uATBAD from 2000 to 2014 were reviewed, and those with computed tomographic angiography imaging were included. Multiplanar reconstruction was used to obtain double orthogonal oblique measurements. All measurements were obtained by a specialized cardiovascular radiologist (D.O.). The maximum aortic diameter, proximal descending thoracic aorta false lumen (FL) diameter, and area were recorded. Outcomes, including the need for intervention and mortality, were tracked over time. Data were analyzed by stratified Kaplan-Meier and multiple Cox regression analysis using SAS v 9.4 (SAS Institute, Cary, NC).

Results During the study period, 294 patients with uATBAD were admitted with 156 having admission computed tomographic angiography imaging available for analysis. The cohort had an average age of 60.6 years (±13.6 years); 60% were males. The average follow-up time was 3.7 years (interquartile range, 2.1–6.9). A stratified analysis demonstrated the most sensitive cutoff for mortality was aortic diameter >44 mm ($P < 0.01$), and it appeared to be a threshold effect with minimal additional information added by finer size stratification. FL diameter did not predict mortality in our series ($P = 0.36$). Intervention-free survival, alternatively, appeared to decrease over the range of diameters from 35 to 44 mm ($P < 0.01$). An FL diameter >22 mm was associated with decreased intervention-free survival ($P < 0.04$). Age >60 years on admission also demonstrated decreased survival compared with those ≤60 years of age (P <0.01). Diameter >44 mm persisted as a risk factor for mortality (hazard ratio, 8.6; P <0.01) after adjustment for diabetes (6.7; P <0.01), age (1.06/y; P <0.01), history of stroke (5.4; P <0.01), connective tissue disorder (2.3; P <0.01), and syncope on admission (9.5; P <0.04). The 1-, 5-, and 10-year intervention rate for patients with admission aortic diameter >44 mm was 18.8%, 29.5%, and 50.3%, respectively, compared with 4.8%, 13.3%, and 13.3% in the ≤44 mm group (P <0.01).

Conclusion Aortic diameter >44 mm is a predictor of mortality after adjustment for other significant risk factors. Age >60 years on admission is a predictor of mortality. An FL diameter >22 mm as well as those with maximum aortic diameter >44 mm on admission were associated with decreased intervention-free survival. Patients with these high-risk criteria may benefit from thoracic endovascular aortic repair. Further studies are needed to further define those patients at highest risk and, thus, most likely to benefit from early intervention.

Relevant Studies Winnerkvist A, Lockowandt U, Rasmussena E, Rådegran K. A prospective study of medically treated acute type B aortic dissection. *Eur J Vasc Endovasc Surg*. 2006 Oct;32(4):349–55. Epub 2006 Jun 6.

Song JM, Kim SD, Kim JH, Kim MJ, Kang DH, Seo JB, Lim TH, Lee JW, Song MG, Song JK. Long-term predictors of descending aorta aneurysmal change in patients with aortic dissection. *J Am Coll Cardiol*. 2007 Aug 21;50(8):799–804. Epub 2007 Aug 6.

Durham CA, Aranson NJ, Ergul EA, Wang LJ, Patel VI, Cambria RP, Conrad MF. Aneurysmal degeneration of the thoracoabdominal aorta after medical management of type B aortic dissections. *J Vasc Surg*. 2015; 62: 900–6.

Estrera AL, Miller CC, Goodrick J, Porat EE, Achouh PE, Dhareshwar J, Meada R, Azizzadeh A, Safi HJ. Update on outcomes of acute type B aortic dissection. *Ann Thorac Surg*. 2007 Feb;83(2):S842–5; discussion S846–50.

AUTHOR COMMENTARY BY H.M. RAY, C.A. DURHAM, D. OCAZIONEZ, K.M. CHARLTON-OUW, ANTHONY L. ESTRERA, CHARLES C. MILLER III, HAZIM J. SAFI, AND ALI AZIZZADEH

Despite low in-hospital mortality, patients with uncomplicated acute type B aortic dissection (uATBAD) remain at high risk of developing subsequent aortic complications and need for intervention.[1] Based on our single-institution series, the rate of in-hospital mortality for this cohort was 1.2%, while the rate of intervention at 10 years ranged from 11.3%–34.4% (Table 15.1). Moreover, the survival rate at 5 years was 75%. We set out to determine predictors of intervention and mortality in this cohort. Proper risk stratification allowed us to intervene in high-risk patients before they developed aortic complications, such as rupture and death. Previously published studies identified maximum aortic diameter >40mm[2] and upper descending thoracic aortic false lumen (FL)

Table 15.1 Intervention Rate (%)

Admission Aortic Diameter (mm)	1 Year	5 Years	10 Years
>44	18.8	29.5	50.3
≤44	4.8	13.3	13.3

Note: Overall Intervention Rate:
- >44 mm: 34.4%
- <44 mm: 11.3%
- (OR 4.12, $p = 0.02$)

diameter ≥22 mm on admission as high-risk criteria for aortic mortality.[3] However, these studies did not describe specific imaging techniques, such as how the measurements were made, who made them, or if advanced reconstruction software was utilized. Given the shortcomings of the research available at the time, we performed a controlled study utilizing modern 3D reconstruction software with double orthogonal oblique measurements taken by a fellowship-trained cardiovascular radiologist.

Our goal was to obtain measurements in a systematic manner at standardized and easily identifiable areas in order to make the findings reproducible and clinically relevant. This study was a retrospective analysis of a single-center cohort data examining patients with uATBAD and adequate admission computed tomography angiography (CTA) imaging for analysis over a 14-year period. In all, 156 patients had admission CTA imaging available for analysis using 3D reconstruction software. We found that maximum aortic diameter on admission >44 mm and age >60 were risk factors for mortality. In addition, maximum aortic diameter >44 and FL diameter >22 mm were associated with decreased intervention-free survival. Moreover, 69% of patients in the cohort had at least one of the following three risk factors: maximum aortic diameter >44 mm; FL diameter >22 mm; and age >60 (Table 15.2). In other words, the majority of the patients with uATBAD would be potential candidates for thoracic endovascular aortic repair (TEVAR).

This study is limited by its retrospective nature as well as the fact that CTA images from the time of admission were no longer available in our hospital's archiving and communication system for a large portion of the cohort.

The significance of this contribution to the vascular surgery literature lies in identifying high-risk criteria for intervention and mortality in patients with uATBAD. The findings support earlier intervention in the form of TEVAR in those deemed high risk

Table 15.2 Risk Factors

TAD >44 mm/FLD >22/Age >60%	
1 Risk Factor	44
2 Risk Factors	19
3 Risk Factors	6
Total	69

for complications: maximum aortic diameter >44 mm; FL diameter >22 mm; and age >60. We hope that risk stratification and earlier intervention, based on the findings of this study, may lead to improved outcomes in patients with uATBAD.

REFERENCES

1. Estrera AL, Miller CC, Goodrick J, Porat EE, Achouh PE, Dhareshwar J, Meada R, Azizzadeh A, Safi HJ. Update on outcomes of acute type B aortic dissection. *Ann Thorac Surg*. 2007 Feb;83(2):S842–5; discussion S846–50.
2. Winnerkvist A, Lockowandt U, Rasmussena E et al. A prospective study of medically treated acute type B aortic dissection. *Eur J Vasc Endovasc Surg*. 2006 Oct;32(4):349–55. Epub 2006 Jun 6.
3. Song JM, Kim SD, Kim JH et al. Long-term predictors of descending aorta aneurysmal change in patients with aortic dissection. *J Am Coll Cardiol*. 2007 Aug 21;50(8):799–804. Epub 2007 Aug 6.

CHAPTER 16

Endovascular Repair of Type B Aortic Dissection: Long-Term Results of the Randomized Investigation of Stent Grafts in Aortic Dissection Trial

Nienaber CA, Kische S, Rousseau H, Eggebrecht H, Rehders TC, Kundt G, Glass A, Scheinert D, Czerny M, Kleinfeldt T et al.
INSTEAD-XL Trial. Circ Cardiovasc Interv. 2013 Aug;6(4):407–16

ABSTRACT

Background Thoracic endovascular aortic repair (TEVAR) represents a therapeutic concept for type B aortic dissection. Long-term outcomes and morphology after TEVAR for uncomplicated dissection are unknown.

Methods and Results A total of 140 patients with stable type B aortic dissection previously randomized to optimal medical treatment and TEVAR (n = 72) versus optimal medical treatment alone (n = 68) were analyzed retrospectively for aorta-specific, all-cause outcomes, and disease progression using landmark statistical analysis of years 2 to 5 after index procedure. Cox regression was used to compare outcomes between groups; all analyses are based on intention to treat. The risk of all-cause mortality (11.1% vs. 19.3%; P = 0.13), aorta-specific mortality (6.9% vs. 19.3%; P = 0.04), and progression (27.0% vs. 46.1%; P = 0.04) after 5 years was lower with TEVAR than with optimal medical treatment alone. Landmark analysis suggested a benefit of TEVAR for all endpoints between 2 and 5 years; for example, for all-cause mortality (0% vs. 16.9%; P = 0.0003), aorta-specific mortality (0% vs. 16.9%; P = 0.0005), and for progression (4.1% vs. 28.1%; P = 0.004); Landmarking at 1 year and 1 month revealed consistent findings. Both improved survival and less progression of disease at 5 years after elective TEVAR were associated with stent graft induced false lumen thrombosis in 90.6% of cases (P < 0.0001).

Conclusions In this study of survivors of type B aortic dissection, TEVAR in addition to optimal medical treatment is associated with improved 5-year aorta-specific survival and delayed disease progression. In stable type B dissection with suitable anatomy, preemptive TEVAR should be considered to improve late outcome.

EXPERT COMMENTARY BY JESUS G. ULLOA AND JUSTIN GALOVICH

Research Question/Objective To evaluate the long-term outcomes; up to 5 years of endovascular treatment for subacute uncomplicated type B aortic dissection with optimal medical therapy (OMT) compared to optimal medical therapy alone.

Study Design Retrospective review of a prospectively collected cohort consisting of consecutive patients with uncomplicated type B dissection randomized to thoracic endovascular aortic repair (TEVAR) in addition to optimal medical therapy or optimal medical therapy alone. Patients were randomized in a 1:1 ratio according to a computer generated sequence and stratified to each center. Mantel-Cox regression was used to calculate hazard ratios for comparison of clinical outcomes. Kaplan-Meier survival curves were constructed for time-to-event variables. Landmark analysis was performed at prespecified breakpoint of 2 years from randomization with hazard ratios calculated from randomization up to 24 months, and from 24 months to end of trial, thus allowing assessment of time dependent response to treatment allocation. Additional landmark analysis was performed at breakpoints of 1 month and 1 year.

Sample Size 597 consecutive patients were screened, 140 of which were randomly assigned. Overall 72 were allocated to TEVAR+OMT and 68 to OMT alone on an intention to treat basis.

Follow-Up Minimum 5 years.

Inclusion/Exclusion Criteria Included patients had an uncomplicated type B aortic dissection in the early chronic phase of dissection (greater than 2 weeks from onset), who were treated at 7 European centers between November 2003 and December 2005. Excluded patients had an aortic diameter greater than 5.5 centimeters or other emerging recurrent complications.

Intervention or Treatment Received TEVAR with optimal medical therapy or optimal medical therapy alone.

Results There were no significant differences between groups with regards to baseline characteristics, comorbidities or dissection morphology. There was no loss to follow-up, with 117 patients alive at the end of 5 years. TEVAR was completed in 70 patients with no periprocedural deaths or conversions. The majority (82.9%) had a single stent graft placed. In both groups, 90% of cases had adjusted antihypertensive regimens and systolic blood pressures equal to or less than 130 mmHg. Among OMT patients, TEVAR was necessary in 14 cases and conversion to open repair in four cases for enlarging false lumen diameter. In the TEVAR group, seven cases required additional stent graft and three cases were converted to open.

Regarding all-cause mortality, a greater than 5-year mortality trended lower among TEVAR patients compared to OMT alone (11% vs. 19%). Survival benefit between 2 and 5 years (100% vs. 83%), but not before 2 years, was found for TEVAR patients with findings of a significant interaction between treatment effect and time on landmark analysis at 2 years, 1 year, and 1 month.

When considering aortic specific mortality (death from documented aortic rupture, malperfusion, proximal dissection, or death within 1-hour onset of signs or symptoms in absence of coronary or valvular heart disease), the TEVAR patients had lower 5-year findings (7% vs. 19%). Survival benefit between 2 and 5 years (100% vs. 83%), but not before 2 years, was found for TEVAR patients with findings of a significant interaction between treatment effect and time on landmark analysis at 2 years, 1 year, and 1 month.

Freedom from progression of aortic pathology (combined endpoint of crossover to stent graft or conversion to open repair, additional endovascular or open surgery for rupture, malperfusion, aortic expansion or enlarging aortic diameter greater than 5.5 cm), among TEVAR patients at 5 years was higher (73% vs. 54%). Survival benefit with freedom from progression of aortic pathology between 2 and 5 years (96% vs. 72%), but not before 2 years, was found for TEVAR patients with findings of a significant interaction between treatment effect and time on landmark analysis at 2 years, 1 year, and 1 month.

All patients in the OMT group who ruptured or crossed over had an entry tear of greater than 10 mm. Complete false lumen thrombosis was documented in 91% at the thoracic level with 79% demonstrating morphologic evidence of remodeling among the TEVAR group. OMT was associated with expansion of maximum aortic diameter and rarely exhibited false lumen thrombosis.

Study Limitations Use of landmark analysis in which findings become observational, confounders may be unaccounted for, and early events may be omitted, making analysis dependent on time-point specific results. Lack of information regarding OMT regimen. Unclear, but likely homogenous racial-ethnic patient study demographics limiting generalizability to heterogenous populations.

Study Impact Nienaber and colleagues, through their work, have helped us understand that there is no such thing as an "uncomplicated" aortic dissection. The ensuing risks of all-cause mortality (20%–40% at 5 years) and aortic specific mortality despite optimal medical therapy are humbling.

The finding that endovascular intervention during the subacute phase of type B aortic dissection presenting without malperfusion decreases mortality and aortic specific morbidity gives the modern vascular surgeon another tool to address a difficult pathology. Findings of aortic remodeling as exhibited by false lumen thrombosis speak to the dynamic nature of dissections and the importance of treating perfusion pressure differentials between the true and false lumen. Prior studies have found an initial aortic diameter greater than 3.5 cm at presentation to be a risk factor for future growth, while 28% of patients will go on to require an operative intervention for aneurysmal degeneration despite medical therapy.[1]

Though there is a trend toward lower morbidity and mortality among TEVAR recipients, we cannot ignore the time dependent nature of these findings. The authors demonstrated no benefit before 2 years and found slightly higher early perioperative risk of complications among the TEVAR group that was offset by the longer survival. This brings into question who should have a TEVAR for subacute dissection without evidence of malperfusion. Should a preemptive TEVAR be offered to a person over 75 years of age with incident end-stage renal disease who has an estimated probability of survival of 37% at 3 years?[2] More recent studies utilizing a state-wide data set found a similar trend toward survival benefit among TEVAR patients.[3] Nonetheless, providing the correct therapy to the correct patient at the correct time remains the central questions for escalating beyond optimal medical therapy.

The timing of treatment in the study was quite variable, ranging from 2 weeks to more than 4 years from dissection diagnosis/symptom onset. Those who treat aortic dissections are aware that subacute and chronic dissections behave very differently. Subacute dissections, 2 weeks to 6 months, are more likely to remodel compared to the chronic dissections, >6 months. The benefit of TEVAR may have been more apparent if only subacute dissections were enrolled. The optimal time for TEVAR is still debatable but likely in the subacute phase.

The importance of referral to high-volume centers with established protocols and systems of care for aortic surgery cannot be overemphasized. We have not established a size threshold for entry aortic tear at which to intervene. However, the author's findings of greater than 10 mm aortic entry tear provide important objective evidence at which one may intervene for preemptive aortic remodeling. Though the authors recommend surveillance may be tapered after 2 years of disease free progression, our practice remains to obtain annual cross-sectional imaging. In addition to the size of the entry tear, the ratio of false and true lumen diameters and flow volume is likely affecting the aortic remodeling in the medical treatment arm. The anatomy of aortic dissections is quite variable, from the simplistic proximal entry tear and distal re-entry tear to the complex with multiple entry and re-entry tears, the latter of which can be much more challenging and unpredictable. The seminal contribution of this study remains the finding that aortic remodeling and decreased all-cause morbidity, as well as aortic specific mortality are improved through elective stent graft repair of type B dissection with optimal medical therapy.

REFERENCES

1. Durham CA, Aranson NJ, Ergul EA, Wang LJ, Patel VI, Cambria RP, and Conrad MF. Aneurysmal degeneration of the thoracoabdominal aorta after medical management of type B aortic dissections. *J Vasc Surg*. 2015 Oct;62(4):900–6.
2. United States Renal Data System. *2018 USRDS annual data report: Epidemiology of kidney disease in the United States*. National Institutes of Health, National Institute of Diabetes and Digestive and Kidney Diseases, Bethesda, MD, 2018.
3. Iannuzzi JC, Stapleton SM, Bababekov YJ, Chang D, Lancaster RT, Conrad MF, Cambria RP, and Patel VI. Favorable impact of thoracic endovascular aortic repair on the survival of patients with acute uncomplicated type B aortic dissection. *J Vasc Surg*. 2018 Dec;68(6):1649–55.

CHAPTER 17

Outcomes from the Gore Global Registry for Endovascular Aortic Treatment in Patients Undergoing Thoracic Endovascular Aortic Repair for Type B Dissection

Tjaden BL Jr, Sandhu H, Miller C, Gable D, Trimarchi S, Weaver F, Azizzadeh A. J Vasc Surg. 2018;68:1314–23

ABSTRACT

Objective The Global Registry for Endovascular Aortic Treatment (GREAT) is a prospective multicenter registry collecting real-world data on the performance of W.L. Gore (Flagstaff, AZ) aortic endografts. The purpose of the present study was to analyze the implementation and outcomes of thoracic endovascular aortic repair (TEVAR) in GREAT patients with type B aortic dissection (TBAD).

Methods From 2010 to 2016, >5,000 patients were enrolled in the GREAT from 113 centers in 14 countries across 4 continents. The study population comprised those treated for TBAD. The primary outcomes of interest were mortality and freedom from aortic events (AEs).

Results A total of 264 patients (80% male; mean age, 62 years) underwent TEVAR for the treatment of 170 (64%) acute and 94 (36%) chronic cases of TBAD. Chronic TBAD patients required significantly longer endograft coverage than did acute TBAD patients ($P = 0.05$). Early postoperative complications occurred in 9% of patients, with no difference in chronic versus acute dissection ($P = 0.11$). The 30-day aortic mortality and all-cause mortality were 1.5% and 2.3%, respectively, with no differences based on chronicity. During a mean follow-up of 26 months, the total aortic mortality was 2.7% and the total all-cause mortality was 12.5%. The all-cause mortality was significantly greater for chronic versus acute TBAD (19.2% vs. 8.8%, respectively; $P = 0.02$). On multivariate analysis, patients with acute uncomplicated dissections had significantly improved overall survival compared with all other categories of dissections (93% vs. 83% at 2 years; $P < 0.05$). A proximal landing zone diameter >40 mm was associated with an increased risk of retrograde type A dissection (18% vs. 2%; $P = 0.02$). Patients undergoing left subclavian artery (LSA) coverage experienced a two-fold greater rate of AEs compared with noncoverage patients ($P < 0.01$). Patients who underwent LSA revascularization experienced a 1.5-fold greater rate of AEs compared with patients covered without revascularization ($P = 0.04$).

Conclusions TEVAR for TBAD using the conformable GORE TAG thoracic endoprosthesis device can be performed with a low incidence of aortic mortality and complications. Acute uncomplicated TBAD patients had a significantly lower mortality rate than that of other patients. Larger proximal landing zones were associated with more frequent retrograde type A dissection. LSA involvement (coverage and/or revascularization) was associated with an increased risk of AEs during follow-up.

AUTHOR COMMENTARY BY GREGORY A. MAGEE AND FRED WEAVER

The treatment of Stanford type B aortic dissections has undergone significant changes since the seminal publications of Dake and Nienaber in 1999, describing the use of thoracic endovascular aortic repair (TEVAR) to cover the proximal entry tear.[1,2] Medical management had been the mainstay of treatment with good short-term results,[3] but a dismal 5-year survival of only 50%–60%.[4,5] On the basis of these encouraging early results, a randomized trial of elective TEVAR for stable type B dissection was conducted, which failed to show a mortality benefit at 2-years compared to medical management but demonstrated much improved aortic remodeling.[6] Further follow-up of the same study demonstrated that at 5 years the all-cause and aortic-specific mortality was lower with TEVAR, negating the early deaths from procedure related complications in the TEVAR group.[7] This survival advantage of TEVAR was corroborated in an analysis from the International Registry of Acute Aortic Dissection (IRAD).[8] These data led to the adoption of TEVAR for type B dissection patients in many centers worldwide, however, the practice remains controversial in patients with acute uncomplicated and chronic type B dissections.

The primary objective for our study was to evaluate mortality and aortic events (AEs) following TEVAR for acute and chronic type B aortic dissections in a real world practice data set. We utilized the Global Registry for Endovascular Aortic Treatment (GREAT), which enrolled 5,014 patients from 113 centers in four countries across four continents who were treated with endovascular aortic repair using a W.L. Gore (Flagstaff, AZ) aortic endograft between 2010 and 2016. AEs were defined as aortic mortality; aneurysm formation or growth; aortic rupture; spinal cord ischemia; stroke; aortic branch vessel complications; complications associated with debranching, retrograde dissection, new distal dissection, endoleak, or persistent false lumen flow; and graft infection. Analysis was performed by an independent academic research team and statistician.

GREAT included 264 patients who underwent TEVAR for type B aortic dissection that were suitable for analysis. Of these, 170 were treated for acute TBAD and 94 for chronic TBAD. The mean patient age was 62 years and 80% were male.

The principal finding of this study was that acute uncomplicated type B aortic dissections had a significantly lower mortality rate than patients with chronic or acute complicated dissections (Figure 17.1). Additionally, we found that patients with proximal landing zones greater than 40 mm were more likely to develop a retrograde type A dissection. Interestingly, left subclavian artery coverage and/or revascularization was associated with an increased rate of AEs during follow-up. This last finding was counter-intuitive and prompted further analyses.

This study was important because a more nuanced understanding of who, when, and how to treat type B aortic dissection with TEVAR is necessary necessary to improve outcomes and long-term results. The limitations of the study were that it was retrospective in design and limited predominantly to postoperative AEs. Furthermore, GREAT did not capture anatomical data to evaluate aortic remodeling or growth over time.

Following this study we performed a more granular analysis of our center's aortic database to evaluate the impact of left subclavian artery coverage. We found that a landing zone in the non-dissected aorta was less likely to cause retrograde type A aortic dissection, and this almost always required coverage of the left subclavian artery.[9] We also queried the Society for Vascular Surgeons Vascular Quality Initiative (VQI) database to evaluate the impact of left subclavian artery coverage and revascularization. This analysis showed that in patients undergoing TEVAR with coverage of the left subclavian artery, the addition of a revascularization procedure was associated

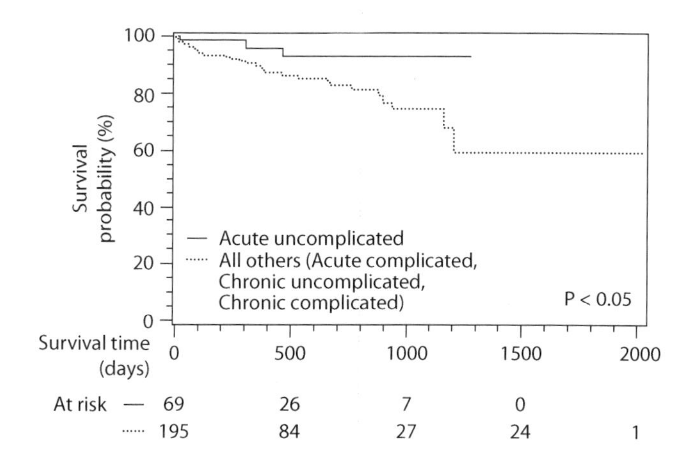

Figure 17.1 Kaplan-Meier curves showing overall survival (freedom from all-cause mortality) stratified by dissection category. The straight line indicates acute uncomplicated dissection, and the dotted line indicates all other dissection types (acute complicated, chronic uncomplicated, chronic complicated).

with a significantly lower spinal cord ischemia rate.[10] These data are somewhat at odds with this secondary analysis of the GREAT data, which is likely a result of different endpoints. Thus, our practice is to routinely revascularize the left subclavian artery when coverage is planned.

We hope this study prompts other aortic endograft manufacturers to evaluate and publish their post-market data, as real world results often differ from those of controlled trials and performance may differ based on design features, which could lead to improved stent designs in the future.

REFERENCES

1. Dake MD, Kato N, Mitchell RS, Semba CP, Razavi MK, Shimono T, Hirano T, Takeda K, Yada I, and Miller DC. Endovascular stent-graft placement for the treatment of acute aortic dissection. *N Engl J Med*. 1999;340(20):1546–52.
2. Nienaber CA, Fattori R, Lund G, Dieckmann C, Wolf W, von Kodolitsch Y, Nicolas V, and Pierangeli A. Nonsurgical reconstruction of thoracic aortic dissection by stent-graft placement. *N Engl J Med*. 1999;340(20):1539–45.
3. Estrera AL, Miller CC, Safi HJ et al. Outcomes of medical management of acute type B aortic dissection. *Circulation*. 2006;114(1 Suppl):I384–9.
4. Elefteriades JA, Hartleroad J, Gusberg RJ, Salazar AM, Black HR, Kopf GS, Baldwin JC, Hammond GL. Long-term experience with descending aortic dissection: The complication-specific approach. *Ann Thorac Surg*. 1992;53(1):11–20; discussion 20-1.
5. Umaña JP, Lai DT, Mitchell RS et al. Is medical therapy still the optimal treatment strategy for patients with acute type B aortic dissections? *J Thorac Cardiovasc Surg*. 2002;124(5):896–910.
6. Nienaber CA, Rousseau H, Eggebrecht H et al. Randomized comparison of strategies for type B aortic dissection: The INvestigation of STEnt Grafts in Aortic Dissection (INSTEAD) trial. *Circulation*. 2009;120(25):2519–28.
7. Nienaber CA, Kische S, Rousseau H et al. Endovascular repair of type B aortic dissection: Long-term results of the randomized investigation of stent grafts in aortic dissection trial. *Circ Cardiovasc Interv*. 2013;6(4):407–16.
8. Fattori R, Montgomery D, Lovato L, Kische S, Di Eusanio M, Ince H, Eagle KA, Isselbacher EM, and Nienaber CA. Survival after endovascular therapy in patients with type B aortic dissection: A report from the International Registry of Acute Aortic Dissection (IRAD). *JACC Cardiovasc Interv*. 2013;6(8):876–82.
9. Kuo EC, Veranyan N, Johnson CE, Weaver FA, Ham SW, Rowe VL, Fleischman F, Bowdish M, and Han SM. Impact of proximal seal zone length and intramural hematoma on clinical outcomes and aortic remodeling after thoracic endovascular aortic repair for aortic dissections. *J Vasc Surg*. 2019 Apr;69(4):987–95.
10. Teixeira PG, Woo K, Beck AW, Scali ST, and Weaver FA, Society for Vascular Surgery V. s. Q. I. V. Association of left subclavian artery coverage without revascularization and spinal cord ischemia in patients undergoing thoracic endovascular aortic repair: A Vascular Quality Initiative® analysis. *Vascular*. 2017;25(6):587–97.

Chapter 18

Placement of Balloon-Expandable Intraluminal Stents in Iliac Arteries: First 171 Procedures

Palmaz JC, Garcia OJ, Schatz RA, Rees CR, Roeren T, Richter GM, Noeldge G, Gardiner GA Jr, Becker GJ, Walker C et al. Radiology. 1990 Mar;174(3 Pt 2):969–75

ABSTRACT

The treatment of aorto-iliac occlusive disease has undergone a marked paradigm shift over the past 30 years with the vast majority of these patients now being treated with endovascular means. The study presented here by Julio Palmaz et al. in 1990 was the first large trial evaluating the safety and efficacy of balloon-expandable stents for the treatment of iliac disease. Prior to this, the standard endovascular therapy had been stand-alone angioplasty. This multicenter study demonstrated that iliac stenting could be performed safely with high technical success and excellent short-term and mid-term clinical outcomes. The positive results from this publication laid the foundation for the transition of the treatment of aorto-iliac occlusive disease from being primarily surgical to being treated with endovascular means.

EXPERT COMMENTARY BY DONALD BARIL

Balloon-expandable intraluminal stents were used to treat iliac artery stenoses or occlusions that failed to respond to conventional balloon angioplasty. One hundred seventy-one procedures were performed in 154 patients, of whom 48 had a limb at risk for amputation. Thirty-six had severe and 70 had moderate intermittent claudication. At the latest follow-up examination (average, 6 months; range, 1–24 months), 137 patients demonstrated clinical benefit, 113 of whom had become asymptomatic. Eleven patients showed no initial benefit, and six improved initially but later developed new vascular symptoms. Complications occurred in 18 patients. In three patients, complications were directly related to the device. Two occlusions were successfully recanalized, and an intramural collection of contrast material secondary to balloon perforation evolved favorably. The remaining patients had groin hematoma (n = 6), distal embolization (n = 4), extravasation (n = 2), transient renal failure (n = 1), pseudoaneurysm at the puncture site (n = 1), or subintimal dissection (n = 1). All stents have remained patent to the latest follow-up examination without evidence of migration or aneurysm formation.

SUMMARY OF RELEVANT STUDY/PAPER BY THE AUTHOR

Research Question/Objective To determine the safety and efficacy of placement of balloon-expandable intraluminal stents for treatment of iliac artery stenoses and occlusions.

Study Design Retrospective review of data collected from a prospective multicenter trial.

Sample Size 154 patients who underwent 261 stent placements during 171 separate procedures. This group included 28 women and 126 men with an average age of 62.7 years. The majority of patients were claudicants (106) with nearly one-third of the patients suffering from limb-threatening ischemia (48).

Follow-Up 6 months (range 1–24 months).

Inclusion/Exclusion Criteria Indications for stent placement were inadequate immediate post-angioplasty response, restenosis after prior iliac balloon angioplasty, and total iliac artery occlusion. Contraindications to stent placement were extravasation of contrast after initial balloon angioplasty, marked tortuosity of the iliac arteries, and dense, extensive arterial calcification. Additional relative contraindications included concomitant iliac artery aneurysms, severe hypertension, impaired pain sensation, stenosis of the common femoral artery, and poor distal arterial outflow.

Intervention or Treatment Received Patients were treated with a stainless steel stent (3.1 × 30 mm) which was crimp-mounted on an 8 × 30 mm angioplasty balloon catheter and delivered via a 10-French sheath, 30 cm in length. Conventional angioplasty was used as first-line therapy with those who did not respond adequately, then undergoing stent placement. Inadequate response was defined as a dissection, recoil leading to a residual stenosis of >30%, and/or a transtenotic mean pressure gradient of >5 mmHg. Additionally, stents were placed for restenotic lesions after prior angioplasty and total occlusions. Patients were pretreated with aspirin (325 mg daily) and dipyridamole (25 mg every 8 hours) starting 48 hours before the procedure and were continued on this regimen for 3 months after the intervention. Patients were systemically heparinized during the procedure.

One-hundred-eighty-one stents were placed in common iliac arteries and 80 stents were placed in external iliac arteries. Seventeen patients underwent bilateral stent placement and 21 patients underwent stent placement in ipsilateral common and external iliac arteries. Twelve patients underwent stent placement in addition to a surgical outflow procedure.

Results The mean intra-arterial pressure gradient improved from 36.4 mmHg to 1.6 mmHg and only five of the treated iliac arteries had a gradient of 10 mmHg or greater after treatment. Procedure related complications occurred in 9.7% of patients. Two patients developed early stent thrombosis within a week of placement and were both subsequently treated successfully percutaneously. Six patients had groin hematomas requiring transfusion of surgical evacuation. Four patients had distal embolization which were all treated with surgical embolectomy. One patient developed transient renal failure which resolved with conservative therapy.

At initial 2-week follow-up, 114 of the 154 patients were asymptomatic, 25 had moderate claudication, seven had severe claudication, four had healing wounds, and four were lost to follow-up. At the latest follow-up (average 6 months), 113 patients were asymptomatic, 25 had moderate claudication, five had severe claudication, two patients had rest pain, and one had undergone a below-knee amputation. There was noted to be a net benefit in 134 patients, no initial improvement in 11 patients, and initial improvement followed by new symptoms in six patients. Ankle-arm indices were noted to improve postprocedure, increases that were maintained at the latest follow-up examination.

Of the 125 patients who were seen at 6 month follow-up, 43 underwent repeat angiography. Patency rates of this group were 100% and based on clinical examination and hemodynamic evaluation, the remaining patients were also determined to have patent stents. No evidence of stent migration or aneurysm formation was seen in the follow-up period.

Study Limitations This study has the limitations of being a retrospective review of prospectively collected data. As such, there was no randomization to compare stenting to angioplasty alone, although the criteria for stenting were well-defined in the study. At the time of publication, angioplasty was the gold standard for endovascular therapy of iliac lesions. Additionally, the length of follow-up is a limiting factor, although, as the first large study of use of balloon-expandable stents for the treatment of iliac occlusive disease, this is certainly understandable.

Study Impact This paper, authored by Julio Palmaz, was the summary report of a multicenter clinical trial evaluating the safety and efficacy of balloon-expandable stent for the treatment of stenoses and occlusions of iliac arteries. At the time of publication, endovascular therapy of iliac artery occlusive disease was limited nearly exclusively to angioplasty alone with only a few case reports of stent usage. This study included a large number of patients with a significant burden disease who underwent procedures with a very high technical success rate, very acceptable complication rates, and excellent short-term and mid-term clinical outcomes. This publication laid the foundation for the transition of the treatment of aorto-iliac occlusive disease from being primarily surgical to being treated with endovascular means. The use of stents allowed for the treatment of more complex disease including more proximally into the aorta and more distally into the external iliac arteries. Open reconstructions, including aorto-bifemoral bypass and aortic endarterectomy, which had been associated with excellent outcomes and patency rates, now had a less invasive rival technique that ultimately was and continues to have excellent long-term outcomes.

Following the initial description of this technique by Dr. Palmaz, the armamentarium of stents for the treatment of aorto-iliac occlusive disease has evolved and expanded. The profile of these devices has decreased over time, allowing for the safe and efficacious percutaneous treatment of most disease. Furthermore, concomitant advances in wires, crossing catheters, and imaging have also allowed for the treatment of more complex lesions which were once only thought to be treatable by conventional surgical techniques.

There have been multiple comparisons between the endovascular and open treatment of complex aorto-iliac disease since this initial description of balloon-expandable stents for the treatment of iliac disease. These have continued to demonstrate that endovascular approaches, primarily the use of balloon expandable stents, offer a safe and less invasive treatment method with early and late results that rival those obtained with conventional open techniques.[1,2]

Over the past decade, further technological advances have been made, including the use of covered stents along with the use of aortic endografts to treat complex aorto-iliac disease.[3,4] Although there is a paucity of data, it appears that covered stents appear to have a patency advantage for the treatment of more advance lesions. Concomitantly, the use of "hybrid" procedures, combining most frequently femoral endarterectomy and reconstruction along with retrograde iliac stenting, has further expanded the patients suitable for endovascular reconstruction of their aorto-iliac disease.[5]

It is evident now that this paper was the foundation for a paradigm shift in the treatment of aorto-iliac disease whereby the standard of care today for most is an endovascular approach. Unlike infra-inguinal disease where endovascular therapies have been plagued by restenosis and occlusion, the use of stents in the aorto-iliac segment have been demonstrated to be durable and efficacious over time. In large part due to this initial publication, the majority of patients today can be treated with a minimally invasive approach for even the most complex of aorto-iliac disease.

REFERENCES

1. Kashyap VS, Pavkov ML, Bena JF, Sarac TP, O'Hara PJ, Lyden SP, and Clair DG. The management of severe aortoiliac occlusive disease: Endovascular therapy rivals open reconstruction. *J Vasc Surg*. 2008 Dec;48(6):1451–7, 1457.
2. Dorigo W, Piffaretti G, Benedetto F, Tarallo A, Castelli P, Spinelli F, Fargion A, and Pratesi C. A comparison between aortobifemoral bypass and aortoiliac kissing stents in patients with complex aortoiliac obstructive disease. *J Vasc Surg*. 2017 Jan;65(1):99–107.

3. Mwipatayi BP, Sharma S, Daneshmand A, Thomas SD, Vijayan V, Altaf N, Garbowski M, and Jackson M; COBEST co-investigators. Durability of the balloon-expandable covered versus bare-metal stents in the Covered versus Balloon Expandable Stent Trial (COBEST) for the treatment of aortoiliac occlusive disease. *J Vasc Surg*. 2016 Jul;64(1):83–94.
4. Maldonado TS, Westin GG, Jazaeri O et al. Treatment of aortoiliac occlusive disease with the Endologix AFX Unibody Endograft. *Eur J Vasc Endovasc Surg*. 2016 Jul;52(1):64–74.
5. Chang RW, Goodney PP, Baek JH, Nolan BW, Rzucidlo EM, and Powell RJ. Long-term results of combined common femoral endarterectomy and iliac stenting/stent grafting for occlusive disease. *J Vasc Surg*. 2008 Aug;48(2):362–7.

CHAPTER 19

The Natural History of Bilateral Aortofemoral Bypass Grafts for Ischemia of the Lower Extremities

Malone JM, Moore WS, Goldstone J. Arch Surg. 1975 Nov;110(11):1300–6

ABSTRACT

Analysis of the immediate and long-term results in 180 patients undergoing bilateral aorto-femoral bypass grafts for occlusive disease of the lower extremities showed the immediate graft limb patency in 360 graft limbs to be 99.2%. The cumulative 10-year graft limb patency was 66%. Factors associated with thrombosis of the graft limb revealed correlations for localized atherosclerotic disease of either the profunda femoris artery or the tibial trifurcation vessels. The highest correlation for graft limb thrombosis was with simultaneous lesions involving both the profunda femoris artery and tibial trifurcation vessels. The acute lower extremity salvage rate was 94%, and the 10-year cumulative extremity salvage for legs at risk of amputation was 85%. Postoperative symptoms correlated well with patency. Overall operative mortality was five patients out of 180 (2.5%).

AUTHOR COMMENTARY BY JERRY GOLDSTONE

For several decades, aorto-bifemoral bypass graft (AFBG) was one of the signature operations performed by vascular surgeons and was the gold standard for treatment of aorto-iliac occlusive disease. It was also favored by some surgeons for the treatment of abdominal aortic aneurysms in order to avoid complex iliac artery anatomy.

At the time this paper was written, in 1975, there was ongoing debate regarding the superiority of aorto-iliac (-femoral) endarterectomy, a debate particularly lively within our own institution, the University of California, San Francisco. Indeed, my first major vascular operation as a resident was a very satisfying aorto-ilio-femoral endarterectomy. Although technically more demanding, endarterectomy's major advantage was/is its absence of prosthetic material and thus freedom from the possibility of prosthetic graft infection. In addition, when confined to the abdomen, it eliminated the late development of anastomotic femoral aneurysms which, at one time, were erroneously attributed, at least in part, to forces of hip flexion on grafts crossing beneath the inguinal ligament. It also became known that aorto-iliac bypass for occlusive disease was associated with a nearly four-fold increase in the need for subsequent down-stream revascularization when compared to aorto-femoral bypass. Thus, the aorto-femoral bypass became the most common operation for the treatment of supra-inguinal (i.e., in-flow) occlusive disease.

Our research and publication were done while these issues were unresolved and actively debated at scientific meetings as well as in publications. The most significant findings of our study were: (1) AFBG could be performed with very low mortality (2.5%) and morbidity rates, even in a population of 100% smokers; (2) even though 40% of the patients had severe ischemia (Rutherford classification 4–6), excellent long-term limb-salvage, graft-limb patency, and symptom improvement were obtained; (3) the graft-limb thrombosis rate was quite low (4%/year) and was uniformly related to either disease in or progression of untreated lesions in vessels distal to the femoral anastomosis (runoff); (4) the importance of treating profunda orifice lesions as part of the femoral anastomosis was highlighted by the significant decrease in graft patency when profunda lesions were not dealt with. In this series, profunda orifice lesions were treated by extending the distal prosthetic graft onto the profunda as a patch angioplasty. However, popliteal and tibial arterial lesions were not treated at the same time. Our analysis also discovered that 61% of the profunda lesions were not appreciated on pre-operative angiograms, emphasizing the importance of obtaining oblique views of the common femoral bifurcation. (5) Graft-limb thrombosis inevitably led to recurrence of symptoms. In contrast, no patient experienced worsening of symptoms in the absence of graft thrombosis. This was emphasized by the cumulative life-table curves for graft patency and maintenance of symptom status which were essentially superimposable for patients whose symptoms were either cured (38%) or improved (53%).

There are several technical details described in the paper that are not considered ideal by today's standards. First, the uniform use of a polyester graft with a 19 mm main body. Several factors should be considered when determining grafts size, and one size is certainly not appropriate for all patients. Similar consideration is appropriate for the diameter of the limbs of the bifurcated graft relative to the size of the recipient femoral arteries. Because narrower grafts result in higher flow velocity, the ideal main body size for most patients is probably 14 or 16 mm. Our study was performed when polyester was the only graft material available in the United States. Today, ePTFE is also available, and there is no evidence proving superiority of one graft material or configuration, so this remains the choice of individual surgeons. My preference has been a gelatin-impregnated, knitted polyester graft soaked in a rifampicin solution immediately prior to implantation.

The use of silk sutures for the femoral anastomoses in the early years of our series is understandable only when it is realized that during those years silk was thought to be a permanent material. The late fragmentation of silk sutures was not elucidated until the mid-1960s after which plastic sutures have been uniformly employed with vascular prosthetics.

Another technical aspect that deserves discussion is the nature of the proximal aortic anastomosis. In this paper, all were performed in an end-side fashion. Again, without convincing evidence of superiority, many surgeons advocate an end-end proximal anastomosis except when ante-grade perfusion of the inferior mesenteric or internal iliac arteries is deemed necessary. In addition, contrary to the description in the paper, the proximal anastomosis, whatever the configuration, should be placed as close to the lowest renal artery as possible to minimize the risk of subsequent impairment of graft flow by progression of aortic disease in the distal aorta. Another issue is that of bilateral lumbar sympathectomy. This was a common routine adjunct thought to improve distal perfusion by lowering peripheral vascular resistance and possibly minimizing tissue damage in the presence of distal microembolization. The absence of any evidence that this is worthwhile has led to its almost uniform abandonment in recent decades.

This study was retrospective in nature, from a single institution using hand-written medical records. The data were analyzed and presented in life-table format, now uniform in vascular reporting but which was just beginning to be used in the vascular literature in the early 1970s. The division of the analysis into two groups, prior to 1966 and after 1966, was somewhat arbitrary but primarily due to changes in perioperative antibiotic management, Over the 15-year span of the of the study, there were considerable improvements in many periprocedural and technical factors but most of these were fairly constant after 1966 when the majority (141/180) of the operations were performed. Nine percent of the patients had no change in their symptom status despite patent arterial reconstructions. The reasons for this were never determined which was disappointing because one of the objectives of the study was to identify factors that would predict successful treatment. We assumed that these patients were incorrectly diagnosed as suffering from arterial occlusive disease.

These limitations notwithstanding, this study, along with others (see Bibliography), was important in establishing the high success rate and durability of aorto-femoral bypass for the treatment of aorto-iliac atherosclerosis, enabling it to become one of the signature operations performed by vascular surgeons. The more recent emergence and ascendency of endovascular techniques has created a new controversy: Is iliac angioplasty and stenting comparable to or possibly even better than AFBG? The advocacy of endo first is popular and has relegated AFBG to very infrequent use. Graduates of Accreditation Council for Graduate Medical Education (ACGME)-approved vascular training programs now perform only a small number of these procedures. Technical expertise gained from repetitive experience is surely being lost and will almost certainly influence surgeons to choose endovascular treatment as the initial option. Will AFBG go the way of open cholecystectomy or other once standard operations? It is unlikely that there will ever be a randomized trial comparing the two treatment modalities and until there is robust data regarding long-term outcomes of endovascular treatment, AFBG should remain as the standard for comparison.

REFERENCES

1. Arnaoutakis DJ, and Belkin M. Surgical management of aortoiliac occlusive disease. In: Moore WS, Lawrence PF, and Oderich GS, (Eds): *Vascular and Endovascular Surgery. A Comprehensive Review*. 9th ed. Elsevier, Philadelphia, 2019, pp. 358–69.
2. Brewster DC, Perler BA, Robison JG et al. Aortofemoral grafts for multi-level occlusive disease: Predictors of success and need for distal bypass. *Arch Surg*. 1982;117:1599–606.
3. Brewster DC, Darling RC. Optimal methods of aortoiliac reconstruction. *Surgery*. 1978;84:817–25.
4. Crawford ES, Bomberger RA, Glaser DH et al. Aortoiliac occlusive disease: Factors influencing survival and function following reconstructive operation over a twenty-five year period. *Surgery*. 1981;90:108–17.
5. Danczyk RC, Mitchell EL, Petersen BD et al. Outcomes of open operation for aortoiliac occlusive disease after failed endovascular therapy. *Arch Surg*. 2012;147:841–5.
6. Jones AF, and Kempczinski RF. Aortofemoral bypass grafting. A reappraisal. *Arch Surg*. 1981;116:301–5.
7. Lee J. Could endo-first strategy really be better? *Arch Surg*. 2012;147:846.
8. Malone JM, Goldstone J, and Moore WS. Autogenous profundaplasty: The key to long-term patency in secondary repair of aortofemoral graft occlusion. *Ann Surg*. 1978;188:817–23.

CHAPTER 20

Supervised Exercise, Stent Revascularization, or Medical Therapy for Claudication Due to Aortoiliac Peripheral Artery Disease: The CLEVER Study

Murphy TP, Cutlip DE, Regensteiner JG, Mohler ER 3rd, Cohen DJ, Reynolds MR, Massaro JM, Lewis BA, Cerezo J, Oldenburg NC et al.
J Am Coll Cardiol. 2015 Mar 12;65(18):2055

ABSTRACT

Background Treatment for claudication that is due to aorto-iliac peripheral artery disease (PAD) often relies on stent revascularization (ST). However, supervised exercise (SE) is known to provide comparable short-term (6-month) improvements in functional status and quality of life. Longer-term outcomes are not known.

Objectives The goal of this study was to report the longer-term (18-month) efficacy of SE compared with ST and optimal medical care (OMC).

Methods Of 111 patients with aorto-iliac PAD randomly assigned to receive OMC, OMC plus SE, or OMC plus ST, 79 completed the 18-month clinical and treadmill follow-up assessment. SE consisted of 6 months of SE and an additional year of telephone-based exercise counseling. Primary clinical outcomes included objective treadmill-based walking performance and subjective quality of life.

Results Peak walking time improved from baseline to 18 months for both SE (5.0 ± 5.4 min) and ST (3.2 ± 4.7 min) significantly more than for OMC (0.2 ± 2.1 min; $p < 0.001$ and $p = 0.04$, respectively). The difference between SE and ST was not significant ($p = 0.16$). Improvement in claudication onset time was greater for SE compared with OMC, but not for ST compared with OMC. Many disease-specific quality-of-life scales demonstrated durable improvements that were greater for ST compared with SE or OMC.

Conclusions Both SE and ST had better 18-month outcomes than OMC. SE and ST provided comparable durable improvement in functional status and in quality of life up to 18 months. The durability of claudication exercise interventions merits its consideration as a primary PAD claudication treatment.

EXPERT COMMENTARY BY ANTHONY COMEROTA

Research Question/Objective Pharmacotherapy, supervised exercise (SE), and lower extremity revascularization are effective therapies for patients with intermittent claudication (IC). The relative benefits of these strategies of care have not been previously examined. Furthermore, there are important differences between patients with IC due to infra-inguinal occlusive disease and those with aorto-iliac occlusive disease. Individuals with aorto-iliac disease have more ischemic muscle mass with walking, are often more symptomatic than those with distal disease, and might experience less improvement with exercise training.[1] Furthermore, outcomes are more favorable with endovascular revascularization of the aorto-iliac segment, with results being more predictable and durable than those observed following endovascular revascularization for infra-inguinal disease.

The objectives of this study were to evaluate the benefits of optimal medical care (OMC), supervised exercise (SE), and stent revascularization (ST) on both walking outcomes and measures of quality of life (QOL) in patients with IC due to aorto-iliac peripheral arterial disease (PAD).

Study Design The CLEVER study was an observer-blinded randomized multicenter clinical trial conducted at 22 sites in North America.[2] The study evaluated three distinct treatment groups: OMC, SE, and ST. Randomization to treatment group was performed with a real-time web-based randomization system in a 2:2:1 ratio (ST: SE: OMC). Half as many were enrolled in OMC because the treatment effect between the other groups and OMC was assumed to be much larger than between SE and ST. Randomization was stratified by geographic region and cilostazol use at baseline.

SE consisted of 26 weeks of exercise, three times a week, for 1 hour at a time. Sites were trained to provide SE using a common protocol, and the progress of each participant was monitored by an oversight committee.

ST was done to relieve significant stenoses (>50% by diameter) in the aorta and iliac arteries with Food and Drug Administration-approved self-expanding or balloon-expandable stents. Intraprocedural or postprocedural platelet inhibition was at the discretion of the treating physician.

Pedometers were supplied to all subjects and were worn for 7 consecutive days immediately before their 6-month treadmill test.

The primary endpoint was changed from baseline to 6 months in the peak walking time (PWT) on a graded treadmill test using the Gardner protocol.[3] This is considered the most objective and reliable endpoint to evaluate improvements in functional status for patients with claudication evaluated in clinical trials.

Secondary endpoints included changes in claudication onset time (COT), change in community-based walking as assessed by pedometer measurements over 7 consecutive days, self-reported walking, and QOL.

The SF-12 was used to assess generic QOL.[4] Claudication related symptoms and functional impairment were assessed with two questionnaires designed for and validated in patients with PAD: the Walking Impairment Questionnaire (WIQ)[5] and the Peripheral Artery Questionnaire (PAQ).[6]

Sample Size 119 study participants were randomized. Enrollment was terminated by the data and safety monitoring board after review of the interim results and due to slow enrollment.

Follow-Up Participants were called monthly to inquire about adverse events, at 3 months to refill their cilostazol medication, and at 6 months to undergo the same testing as at baseline. Pedometers were worn for 7 consecutive days immediately before the 6-month treadmill test.

Patients in the SE group received telephone support from the beginning of month 7 to the end of month 18.

Inclusion/Exclusion Criteria Subjects were required to have moderate to severe IC (ability to walk 2 min. but not more than 12 min. on a graded treadmill test) and objective evidence of hemodynamically significant aorto-iliac arterial stenosis involving the most symptomatic limb. Two treadmill exercise tests were completed at baseline to confirm reproducibility of results; those who deviated by more than 25% were excluded. Patients were also excluded if: they had critical limb ischemia, comorbid conditions that limited their walking, or aortic occlusion from the renal arteries to the inguinal ligament.

Intervention OMC was established by the 2005 ACC/AHA Guidelines for the management of patients with peripheral artery disease to promote best practices for risk factor management, use of antiplatelet therapy and use of claudication pharmacotherapy.[7] All participants received cilostazol 100 mg by mouth twice daily. In addition, OMC included advice about home exercise and diet in the form of standardized verbal instruction and printed material. Cardiovascular risk factor data were collected and feedback was provided to the sites by a central risk factor committee. Risk factors were managed directly by the local study site.

SE consisted of 26 weeks of exercise, three times a week, for 1 hour at a time. Sites were trained to provide SE using a common protocol. The progress of each participant was monitored by an oversight committee. Patients in the SE group received quarterly contact by research coordinators during the supervised phase and then participated in a telephone-based maintenance program designed to promote exercise adherence during the unsupervised phase of the study. This telephone support system was provided to SE patients from the beginning of month 7 to the end of month 18.

ST was done to relieve hemodynamically significant stenoses (>50% by diameter) in the aorta and iliac arteries with approved self-expanding or balloon-expandable stents. Intraprocedural or postprocedural platelet inhibition was at the discretion of the treating physician.

Results Baseline anthropomorphic, physiological, and biochemical characteristics were similar at baseline across the treatment groups. All three groups were well matched in terms of baseline demographics and performance variables, except for a higher prevalence of male sex and prior stroke in the SE group.

In the ST group, no patient underwent a concomitant femoral-popliteal revascularization procedure. Only one patient underwent aortic stenting. The mean lesion length was 3.9 ± 3.4 cm and the mean preprocedural stenosis was 83 ± 19%. The average number of stents used per patient was 1.8 ± 1.2. An evaluation for restenosis was not indicated by recurrent leg symptoms during follow-up in any study participant.

Adherence to cilostazol was >90% and similar across all three treatment groups.

Primary Endpoint The primary endpoint of change in PWT at 6 months and extended to 18 months is presented in the following table. Improvement in PWT was greatest for SE, intermediate for ST, and least with OMC.

Change in PWT at 6 Mos. and 18 Mos. (min.)

Group	6 Mos.[1]	18 Mos.[8]
Supervised Exercise (SE)	5.8 ± 4.6	5.0 ± 5.4
Stent (ST)	3.7 ± 4.9	3.2 ± 4.7
Optimal Medical Care (OMC)	1.2 ± 2.6	0.2 ± 2.1
Between Group Comparison of PWT at 6 Mos. and 18 Mos.		
SE vs. OMC	$p < 0.001$	$P < 0.001$
ST vs. OMC	$p = 0.02$	$P = 0.04$
SE vs. ST	$P = 0.04$	$P = 0.16$

Secondary Endpoints At 6 and 18 months there were no significant changes in ABIs compared to baseline in either the OMC or SE groups, whereas the resting ABI improved by 0.29 ± 0.33 in the ST group, which was significantly greater than OMC and SE at 6 and 18 months ($p < 0.0001$).

For COT, both the SE and ST groups demonstrated significantly greater improvement compared with OMC, but no significant difference was observed between SE and ST.

There were no baseline differences in QOL. However, at 6 months there were significant differences in QOL in the ST and SE groups compared to the OMC group. Compared with SE, ST was associated with significantly greater benefit across most of the disease specific QOL measures but not for generic scales. These observations persisted at 18 months.

Study Limitations The study had a smaller sample size than originally planned, predominantly due to slow enrollment. This is a challenge faced by most comparative effectiveness clinical trials, in which recruitment is typically hampered by clinician bias in favor of one treatment strategy or a reimbursement bias that is not comparable across the tested interventions. Of the 111 patients evaluable for the primary endpoint, only 79 (71%) were available for their 18-month treadmill.

Relevant Studies This study shows that for a population with advanced aorto-iliac PAD, changes in PWT over 6–18 months were greater among those who received SE than those receiving OMC and those revascularized with ST, despite higher ABIs in the ST group. These results demonstrate preservation of the benefits of SE for a full year after formal SE ended.

The improvements in treadmill measures of functional status were not observed in the pedometer-derived measurements of community walking. It is possible that improved leg function, even with a reduction in claudication symptoms, may not lead to an increase in a patient's ambulatory behavior.[9]

An apparent paradox was the uniformly improved QOL in the ST group compared to SE, despite longer PWTs in the SE group. This may reflect a subjective overestimation of benefit in revascularized patients. This was recently addressed by Henni et al.[10], where they demonstrated that patients overestimated their improvement of objectively measured treadmill walking distance following revascularization.

The CLEVER data provide strong evidence of benefit of SE and comparable durability of SE and ST to improve the ischemic symptoms and walking distance of patients with IC.

REFERENCES

1. Pernow B, and Zetterquist S. Metabolic evaluation of the leg blood flow in claudicating patients with arterial obstruction at different levels. *Scand J Clin Lab Invest.* 1968;21:277–87.
2. Murphy TP, Cutlip DE, Regensteiner JG et al. Supervised exercise, stent revascularization, or medical therapy for claudication due to aortoiliac peripheral artery disease: The CLEVER study. *Circulation.* 2012;125:130–9.
3. Hiatt WR, Hirsch AT, Regensteiner JG, and Brass EP. Clinical trial for claudication: Assessment of exercise performance, functional status, and clinical endpoints: Vascular clinical trialists. *Circulation.* 1995;92:614–21.

4. Ware J Jr, Kosinski M, and Keller SD. A 12-item short-form health survey: Construction of scales and preliminary tests of reliability and validity. *Med Care*. 1996;34:220–33.
5. Regensteiner JG, Steiner JF, and Hiatt WR. Exercise training improves functional status in patients with peripheral arterial disease. *J Vasc Surg*. 1996;23:104–15.
6. Spertus J, Jones P, Poler S, and Rocha-Singh K. The peripheral artery questionnaire: A new disease-specific health status measure for patients with peripheral arterial disease. *Am Heart J*. 2004;147:301–8.
7. Hirsch AT, Haskal ZJ, Hertzer NR et al. ACC/AHA 2005 Practice guidelines for the management of patients with peripheral arterial disease (lower extremity, renal mesenteric, and abdominal aortic). *Circulation*. 2006;113:e113–654.
8. Murphy TP, Cutlip DE, Regensteiner JG et al. Supervised exercise, stent revascularization, or medical therapy for claudication due to aortoiliac peripheral artery disease: The CLEVER study. *J Am Coll Cardiol*. 2015;65:999–1099.
9. McDermott MM, Ades P, Guralinik JM et al. Treadmill exercise and resistance training in patients with peripheral arterial disease with and without intermittent claudication: A randomized controlled trial. *JAMA*. 2009;301:165–74.
10. Henni S, Ammi M, Sempore Y et al. Treadmill measured vs. questionnaire estimated changes in walking ability in patients with peripheral artery disease. *Eur J Vasc Endovasc Surg*. 2019;57:676–84.

CHAPTER 21

Thirty-Year Trends in Aortofemoral Bypass for Aortoiliac Occlusive Disease

Sharma G, Scully RE, Shah SK, Madenci AL, Arnaoutakis DJ, Menard MT, Ozaki CK, Belkin M. *J Vasc Surg. 2018 Jul 9. pii: S0741–5214(18)30857–7*

ABSTRACT

Objective Endovascular intervention has supplanted open bypass as the most frequently used approach in patients with aorto-iliac segment atherosclerosis. We sought to determine whether this trend together with changing demographic and clinical characteristics of patients undergoing aorto-bifemoral bypass (ABFB) for aorto-iliac occlusive disease (AOD) has an association with postoperative outcomes.

Methods Using a prospectively maintained institutional database, we identified patients who underwent ABFB for AOD from 1985 to 2015. Patients were divided into two cohorts: the historical cohort (HC) included patients who underwent ABFB for AOD from 1985 to 1999 and the contemporary cohort (CC) who underwent ABFB for AOD from 2000 to 2015. Medical and demographic data, procedural information, postoperative complications, and follow-up data were extracted. Cox proportional hazards regression was used to evaluate associations with the endpoint of primary patency. A similar analysis was performed for major adverse limb events (MALEs; the composite of above-ankle amputation, major re-intervention, graft revision, or new bypass graft of the index limb) in the subset of patients with critical limb ischemia.

Results There were a total of 359 cases: 226 in the HC and 133 in the CC. The CC had more women (56.4% vs. 43.8%; P <0.02), smokers (87.2% vs. 67.7%; P <0.001), and patients who failed prior aorto-iliac endovascular intervention (17.3% vs. 4.8%; P <0.0001), but fewer patients with coronary artery disease (32.3% vs. 47.3%; P <0.005). 30-day mortality was less than 1% in both cohorts, but 10-year survival was higher in the CC (67.7% vs. 52.6%; P <0.02). 5-year primary, primary-assisted, and secondary patency were higher in the HC (93.3% vs. 82.2%; P <0.005; 93.8% vs. 85.7%; P <0.02; 97.5% vs. 90.4%; P <0.02, respectively). CC membership, decreasing age, prior aortic surgery, and decreasing graft diameter were significant independent predictors of loss of primary patency after adjustment (hazard ratio [HR], 7.03; 95% confidence interval [CI], 2.80–17.63; P <0.0001; HR, 0.93; 95% CI, 0.90–0.96; P <0.0001; HR, 18.80; 95% CI, 5.94–59.58; P <0.0001; and HR, 0.73; 95% CI, 0.55–0.95; P <0.02, respectively). Similarly, CC membership, prior aortic surgery, and decreasing graft diameter were significant independent predictors of MALE in the critical limb ischemia cohort after adjustment (HR, 21.13; 95% CI, 4.20–106.40; P <0.0002; HR, 40.40; 95% CI, 3.23–505.61; P <0.004; and HR, 0.51; 95% CI, 0.30–0.86; P <0.01, respectively).

Conclusions Compared with the pre-endovascular era, demographic and clinical characteristics of patients undergoing ABFB for AOD in the CC have changed. Although long-term patency is slightly lower among patients in the CC during which a substantial subset of AOD patients are being treated primarily via the endovascular approach, durability remains excellent and limb salvage unchanged. After adjustment, the time period of index ABFB independently predicted primary patency and MALE, as did graft diameter and prior aortic surgery. These changing characteristics should be considered when counseling patients and benchmarking for re-intervention rates and other outcomes.

AUTHOR COMMENTARY BY MICHAEL BELKIN AND GAURAV SHARMA

Research Question/Objective See abstract.

Study Design Retrospective, single center, cohort study.

Sample Size See abstract.

Follow-Up Median follow-ups were 107 and 41 months in the HC and CC, respectively.

Inclusion/Exclusion Criteria The study included all patients undergoing aorto-femoral bypass for aorto-iliac occlusive disease as determined by preoperative conventional aortography, computed tomographic imaging, or magnetic resonance angiography at our tertiary referral, academic medical center from 1985 to 2015. Patients had peripheral arterial disease manifest either as claudication or critical limb ischemia. There were no *acute* limb ischemia patients.

Intervention or Treatment Received All patients underwent aorto-bifemoral bypass (ABFB). Nearly 100% of procedures were performed with woven polyester conduit. Both end-to-side and end-to-end proximal anastomotic configurations were used. Approximately 85% of patients had distal anastomoses constructed to each common femoral artery, with the remaining 15% distributed across permutations of common, superficial, and profunda femoris arteries. Less than 10% underwent concomitant visceral revascularization, and there were shifts in the number undergoing femoral endarterectomy at the time of index ABFB, as discussed in the following sections.

Results See abstract.

Study Limitations This represents a single center experience, thus potentially limiting the generalizability. Although all analyses were based on prospectively collected data, the study itself was retrospective in nature. All lesions were Trans-Atlantic Inter-Society Consensus (TASC) C or D, but the specific classification could not be determined for a significant percentage of patients and thus was omitted from analysis.

Relevant Studies A discussion of studies that came before or after the discussed article that are of relevance and provide additional context follows.

McPhee et al. (*J Vasc Surg* 2016;64:1660–6.): In this retrospective cohort study of the Veterans Affair population, the authors compared ABFB to "alternative inflow procedures" (e.g., femoral endarterectomy and iliac angioplasty/stenting) for claudication. They did not include patients with critical limb ischemia (CLI). On unadjusted and adjusted analyses, mortality beyond 30 days was similar in both groups. 30-day mortality in the data set was higher than in our institutional series (2.7% vs. <1%).

Madenci et al. (2016;212: 461–7.e2.): In a similar American College of Surgeons National Surgical Quality Improvement Program (ACS-NSQIP)-based study of claudicants undergoing ABFB versus inflow procedures ranging from femoral endarterectomy to nonanatomic reconstructions (e.g., femoro-femoral bypass, axillo- or ilio-femoral bypass), the authors found that ABFB patients had more short-term medical complications (renal, cardiorespiratory, venous thromboembolism) as well as graft-related and other complications requiring unplanned re-operation after propensity-score matching.

Indes et al. (*J Endovasc Ther* 2013;20:443–55.): In a pooled analysis of multiple databases, the authors compared 3,733 patients undergoing open surgical revascularization for AOD with 1,625 patients undergoing endovascular intervention. The open bypass group had higher morbidity and 30-day mortality but increased patency at 1-, 3-, and 5-year follow-up—the latter being 83% for open bypass versus 71% for endovascular intervention.

Hertzer et al. (*J Vasc Surg* 2007;45:527–35; discussion: 535.): In a nearly three-decade, retrospective, single-institution, single-surgeon series of 355 anatomic repairs for AOD manifesting as claudication or advanced ischemia in nearly equal numbers, the authors report impressive results including limb-based primary patency of approximately 90% at 10 years and exceeding 80% at 15 years for ABFB. Female sex was associated with increased odds of short-term graft thrombosis and major amputation. In addition, decreased age and prior inflow procedures were predictors of late graft failure.

Reed et al. (*J Vasc Surg* 2003;37:1219–25.): In an analysis of the predictors of durability of ABFB at the current authors' institution, smaller aortic diameter and younger age at time of index ABFB were independently linked to decreased long-term patency.

Study Impact The rapid and continuing expansion of endovascular technology over the last three decades has been one of the major trends defining the care of vascular disease in the modern era. Perhaps the greatest success and proliferation of these techniques has occurred in the aorto-iliac segment, where many now consider endovascular therapy to be first-line in the treatment of occlusive disease. However, open surgery will continue to remain a critical tool in the management of AOD in the future. Long-term durability remains lower with endovascular modalities than open reconstruction. Primary patency of stenting in this anatomic territory has been reported to be 66% at 5 years and 46% at 10 years in longitudinal series, with notably diminished patency in Trans-Atlantic Inter-Society Consensus (TASC) C and D lesions. This stands in contrast to historic ABFB primary patency of 85% to 97% at 5 years and exceeding 80% at 10 and 15 years. Treatment of endovascular failure will continue to include ABFB, which has superior durability when compared to extra-anatomic open surgical options.

Given this continued importance of ABFB, the work described herein highlights several issues that will be pertinent to current and future generations of vascular specialists who endeavor to provide care to patients with AOD. First, as medical and endovascular therapies have evolved, shifts in patient demographics, clinical characteristics, and anatomic features have occurred. These changes often result in increasing patient complexity, with more patients on dialysis, with a presenting indication of critical limb ischemia, and with previous interventions for AOD undergoing ABFB. Anatomic complexity was further suggested by a rise in the number of end-to-side anastomoses and concomitant femoral endarterectomies that are now required, suggesting ilio-femoral outflow disease. Not surprisingly, there are more 30-day re-admissions, more short-term re-interventions, and reduced patency in the contemporary era. It is critical that vascular surgeons consider these facts as they formulate their operative and postoperative approaches and counsel patients requiring intervention for AOD. To this end, independent predictors of loss of primary patency are younger age, prior open aortic surgery history (but not aorto-iliac endovascular intervention), and decreasing graft diameter; the latter two predict major adverse limb events (defined as the composite of above-ankle amputation or major re-intervention such as thrombectomy/thrombolysis, graft revision, or new bypass graft of the index limb) in the CLI subset as well. These features should further guide patient selection and allow surgeons and patients to anticipate challenges in the postoperative period.

In spite of this increasing complexity, excellent mortality, patency, and, in the case of CLI patients, limb-salvage outcomes remain achievable. 30-day mortality was 0.8% in the contemporary cohort. Secondary patency exceeded 90% at 5 years. Limb salvage was 98%. Thus facility with the execution of ABFB and postoperative care of patients undergoing the operation will continue to be relevant for the next generation of vascular specialists. Another trend notable from this and other work has been the decline in the number of open aortic surgical procedures being performed with predicted shortfalls in volume during training. It is critical that the vascular surgical leadership and those who take on the responsibility of training future generations of vascular surgeons are vigilant in maintaining a pipeline of surgeons facile in direct anatomic reconstructive options such as ABFB.

BIBLIOGRAPHY

Bosch JL, and Hunink MG. Meta-analysis of the results of percutaneous transluminal angioplasty and stent placement for aortoiliac occlusive disease. *Radiology*. 1997;204:87–96.

Chiesa R, Marone EM, Tshomba Y, Logaldo D, Castellano R, and Melissano G. Aortobifemoral bypass grafting using expanded polytetrafluoroethylene stretch grafts in patients with occlusive atherosclerotic disease. *Ann Vasc Surg*. 2009;23:764–9.

de Vries SO, Hunink MG. Results of aortic bifurcation grafts for aortoiliac occlusive disease: A meta-analysis. *J Vasc Surg*. 1997;26:558–69.

Dua A, Upchurch GR Jr, Lee JT, Eidt J, and Desai SS. Predicted shortfall in open aneurysm experience for vascular surgery trainees. *J Vasc Surg*. 2014;60:945–9.

Farber A, and Eberhardt RT. The current state of critical limb ischemia: A systematic review. *JAMA Surg*. 2016;151:1070–7.

Hertzer NR, Bena JF, and Karafa MT. A personal experience with direct reconstruction and extra-anatomic bypass for aortoiliofemoral occlusive disease. *J Vasc Surg*. 2007;45:527–35; discussion: 535.

Indes JE, Mandawat A, Tuggle CT, Muhs B, and Sosa JA. Endovascular procedures for aorto-iliac occlusive disease are associated with superior short-term clinical and economic outcomes compared with open surgery in the inpatient population. *J Vasc Surg*. 2010;52:1173–9.

Indes JE, Pfaff MJ, Farrokhyar F et al. Clinical outcomes of 5358 patients undergoing direct open bypass or endovascular treatment for aortoiliac occlusive disease: A systematic review and metaanalysis. *J Endovasc Ther*. 2013;20:443–55.

Kashyap VS, Pavkov ML, Bena JF et al. The management of severe aortoiliac occlusive disease: Endovascular therapy rivals open reconstruction. *J Vasc Surg*. 2008;48:1451–7.

Madenci AL, Ozaki CK, Gupta N, Raffetto JD, Belkin M, and McPhee JT. Perioperative outcomes of elective inflow revascularization for lower extremity claudication in the American College of Surgeons National Surgical Quality Improvement Program database. *Am J Surg*. 2016;212:461–7.e2.

McPhee JT, Madenci A, Raffetto J, Martin M, and Gupta N. Contemporary comparison of aortofemoral bypass to alternative inflow procedures in the Veteran population. *J Vasc Surg*. 2016;64:1660–6.

Powell RJ, Fillinger M, Walsh DB, Zwolak R, and Cronenwett JL. Predicting outcome of angioplasty and selective stenting of multisegment iliac artery occlusive disease. *J Vasc Surg*. 2000;32:564–9.

Schurmann K, Mahnken A, Meyer J et al. Long-term results 10 years after iliac arterial stent placement. *Radiology*. 2002;224:731–8.

Sharma G, Farber A, and Menard MT. Endovascular or open surgical therapy for critical limb ischemia. *Amer Coll Cardiology Expert Analysis*. 24 August 2017. https://www.acc.org/latest-in-cardiology/articles/2017/08/24/07/20/endovascular-or-open-surgical-therapy-for-critical-limb-ischemia

Sharma G, Scully RE, Shah SK, Madenci AL, Arnaoutakis DJ, Menard MT, Ozaki CK, and Belkin M. *J Vasc Surg*. 2018;68:1796–805.

CHAPTER 22

Shifting Paradigms in the Treatment of Lower Extremity Vascular Disease: A Report of 1000 Percutaneous Interventions

DeRubertis BG, Faries PL, McKinsey JF, Chaer RA, Pierce M, Karwowski J, Weinberg A, Nowygrod R, Morrissey NJ, Bush HL et al.

Ann Surg. 2007 Sep;246(3):415–22; discussion 422–4

ABSTRACT

Objectives Catheter-based revascularization has emerged as an alternative to surgical bypass for lower extremity vascular disease and is a frequently used tool in the armamentarium of the vascular surgeon. In this study we report contemporary outcomes of 1,000 percutaneous infra-inguinal interventions performed by a single vascular surgery division.

Methods We evaluated a prospectively maintained database of 1,000 consecutive percutaneous infra-inguinal interventions between 2001 and 2006 performed for claudication (46.3%) or limb-threatening ischemia (52.7%; rest pain in 27.7% and tissue loss in 72.3%). Treatments included angioplasty with or without stenting, laser angioplasty, and atherectomy of the femoral, popliteal, and tibial vessels.

Results Mean age was 71.4 years, and 57.3% were male; comorbidities included hypertension (84%), coronary artery disease (51%), diabetes (58%), tobacco use (52%), and chronic renal insufficiency (39%). Overall 30-day mortality was 0.5%. Two-year primary and secondary patencies and rate of amputation were 62.4%, 79.3%, and 0.5%, respectively, for patients with claudication. Two-year primary and secondary patencies and limb-salvage rates were 37.4%, 55.4%, and 79.3% for patients with limb-threatening ischemia. By multivariable Cox PH modeling, limb threat as procedural indication (P = 0.0001), diabetes (P = 0.003), hypercholesterolemia (P = 0.001), coronary artery disease (P = 0.047), and Transatlantic Inter-Society Consensus D lesion complexity (P = 0.050) were independent predictors of recurrent disease. For patients that developed recurrent disease, 7.5% required no further intervention, 60.3%

underwent successful percutaneous re-intervention, 11.7% underwent bypass and 20.5% underwent amputation. Patency rates were identical for the initial procedure and subsequent re-interventions (P = 0.97).

Conclusion Percutaneous therapy for peripheral vascular disease is associated with minimal mortality and can achieve 2-year secondary patency rates of nearly 80% in patients with claudication. Although patency is diminished in patients with limb-threat, limb-salvage rates remain reasonable at close to 80% at 2 years. Percutaneous infra-inguinal revascularization carries a low risk of morbidity and mortality and should be considered first-line therapy in patients with chronic lower extremity ischemia.

AUTHOR COMMENTARY BY BRIAN DERUBERTIS

"Shifting Paradigms in the Treatment of Lower Extremity Vascular Disease: A Report of 1,000 Percutaneous Interventions" was a report of contemporary outcomes following 1,000 percutaneous infra-inguinal interventions on patients with peripheral arterial occlusive disease presenting with either claudication or chronic limb-threatening ischemia. It was a notable publication and a significant contribution to the management of PAD due to its scope and its impact, and the original data were presented at the 127th Annual Meeting of the American Surgical Association in Boulder Springs, Colorado. A number of factors contributed to the impact of this paper on the field of vascular surgery, including the size of the study population, the completeness of follow-up with clinically relevant patency and limb-salvage data, the inclusion of both claudicants and patients with chronic limb-threatening ischemia, and the fact that to date the amount of data to support percutaneous intervention for PAD in the medical literature was significantly lacking. Perhaps most importantly, however, this manuscript both heralded and reflected an emerging trend toward percutaneous management of PAD, especially among the surgical community that had always recognized the clinical utility of open surgical approaches to lower leg revascularization.

This manuscript includes 1,000 consecutive percutaneous lower extremity arterial interventions that were collected in a prospectively maintained database and analyzed retrospectively. Seven-hundred and thirty patients underwent 856 primary interventions and 144 re-interventions over the study period. Interventions were performed for claudication in 46% and for rest pain or tissue loss in 53%. Patency outcomes were assessed postoperatively and at 6-month intervals thereafter and were reported as primary and secondary patency rates out to 36 months for both patient groups, while limb-salvage rates over the same follow-up period were reported for patients with chronic limb-threatening ischemia. Lesion distribution and TASC classification were carefully recorded for all patients, and outcomes were analyzed according to lesion type and location.

Complication rates were quite low, with 5% hematoma rate (0.8% operative) and 2% renal dysfunction (with only 2 of the 730 patients requiring dialysis and only in those with baseline creatinine >2.6), suggesting that percutaneous intervention is very safe in this relatively ill patient population. Primary patency rates at 12 and 30 months were 61% and 48%, respectively, although secondary patency rates were significantly higher at 77% and 66% for all interventions. The limb-salvage rate in patients with rest pain and tissue loss was 79% at 30 months. The most significant predictor of loss of patency was indication for intervention, with chronic limb-threatening ischemia patients having worse patency rates than claudicants, although additional predictors on multivariate analysis included diabetes, coronary artery disease, hypercholesterolemia, and increasing TASC classification. Tibial patency following intervention at the infra-geniculate level was significantly worse than more proximal interventions, with primary patency of tibial segments ranging from 34%–38% at 24 months depending on type of treatment modality used. Patency rates following the 144 re-interventions were equivalent to those of the primary interventions.

This manuscript provided a significant contribution to the existing medical literature on treatment of arterial occlusive disease for several reasons. The size of the patient population and the robustness of the clinically relevant follow-up data are among the most important of these. In the BASIL trial, published in *Lancet* in 2005, the authors found that an endovascular-first approach resulted in equivalent amputation-free survival and improved short-term cost effectiveness compared to bypass surgery and thereby provided data to support this endovascular-first strategy for most patients with arterial occlusive disease of the lower extremities.[1] However, with the exception of this important randomized trial, data to support the use of percutaneous intervention in these patients were generally lacking at the time. Although we now have a growing number of manuscripts detailing the results of randomized device trials in lower extremity arterial occlusive disease and analyses of large clinically impactful databases (i.e., Vascular Quality Initiative), this was not the case in 2007 when our data were initially presented and published.[2–4] Most published manuscripts on percutaneous intervention at the time included small patient populations and, especially in the case of manuscripts published in nonsurgical journals, limited follow-up data characterized by lack of clinically relevant endpoints (i.e., reporting of target lesion revascularization rates rather than patency and limb-salvage rates). These limitations to the existing literature made detailed analysis of patient-specific outcomes and the impact of lesion location/type on outcome difficult. The robustness of the patient population and clinically relevant follow-up data in our manuscript allowed us to perform more detailed analysis of the impact of patient characteristics and lesion location/severity on outcome, and these results were reported in this manuscript and subsequent publications by our group.[5–7] Additionally, we were able to characterize the differences between claudicants and limb-threat patients in terms of the type of interventions required by each as well as the respective results of these interventions. For example, limb-threat patients were more likely to require more distal interventions (tibial vs. femoropopliteal) and multilevel intervention than claudicants. Furthermore, the size of our data set allowed us to compare the results of different types of treatment modalities (angioplasty vs. atherectomy) or treatment levels (femoropopliteal vs. tibial).

Included among some of the more important findings in this analysis are the results of tibial interventions and the results of re-interventions. Regarding tibial interventions, these distal interventions were relatively uncommon at the time of our manuscript based on the representation of these procedures in the existing literature. Based on our analysis, we reported a 2-year primary patency rate ranging from 34%–38% depending on treatment modality and noted no statistically significant difference in patency rates between different modalities (i.e., angioplasty vs. atherectomy). This was an important finding as it highlighted an ongoing clinical need, which still exists to date in 2019, for modalities that have a durable effect in the infra-geniculate circulation. Currently, there is a diverse range of devices available for the femoropopliteal segment, with 12-month patency rates in the 80%–90% range, but this is not the case for the tibial arteries, and therefore patients undergoing tibial intervention who need long-term patency for durable relief of rest pain or for healing of large wounds should expect a high likelihood of requiring re-intervention. This finding underscores the continued need to explore emerging technologies for the tibial arteries, including drug-coated balloons and bioresorbable scaffold technology.

Regarding re-interventions, one of the notable findings in this manuscript was the fact that re-interventions fared as well as index interventions in terms of complication rates, patency rates, and limb-salvage rates. This finding is seemingly contradictory to recent reports that suggest poorer limb outcomes following prior failed vascular procedures (both open and percutaneous) and supports the authors' belief that properly performed percutaneous interventions, in which bypass target arteries are respected and all runoff vessels are maintained, do not negatively impact limb patency rates nor harm subsequent options for limb salvage.[8]

Another important contribution of this manuscript included the fact that it was published in the surgical literature and all interventions were performed by the Division of Vascular Surgery at New York Presbyterian Hospital rather than by nonsurgical interventionalists, as this reflected the growing support for percutaneous intervention among a medical specialty that traditionally favored open surgical bypass for complex arterial occlusive disease. The procedures in this series included many patients with multilevel disease, tissue loss, and other challenging clinical presentations and oftentimes required distal tibial interventions with 0.014-inch wire platforms, a variety of crossing and re-entry devices, and treatment modalities that included atherectomy rather than more straightforward angioplasty or stenting. This speaks to the complexity of the procedures and the vascular surgical community's consistent ability to adapt to the changing technology and techniques required to offer vascular patients the full spectrum of treatment options and comprehensive vascular disease care.

Overall, the favorable clinical outcome results and the low periprocedural complication rates in this large data set significantly contributed to the support in the existing literature for an endovascular-first strategy and helped to set expectations for patency rates and need for re-intervention in different populations. The robust nature of the data set allowed for detailed analysis of patient factors and lesion characteristics that impacted outcome. Finally, this manuscript reflected the growing expertise with techniques by the vascular surgical community, who continue to strive for the proper balance between emerging technology and time-proven treatment modalities such as surgical bypass.

REFERENCES

1. Adam DJ, Beard JD, Cleveland T, Bell J, Bradbury AW, Forbes JF, Fowkes FG, Gillepsie I, Ruckley CV, Raab G, Storkey H; BASIL trial participants. Bypass versus angioplasty in severe ischaemia of the leg (BASIL): Multicentre, randomised controlled trial. *Lancet.* 3 Dec 2005;366(9501):1925–34.
2. Schneider PA, Laird JR, Tepe G et al. Treatment effect of drug-coated balloons is durable to 3 years in the femoropopliteal arteries: Long-term results of the IN.PACT SFA randomized trial. *Circ Cardiovasc Interv.* Jan 2018;11(1):e005891
3. Dake MD, Ansel GM, Jaff MR et al. Durable clinical effectiveness with paclitaxel-eluting stents in the femoropopliteal artery: 5-Year Results of the Zilver PTX randomized trial. *Circulation.* 12 Apr 2016;133(15):1472–83.
4. Lu K, Farber A, Schermerhorn ML et al. The effect of ambulatory status on outcomes of percutaneous vascular interventions and lower extremity bypass for critical limb ischemia in the Vascular Quality Initiative. *J Vasc Surg.* Jun 2017;65(6):1706–12.
5. DeRubertis BG, Peirce M, Chaer RA et al. Lesion severity and treatment complexity are associated with outcome after percutaneous infra-inguinal intervention. *J Vasc Surg.* Oct 2007;46(4):709–16.
6. DeRubertis BG, Chaer RA, Hynecek RL, Benjelloun R, Trocciola SM, Karwowski J, Bush H, McKinsey JF, Kent KC, Faries PL. Reduced primary patency rate in diabetic patients after percutaneous intervention results from more frequent presentation with limb-threatening ischemia. *J Vasc Surg.* Jan 2008;47(1):101–87.
7. DeRubertis BG, Vouyouka A, Rhee S, Karwowski J, Angle N, Faries PL, and Kent KC. Percutaneous intervention for infra-inguinal occlusive disease in women: Equivalent outcomes despite increased severity of disease compared to men. *J Vasc Surg.* Jul 2008;48(1):150–7.
8. Hossain S, Leblanc D, Farber A et al. Infrainguinal bypass following failed endovascular intervention compared with primary bypass: A systematic review and meta-analysis. *Eur J Vasc Endovasc Surg.* Mar 2019;57(3):382–91.

CHAPTER 23

Durable Clinical Effectiveness with Paclitaxel-Eluting Stents in the Femoropopliteal Artery: 5-Year Results of the Zilver PTX Randomized Trial

Dake MD, Ansel GM, Jaff MR, Ohki T, Saxon RR, Smouse HB, Machan LS, Snyder SA, O'Leary EE, Ragheb AO et al. Zilver PTX Investigators. Circulation. 2016 Apr 12;133(15):1472–83; discussion 1483

EXPERT COMMENTARY BY NINA BOWENS AND MARK ARCHIE

Research Question/Objective This study sought to evaluate whether paclitaxel (PTX)-coated stents outperform percutaneous transluminal angioplasty (PTA) and bare metal stenting (BMS) of symptomatic femoropopliteal artery lesions.

Study Design Prospective, multinational, randomized controlled trial (RCT). Patients with symptomatic disease of the above-the-knee femoropopliteal artery were randomized to primary paclitaxel-coated self-expanding drug-eluting stents (DESs) versus PTA. Due to early failure of PTA, there was a second randomization to provisional BMS or provisional DES. Primary endpoints included primary patency and event-free survival at 1 and 5 years. Events were classified as major adverse events including death, amputation, clinically driven revascularization of the target lesion, target limb ischemia requiring surgical intervention, and worsening of the Rutherford class to 5 or 6. Secondary endpoints included comparison of the provisionally stented groups.

Sample Size 479 patients were enrolled from 55 sites in the United States, Japan, and Germany. 241 patients were included in the DES group and 238 in the PTA group. 120 patients experienced acute failure of PTA, 59 of whom were randomized to provisional BMS and 61 to DES.

Follow-Up The study was designed with planned 5-year follow-up.

Inclusion/Exclusion Criteria The study included patients with up to two lesions of the femoropopliteal artery (*de novo* or restenotic). Clinical inclusion criteria were Rutherford Score ≥ 2 and ankle brachial index of <0.9. Clinical exclusion criteria included untreated

>50% stenosis of the arterial inflow, pre-treatment of the lesion of interest, and prior stenting. Angiographic inclusion criteria consisted of lesions ≤14 cm, ≥50% stenosis, vessel diameter 4–9 mm, and at least one runoff vessel with nonsignificant disease.

Intervention or Treatment Received Patients received either PTA, DES, or BMS as described according to the randomization protocol outlined previously.

Results 1-year and 5-year patency demonstrated superiority of DES compared to PTA group (optimal PTA and provisional BMS or DES) when the primary endpoint of event-free survival (81.4% vs. 70.1%) was considered. Primary patency for overall DES (primary DES + provisional DES) was 66.4% versus 43.4% for standard of care, defined as optimal PTA and provisional BMS. Similarly, when these groups were compared evaluating freedom from TLR, DES outperformed standard of care (83.1% vs. 67.6%). Comparisons of provisional stenting continued to reflect superiority of DES with primary patency (72.4% vs. 53%) and freedom from TLR (84.9% vs. 71.6%). The study concludes an overall 5-year relative risk reduction of >40% for restenosis and target lesion revascularization with use of DES.

Study Limitations This study was the first RCT evaluating endovascular devices within the femoropopliteal space with long-term follow-up. Furthermore, there is a scarcity of comparative data. The study failed to evaluate primary DES as compared to primary BMS. The trial also did not consider alternative technology including drug-coated balloons and atherectomy. Similar to other RCTs of this nature, there was a reported 6.4% per year combined withdrawal and loss to follow-up.

The trial, while pivotal, did have significant clinical limitations. Interventions within this study were performed primarily on claudicants (Rutherford 2–3) as opposed to patients with chronic limb-threatening ischemia (91% vs. 9%). The cited lesion length was also relatively short with a mean of slightly more than 6 cm. Moreover, the generalizability of the results to the PAD population as a whole may be limited.

Relevant Studies The RESILIENT trial established the superiority of stenting over PTA for interventions in the SFA.[1] However, both PTA and BMS perform poorly due to early restenosis.[1,2] Drug-eluting, antiproliferative technology was initially introduced in the coronary arteries and expanded to lower extremity vasculature with the objective of prolonging patency.[3] Initial use of Sirolimus-coated stents in the femoral artery failed to show significant improvement over BMS.[4] Tepe et al. demonstrated reduction in restenosis and TLR with use of PTX-coated balloons compared to plain angioplasty.[5] Similar results were reported in the LEVANT I trial.[6] Prior to the Zilver PTX trial, the DEBATE-SFA trial demonstrated improved patency with use of drug-coated balloons + BMS when compared to PTA + BMS.[7]

The widespread adoption of DES for the treatment of PAD has led to critical evaluation of patient outcomes. Interestingly, PTX technology in the coronary circulation has been largely abandoned due to superior results of limus-based platforms including reduction in all-cause death.[8] Notably, this transition has not occurred in the application of drug technology to the peripheral vascular system.

Perhaps one of the most controversial topics in the modern era of vascular surgery has been the meta-analysis of RCTs reporting increased risk of death following application of PTX drugs in the femoropopliteal space.[9] The study evaluated 28 RCTs with the findings of increased all-cause mortality at 2 years and called for further investigations. The FDA issued a warning recommending extreme caution and informed consent with the use of PTX balloons or stents with a strong suggestion for alternative therapies.[10] Numerous responses followed this publication. The trial was criticized for lack of plausible biological and pharmacokinetic mechanism, patient-level data, and disparate patient populations.

Dake et al. examined patient-level data from the Zilver PTX RCT in addition to the Japanese post-surveillance studies evaluating Zilver PTX versus BMS. This analysis failed to show a difference in all-cause mortality between DES and non-DES groups.[11] Additional investigation is warranted to verify the true relationship of peripheral arterial treatment technologies utilizing PTX.

Study Impact The Zilver PTX randomized trial is one of the largest randomized trials to evaluate an endovascular device within the femoropopliteal artery. The scaffolding properties of the self-expanding nitinol stent allow for luminal gain and overcome the common failure modes of angioplasty such as flow-limiting dissection and recoil. The addition of paclitaxel increases durability and reduces stenosis secondary to intimal hyperplasia. Moreover, these data demonstrate long-term results that approximate lower extremity surgical bypass and arguably outperform the use of prosthetics.[12] By providing a minimally invasive option with good patency, the results helped to revolutionize the treatment of symptomatic PAD.

The Zilver PTX data along with favorable data for drug-coated balloons and the expansion of atherectomy led to the adoption of a largely "endo-first" strategy for the treatment of symptomatic femoropopliteal artery disease. This paradigm shift, however, was predicated on both the durability and long-term safety of the procedure. Recent data linking increased all-cause mortality with the use of paclitaxel in the femoropopliteal artery have led to a significant decline in the use of drug-eluting technologies in the lower extremity. Further studies are needed to clarify the association.

REFERENCES

1. Laird JR, Katzen BT, Scheinert D et al. Nitinol stent implantation versus balloon angioplasty for lesions in the superficial femoral artery and proximal popliteal artery: Twelve-month results from the RESILIENT randomized trial. *Circ Cardiovasc Interv.* 2010;3(3):267–76.
2. Schillinger M, Sabeti S, Loewe C et al. Balloon angioplasty versus implantation of nitinol stents in the superficial femoral artery. *N Engl J Med.* 2006;354(18):1879–88.

3. Park SJ, Shim WH, Ho DS et al. A paclitaxel-eluting stent for the prevention of coronary restenosis. *N Engl J Med.* 2003;348(16):1537–45.
4. Duda SH, Pusich B, Richter G et al. Sirolimus-eluting stents for the treatment of obstructive superficial femoral artery disease: Six month results. *Circulation.* 2002; 106(12):1505–9.
5. Tepe G, Schnoor B, Albrecht T et al. Angioplasty of femoral-popliteal arteries with drug-coated balloons: 5-year follow-up of the THUNDER trial. *JACC Cardiovasc Interv.* 2015;8(1 PT A):102–8.
6. Scheinert D, Duda S, Zeller T et al. The LEVANT I (Lutonix paclitaxel-coated balloon for the prevention of femoropopliteal restenosis) trial for femoropopliteal revascularization: First-in-human randomized trial of low-dose drug-coated balloon versus uncoated balloon angioplasty. *JACC Cardiovasc Interv.* 2014;7(1):10–9.
7. Liistro F, Grotti S, Porto I et al. Drug-eluting balloon in peripheral intervention for the superficial femoral artery the DEBATE-SFA randomized trial (drug eluting balloon in peripheral intervention for the superficial femoral artery). *JACC Cardiovasc Interv.* 2013;6(12):1295–302.
8. Gada H, Kirtane AJ, Newman W et al. 5-year results of a randomized comparison of XIENCE V everolimus-eluting and TAXUS paclitaxel-eluting stents: Final results from the SPIRIT III trial (clinical evaluation of the XIENCE V everolimus eluting coronary stent system in the treatment of patients with *de novo* native coronary artery lesions). *JACC Cardiovasc Interv.* 2013;6(12):1263–6.
9. Kastanos K, Spiliopoulos S, Kitrou P et al. Risk of death following application of paclitaxel-coated balloons and stents in the femoropopliteal artery of the leg: A systematic review and meta-analysis of randomized controlled trials. *J Am Heart Assoc.* 2018;7(24):e011245.
10. Update: U.S. Food & Drug Administration. Treatment of peripheral arterial disease with paclitaxel-coated balloons and paclitaxel-eluting stents potentially associated with increased mortality-letter to health care providers. https://www.fda.gov/medical-devices/letters-health-care-providers/august-7-2019-update-treatment-peripheral-arterial-disease-paclitaxel-coated-balloons-and-paclitaxel.
11. Dake MD, Ansel GM, Bosiers M et al. Paclitaxel-coated Zilver PTX drug-eluting stent treatment does not result in increased long-term all-cause mortality compared to uncoated devices. *Cardiovasc Intervent Radiol.* 2020;43:8–19.
12. Green RM, Abbott WM, Matsumoto T et al. Prosthetic above-knee femoropopliteal bypass grafting: Five-year results of a randomized trial. *J Vasc Surg.* 2000;31(3):417–25.

CHAPTER 24

Drug-Eluting Balloon versus Standard Balloon Angioplasty for Infrapopliteal Arterial Revascularization in Critical Limb Ischemia: 12-Month Results from the IN.PACT DEEP Randomized Trial

IN.PACT DEEP Trial Investigators, Zeller T, Baumgartner I, Scheinert D, Brodmann M, Bosiers M, Micari A, Peeters P, Vermassen F, Landini M, Snead DB et al. J Am Coll Cardiol. 2014 Oct 14;64(15):1568–76

EXPERT COMMENTARY BY STEVEN TOHMASI AND NII-KABU KABUTEY

ABSTRACT

Research Question/Objective Percutaneous transluminal angioplasty (PTA) of the infrapopliteal vessels is routinely performed to restore distal perfusion in patients with critical limb ischemia (CLI). The effectiveness of plain old balloon angioplasty (POBA) of the infrapopliteal arterial system has been limited due to high rates of restenosis and atherosclerotic disease progression. The central goal of this trial was to assess whether the use of drug-eluting balloons (DEBs) for infrapopliteal revascularization in CLI would result in improved safety and efficacy in comparison to traditional PTA.

Study Design The IN.PACT DEEP (RandomIzed AmPhirion DEEP DEB versus Standard PTA for the treatment of below-the-knee CriTical limb ischemia) trial was a prospective, multicenter, patient-blinded, randomized, controlled trial conducted across 13 European sites. The study investigated the efficacy and safety of the paclitaxel-coated IN.PACT Amphirion DEB (IA-DEB) for the treatment of infrapopliteal arterial disease in patients with CLI. The authors assessed two primary efficacy endpoints through a 12-month period: clinically driven target lesion revascularization (CD-TLR; defined as any revascularization associated with deterioration of Rutherford category and/or increasing size of pre-existing wounds and/or occurrence of new wounds) and late lumen loss (LLL; assessed by angiography at 12 months postintervention). The primary safety endpoint studied was a composite of all-cause death, major amputation, and CD-TLR at 6 months postintervention.

Sample Size From September 2009 to July 2012, 358 patients with CLI were enrolled and randomized 2:1 to undergo IA-DEB (n = 239) or PTA (n = 119). The majority of the patients presented with Rutherford category 5 disease (84.1% in the IA-DEB arm vs. 77.3% in the PTA arm).

Follow-Up All subjects were followed for 5 years. Follow-up visits, routine lab testing, vascular diagnostics, wound assessment/care were planned for the following time periods postintervention: 1 month, 6 months, 1 year, 2 years. To examine LLL, a 12-month follow-up angiography was performed on a select cohort of patients (n = 167) who met specific eligibility criteria: a maximum lesion length of 10 cm and consented for angiography at 12-month follow-up.

Inclusion/Exclusion Criteria The inclusion and exclusion criteria of the trial protocol is shown in Table 24.1.

Intervention or Treatment Received Enrolled patients were randomized 2:1 to receive either the paclitaxel-coated IA-DEB (Medtronic, Santa Rosa, California) or standard PTA.

Results Baseline clinical and angiographic characteristics were similar between the IA-DEB and PTA groups with the exceptions of mean lesion length (10.2 vs. 12.9 cm; p = 0.002), impaired inflow (40.7% vs. 28.8%; p = 0.035), prior target limb revascularization (32.2% vs. 21.8%; p = 0.047), and wound depth (0.8 and 1.8 mm; p = 0.040). The clinical trial failed to prove its study hypothesis of superior efficacy of IA-DEB versus PTA. The reported 12-month CD-TLR rates were not statistically significant between the IA-DEB and PTA arms (9.2% vs. 13.1%; p = 0.291) when assessed in the amputation-free surviving cohort. 12-month angiographic follow-up also revealed no significant differences in LLL (0.61 vs. 0.62 mm; p = 0.950), binary restenosis rates (41.0% vs. 35.5%; p = 0.609), and reocclusion rates (11.5% vs. 16.1%; p = 0.531) between the IA-DEB and PTA arms, respectively. The composites of all-death mortality, major amputation, and CD-TLR rates through 6 months were 17.7% in the IA-DEB group and 15.8% in the PTA group. Although the trial's primary safety endpoint was statistically met through noninferiority analysis (p = 0.021), an increased rate of major amputations through 12 months was observed in the IA-DEB group in comparison to the PTA group (8.8% vs. 3.6%; p = 0.080). The combined safety endpoint, including all-cause mortality/major or minor amputation rate, was also higher in the IA-DEB treatment arm (35.2% vs. 25.2%; p = 0.064). Overall, despite having significantly longer lesions and deeper ulcers, the PTA arm demonstrated similar angiographic findings at 12 months and a lower major amputation rate in comparison to the IA-DEB arm. These findings raised safety concerns, resulting in the study being interrupted and the IA-DEB device being withdrawn from the market.

Study Limitations In the manuscript, the authors self-reported the following study limitations (see Table 24.1).

Table 24.1 IN.PACT DEEP inclusion and exclusion criteria

A.	General inclusion criteria
i.1	Age $\geq$18 years and $\leq$85 years
i.2	Patient or patient's legal representative has been informed of the nature of the study, agrees to participate, and has signed an EC-approved consent form
i.3	Female patients of childbearing potential have a negative pregnancy test $\leq$7 days before the procedure and are willing to use a reliable method of birth control for the duration of study participation
i.4	Patient has documented chronic critical limb ischemia (CLI) in the target limb prior to the study procedure with Rutherford category 4, 5, or 6
i.5	Life expectancy >1 year in the investigator's opinion
B.	General exclusion criteria
e.1	Patient unwilling or unlikely to comply with follow-up schedule
e.2	Planned major index limb amputation
C.	General angiographic inclusion criteria
i.6	Reference vessel diameter(s) between 2 and 4 mm
i.7	Single or multiple lesions with $\geq$70% DS of different lengths in one or more main afferent crural vessels including tibioperoneal trunk
i.8	At least one non-occluded crural vessel with angiographically documented runoff to the foot either directly or through collaterals
D.	General angiographic exclusion criteria
e.3	Lesion and/or occlusions located in or extending to the popliteal artery or below the ankle joint space
e.4	Inflow lesion or occlusion in the ipsilateral iliac, SFA, or popliteal arteries with length $\geq$15 cm
e.5	Significant ($\geq$50% DS) Inflow lesion or occlusion in the ipsilateral iliac, SFA, or popliteal arteries left untreated
e.6	Previously implanted stent in the TL(s)
e.7	Aneurysm in the target vessel
e.8	Acute thrombus in the TL
E.	General procedural exclusion criteria
e.9	Failure to obtain <30% residual stenosis in pre-existing, hemodynamically significant ($\geq$50% DS and <15 cm length) inflow lesions in the ipsilateral iliac, SFA, or popliteal artery. DES and/or DEB was not allowed for the treatment of inflow lesions
e.10	Failure to cross the TL with a 0.014′ guide wire
e.11	Use of alternative therapy, e.g., atherectomy, cutting balloon, laser, radiation therapy, DES as part of the index procedure
F.	Angiographic cohort angiographic inclusion criteria
a.i.1	Angio-TL is one identifiable single solitary or a series of multiple adjacent lesions with a DS $\geq$70% and a cumulative length $\leq$100 mm that can be covered by a single IN.PACT Amphirion™ (10-mm balloon landing zone in both edges is mandatory)
a.i.2	Angio-TL is the only lesion in that vessel (only 1 Angio-TL per patient is allowed)
G.	Angiographic cohort general exclusion criteria
a.e.1	GFR <30 mL/min except for patients with renal end-stage disease on chronic hemodialysis

Source: From Zeller T, Baumgartner I, Scheinert D et al. for the IN.PACT DEEP Trial Investigators. IN.PACT Amphirion paclitaxel-eluting balloon versus standard percutaneous transluminal angioplasty for infrapopliteal revascularization of critical limb ischemia: Rationale and protocol for an ongoing randomized controlled trial. *Trials*. 2014;15:63.

1. The study design was not adequately powered to assess major amputation as an endpoint.
2. Procedural operators were unable to be blinded to the assigned treatment.
3. There were no standardized protocols in place for decision-making involving amputations and for the intensity and surveillance of wound care.
4. Low angiographic and wound imaging compliance may have resulted in incomplete assessment of the treatment effect.

Relevant Studies Prior to the IN.PACT DEEP trial, published reports from single-institution studies suggested that using the IA-DEB for infrapopliteal revascularization may reduce rates of vessel restenosis and re-intervention.[1,2] In 2011, Schmidt et al. conducted a retrospective review of 104 patients who underwent IA-DEB for CLI or severe claudication.[1] The investigators found that treated lesions (mean lesion length: 176 mm) had a 3-month angiographic restenosis rate of 27.4%, which is significantly lower than previously published data from the same group using uncoated balloons.[1,3] In a randomized trial of 132 diabetic patients with CLI (mean lesion length: 130 mm), Liistro et al. reported statistically significant differences in the rates of binary restenosis (27% vs. 74%; $p < 0.001$), occlusion (17% vs. 55%; $p < 0.001$), and TLR (18% vs. 43%; $p = 0.002$) at 12 months between the IA-DEB and PTA trial arms, respectively.[2] Despite the promising results from both of these aforementioned studies, the findings from the IN.PACT DEEP trial raised safety concerns and resulted in the IA-DEB device being withdrawn from the market.

Following the IN.PACT DEEP trial, Zeller et al. conducted the BIOLUX P-II multicenter, randomized, controlled trial in which 72 patients were randomized in a 1:1 ratio to undergo treatment with either the paclitaxel-coated Passeo-18 LUX DEB (Biotronik AG, Buelach, Switzerland) or PTA.[4] There was no significant difference between the DEB group and PTA group in the primary performance endpoint of lesion-based patency loss at 6 months (17.1% vs. 26.1%, respectively; $p = 0.298$) and major amputations at 12 months (3.3% vs. 5.6%, respectively).[4] However, in comparison to the IN.PACT DEEP trial, the results of the BIOLUX P-II trial were more favorable as they included less major amputations of the target extremity. Additionally, the primary safety endpoint, a composite of all-cause mortality, target extremity major amputation, target lesion thrombosis, and target vessel revascularization at 30 days, was 0% in the DEB group versus 8.3% in the PTA group.[4]

The critical need for further research on the endovascular management of below-the-knee CLI has led to the design and implementation of additional trials using the paclitaxel-coated Lutonix DEB. In a large, multicenter trial consisting of 314 patients with CLI undergoing infrapopliteal revascularization with the Lutonix 014 DEB device, the reported freedom at 6 months from all-cause death was 91.2%, above-ankle amputation was 97.1%, and target vessel revascularization was 88.0%.[5] While the 6-month outcome data reported appear promising, the 12-month data from this trial have yet to be published.[5] Most recently, Mustapha et al. also conducted a prospective, multicenter, randomized, controlled trial evaluating the efficacy and safety of the Lutonix DEB.[6] The investigators randomly assigned 442 patients with CLI or severe claudication in a 2:1 fashion to undergo infrapopliteal angioplasty with a Lutonix DEB or PTA.[6] The investigators found similar rates of freedom from major adverse limb events and perioperative death at 30 days between both groups (99.3% vs. 99.4%). Freedom from vessel occlusion, CD-TLR, and above-ankle amputation at 6 months was also statistically better for the proximal-segment (the proximal two-thirds of the below-knee arterial pathways) DEB group (76%) versus PTA (62.9%; $p = 0.0079$).[6] Rates of primary patency and CD-TLR at 6-month follow-up statistically favored the DEB group at 6 months.[6] These early findings from studies of the Lutonix DEB appear promising, but additional long-term follow-up data are necessary to fully understand the efficacy and safety of DEBs in treating infrapopliteal arterial lesions.

Study Impact Infrapopliteal atherosclerotic arterial disease is the most common cause of CLI. Patients with CLI often have multiple comorbidities and poor venous conduits, making them poor open surgical candidates. As such, endovascular therapy is commonly preferred for management of challenging infrapopliteal lesions in these patients. DEBs have been shown to have favorable results in the treatment of femoropopliteal lesions, but there are currently limited data on the efficacy and safety of this treatment for infrapopliteal lesions in CLI.

REFERENCES

1. Schmidt A, Piorkowski M, Werner M et al. First experience with drug-eluting balloons in infrapopliteal arteries: Restenosis rate and clinical outcome. *J Am Coll Cardiol.* 2011;58:1105–9.
2. Liistro F, Porto I, Angioli P et al. Drug-eluting balloon in peripheral intervention for below the knee angioplasty evaluation (DEBATE-BTK): A randomized trial in diabetic patients with critical limb ischemia. *Circulation.* 2013;128:615–21.
3. Schmidt A, Ulrich M, Winkler B et al. Angiographic patency and clinical outcome after balloon-angioplasty for extensive infrapopliteal arterial disease. *Catheter Cardiovasc Interv.* 2010;76:1047–54.
4. Zeller T, Beschorner U, Pilger E, Bosiers M, Deloose K, Peeters P, Scheinert D, Schulte KL, Rastan A, and Brodmann M. Paclitaxel-coated balloon in infrapopliteal arteries: 12-month results from the BIOLUX P-II randomized trial (BIOTRONIK'S-first in man study of the Passeo-18 LUX drug releasing PTA balloon catheter vs. the uncoated Passeo-18 PTA balloon catheter in subjects requiring revascularization of infrapopliteal arteries). *JACC Cardiovasc Interv.* 2015;8:1614–22.
5. Thieme M, Lichtenberg M, Brodmann M, Cioppa A, and Scheinert D. Lutonix 014 DCB global below the knee registry study: Interim 6-month outcomes. *J Cardiovasc Surg (Torino).* 2018;59(02):232–6.
6. Mustapha JA, Brodmann M, Geraghty PJ, Saab F, Settlage RA, and Jaff MR. Drug-coated vs uncoated percutaneous transluminal angioplasty in infrapopliteal arteries: Six-month results of the Lutonix BTK trial. *J Invasive Cardiol.* 2019;31(8)205–11.

CHAPTER 25

Bypass versus Angioplasty in Severe Ischaemia of the Leg (BASIL): Multicentre, Randomised Controlled Trial

Adam DJ, Beard JD, Cleveland T, Bell J, Bradbury AW, Forbes JF, Fowkes FG, Gillepsie I, Ruckley CV, Raab G, BASIL Trial Participants et al. Lancet. 2005 Dec 3;366(9501):1925–34

ABSTRACT

Background The treatment of rest pain, ulceration, and gangrene of the leg (severe limb ischaemia) remains controversial. We instigated the BASIL trial to compare the outcome of bypass surgery and balloon angioplasty in such patients.

Methods We randomly assigned 452 patients, who presented to 27 UK hospitals with severe limb ischaemia due to infra-inguinal disease, to receive a surgery-first (n = 228) or an angioplasty-first (n = 224) strategy. The primary endpoint was amputation (of trial leg)-free survival. Analysis was by intention to treat. The BASIL trial is registered with the National Research Register (NRR) and as an International Standard Randomised Controlled Trial, number ISRCTN45398889.

Findings The trial ran for 5.5 years, and follow-up finished when patients reached an endpoint (amputation of trial leg above the ankle or death). Seven individuals were lost to follow-up after randomisation (three assigned angioplasty, two surgery); of these, three were lost (one angioplasty, two surgery) during the first year of follow-up. 195 (86%) of 228 patients assigned to bypass surgery and 216 (96%) of 224 to balloon angioplasty underwent an attempt at their allocated intervention at a median (IQR) of 6 (3–16) and 6 (2–20) days after randomisation, respectively. At the end of follow-up, 248 (55%) patients were alive without amputation (of trial leg), 38 (8%) alive with amputation, 36 (8%) dead after amputation, and 130 (29%) dead without amputation. After 6 months, the two strategies did not differ significantly in amputation-free survival (48 vs. 60 patients; unadjusted hazard ratio 1·07, 95% CI 0·72–1·6; adjusted hazard ratio 0·73, 0·49–1·07). We saw no difference in health-related quality of life between the two strategies, but for the first year the hospital costs associated with a surgery-first strategy were about one-third higher than those with an angioplasty-first strategy.

Interpretation In patients presenting with severe limb ischaemia due to infra-inguinal disease and who are suitable for surgery and angioplasty, a bypass surgery-first and a balloon angioplasty-first strategy are associated with broadly similar outcomes in terms of amputation-free survival, and in the short term, surgery is more expensive than angioplasty.

EXPERT COMMENTARY BY RAMEEN MORIDZADEH AND PETER F. LAWRENCE

The Bypass versus Angioplasty in Severe Ischaemia of the Leg (BASIL) trial, published in *Lancet* in 2005, remains to date one of the most pivotal studies in the field of vascular surgery. Spanning more than 5 years across 27 hospitals in the United Kingdom, the study remains the only published trial offering level 1 evidence for the comparison of endovascular therapy versus surgical bypass in the treatment of infra-inguinal critical limb ischemia (CLI).

By the late 1990s, two main strategies emerged for the treatment of patients with critical limb ischemia, defined as rest pain, tissue loss, or gangrene. Surgical bypass with vein was the accepted standard prior to advances in endovascular therapies. However, surgical complications and mortality were significant in patients with CLI, given their burden of systemic disease. Furthermore, a significant proportion of patients did not have a suitable vein available, with prosthetic bypass yielding less favorable results. Endovascular therapy, which at the time was predominately plain-balloon angioplasty, offered a minimally invasive alternative with less morbidity and mortality. However, the durability and technical feasibility of the endovascular option, particularly in patients with long segment occlusions requiring subintimal recanalization, were of concern. Prior studies attempted to address these issues but had significant flaws, including their retrospective nature, small cohorts, and combined analysis with claudication patients.

The BASIL trial compared an endovascular-first to a surgical bypass-first strategy for patients with infra-inguinal disease, with a total of 452 participants with severe limb ischemia (SLI, defined as rest pain and/or tissue loss) randomised to either arm. Both a vascular surgeon and interventional radiologist had to deem patients suitable for both endovascular treatment and open surgical bypass prior to study inclusion. Patients with supra-inguinal disease (i.e., aorto-iliac disease) were excluded from randomisation. The primary outcome was time to amputation of the index limb or death from any cause, whichever occurred first. Secondary outcomes examined included all-cause mortality, 30-day morbidity and mortality, re-interventions, quality of life, and cost.

Although no difference in 30-day mortality was found between the two arms, the surgical bypass group had significantly higher rates of morbidity, the majority of which were wound complications, infections, or cardiovascular events. Endovascular treatment had a higher rate of re-intervention compared to surgical bypass (26% vs. 18%, difference 8%, 95% CI 0.04-15%). Amputation-free survival was not statistically significant between the two groups at 1 year or 3 years. However, a post hoc analysis demonstrated a benefit for surgery over angioplasty beyond 2 years, with a reduction in the hazard for amputation-free survival (HR 0.37, CI 95% 0.17–0.77) and all-cause mortality (HR 0.34 CI 95% 0.17–0.71). Although there was no difference in readmissions, patients in the surgical arm had longer hospital stays, including longer days spent in units requiring higher levels of care up to 1 year. At 12 months, the surgical strategy was about a third higher than the endovascular-first approach (£23,322 vs. £17,419). There was no difference between the two groups in terms of standardized quality of life scores.

The BASIL trial is a seminal work, which sought to address pressing issues in the treatment of patients with limb-threatening ischemia. Published in 2005, it remains to date the only completed randomised clinical trial comparing open and endovascular therapies for the treatment of critical limb ischemia.

To understand the impetus for this study, one must examine the landscape of treatment strategies for peripheral arterial disease (PAD) at the time. Limited consensus for the treatment of PAD existed, and the only level 1 evidence was comparing vein and prosthetic conduit available to guiding clinicians in their treatment strategies.[1] Rapid expansion, adoption, and availability of catheter-based therapies offered an attractive alternative to bypass surgery, which was viewed as more durable but carried significant risk of morbidity and mortality.

Within this broad context, the BASIL trial pitted an endovascular-first against an open surgery-first strategy in the treatment of advanced limb ischemia. Although there was no difference between the two arms in the primary outcome of amputation-free survival (AFS), a post hoc analysis revealed that patients randomised to open surgery had superior outcomes, namely increased overall survival and a trend toward improved AFS. In a follow-up of the study, an analysis of outcomes by treatment received demonstrated that patients with surgical bypass with prosthetic conduit fared much worse than patients treated with autologous conduit.

Although the BASIL trial aimed to settle a pressing area of clinical equipoise, its results and study limitations generated many additional questions. In terms of applicability to contemporary practice, modern endovascular therapies have evolved considerably from plain balloon angioplasty stand-alone therapy that was implemented in the trial. The armamentarium for endovascular therapy is much broader today and includes stenting, atherectomy, and drug-coated technology. In addition, endovascular techniques have improved along with operators' abilities to perform challenging revascularization procedures in CLI patients with complex and diffuse disease burdens. Another limitation of the study is the requirement for clinical equipoise between the two treatment modalities for a given patient. This results in only approximately 10% of patients being ultimately randomised to the study, which limited its applicability to a general population.

Despite its limitations, the BASIL trial has had a lasting impact in the care of vascular patients with advanced limb ischemia. In modern practice, CLI patients who have a greater than 2-year life expectancy and with a suitable autogenous vein conduit should be strongly considered for open surgical bypass. More significantly, the BASIL trial ushered in an era of evidence-based practice in the management of advanced limb ischemia and offers the only level 1 evidence to guide therapeutic decision-making.

REFERENCE

1. Veith FJ, Gupta SK, Ascer E et al. Six-year prospective multicenter randomized comparison of autologous saphenous vein and expanded polytetrafluoroethylene grafts in infrainguinal arterial reconstructions. *J Vasc Surg*. 1986 Jan;3(1):104–14.

CHAPTER 26

Six-Year Prospective Multicenter Randomized Comparison of Autologous Saphenous Vein and Expanded Polytetrafluoroethylene Grafts in Infrainguinal Arterial Reconstructions

Veith FJ, Gupta SK, Ascer E, White-Flores S, Samson RH, Scher LA, Towne JB, Bernhard VM, Bonier P, Flinn WR et al. J Vasc Surg. 1986 Jan;3(1):104–14

ABSTRACT

This chapter reviews our seminal contributions to lower limb salvage over a 30-year period. The article on the 6-year randomized controlled trial comparing lower extremity vein and prosthetic grafts was one of more than 200 scientific papers my colleagues and I wrote describing various aspects of our pioneering contributions to the field of saving lower limbs threatened by arteriosclerotic ischemia.

AUTHOR COMMENTARY BY FRANK J. VEITH, NEAL S. CAYNE, AND ENRICO ASCHER

This article was part of a series of articles describing an aggressive limb-salvage approach, which we originated and popularized over a 30-year period.[1,2] This approach featured mostly arterial bypasses, but included also percutaneous angioplasties as these became available. Our limb-salvage efforts and many of their elements were first treated with skepticism and disdain, but they are now generally accepted and utilized around the world.

In the late 1960s and 1970s, we cautiously began to challenge the wisdom of the day that a primary below-knee amputation was the best treatment for ischemic lower extremity gangrene and ulceration due to infra-inguinal arterial occlusive disease. Because we had surprising early success in saving many of these ischemic limbs by performing bypasses to patent popliteal and more distal arteries in the leg and foot, we became more emboldened in our efforts to salvage severely ischemic limbs.

Continued successes in these procedures, which were clearly "against the grain" of the times, prompted us to develop an aggressive approach to salvaging almost all ischemic limbs. Nearly all our patients with what is now considered critical limb ischemia were subjected to arteriography. Many of these patients had very distal occlusive disease restricted to the leg and foot and were considered only suitable for a major amputation by others.[2] However, if a patent artery distal to occlusions was visualized, we would perform a bypass to it. In our institution we had unusually good arteriography, which enabled us to visualize patent arteries in the lower leg and foot.[2,3] This allowed us to perform effective revascularization procedures (bypasses or angioplasty) on patients considered unreconstructable in other institutions. Many of our procedures were considered by most vascular surgeons to be excessively aggressive and heretical at the time. In addition, when one of our limb-salvage procedures failed, early or late, we repeated our arteriography and performed a re-operation—another treatment initially considered heretical.[4]

When we presented some of our early cases at surgical meetings, we were considered wrongheaded and excessively radical. Our successful cases were deemed anecdotal and our overall aggressive approach excessively risky and unworthy. We therefore examined the overall results of our aggressive limb-salvage approach in more than 2,800 patients.[1,2] These analyses showed several interesting findings. The procedural 30-day mortality of these limb-salvage procedures was low (~3%). However, by 5 years after their first procedure, 52% of these patients had succumbed from conditions unrelated to their limb-salvage procedures—mostly myocardial infarctions. In the 48% of patients who lived longer than 5 years, 66% of them retained a functional limb for that period of time. Of those who died within the 5 years of their index procedure, 81%–95% retained a functional limb until they died. Moreover, our major amputation rate for critical limb ischemia fell over a 16-year period from 49% to 14%. Clearly, our limb-salvage efforts, with all their adjunctive procedures and re-operations when necessary, were worthwhile.[1,2]

Although we favored the use of the autologous vein as a conduit for our bypasses, many patients had their veins used by others or us for previous procedures, and many others had damaged or diseased veins. So, we were forced to use an alternative conduit for our limb-salvage bypasses in many of our cases. PTFE grafts became available to us in 1978, and we used them mostly when the autologous vein was unavailable or unsuitable for use. These PTFE grafts performed remarkably well for us, unlike for others. These PTFE grafts sometimes even worked reasonably well for bypasses to tibial arteries.[5,6]

However, once again our results were greeted with skepticism and occasionally with derision. So, we undertook a three-center randomized controlled trial comparing autologous saphenous vein grafts to PTFE grafts in limb-salvage infra-inguinal arterial reconstructions. We had no outside or industry funding for this trial. The three groups (Bronx, NY; Chicago, IL; Milwaukee, WI) doing it just did it using their clinical resources. The 6-year results are presented in the abstract and article referenced previously.

The PTFE graft bypasses to the popliteal artery performed remarkably well and equally well compared to vein graft bypasses for 2 years, and then there was a deterioration in primary patency. However, with re-operative and other procedures, the limb-salvage results with the two grafts approached parity. With bypasses to tibial or peroneal arteries, vein grafts achieved clearly superior primary patency. However,

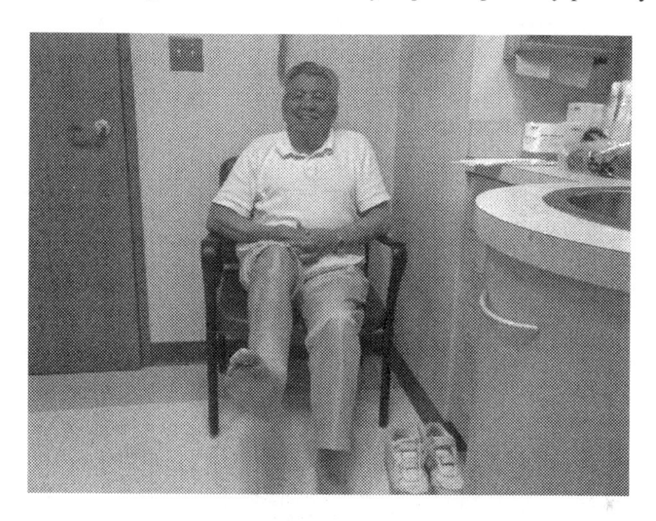

Figure 26.1

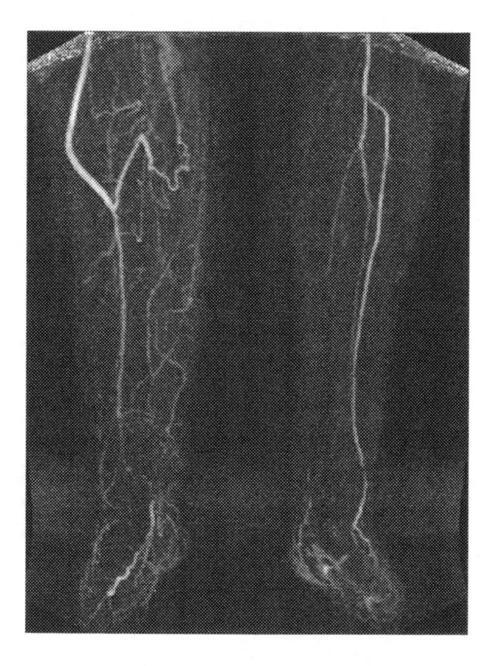

Figure 26.2

with repeat operations and healing of foot wounds, limb-salvage results were equally good with PTFE and vein grafts. So, we still believe—again against the grain—that PTFE tibial bypasses for limb-salvage are worthwhile when a patient is facing an amputation and no other alternative is available. And we have dozens of anecdotal cases to prove this still heretical opinion. Shown in the Figures 26.1 and 26.2 are a photo and an angiogram of one such patient with a common iliac to peroneal artery PTFE bypass patent 13 years after it was performed.

REFERENCES

1. Veith FJ, Gupta SK, Samson RH et al. Progress in limb salvage by reconstructive arterial surgery combined with new or improved adjunctive procedures. *Ann Surg*. 1981;194:386–9.
2. Veith FJ, Gupta SK, Wengerter KR, Goldsmith J, Rivers SP, Bakal CW, Dietzak AM, Cynamon J, Sprayragen SL, and Gliedman ML. Changing arteriosclerotic disease patterns and management strategies in lower-limb-threatening ischemia. *Ann Surg*. 1990;212:402–12.
3. Veith FJ, Ascer E, Gupta SK, White-Flores S, Sprayragen S, Scher LA, and Samson RH. Tibiotibial vein bypass grafts: A new operation for limb salvage. *J Vasc Surg*. 1985;2:552–7.
4. Veith FJ, Gupta SK, Ascer E et al. Improved strategies for secondary operations on infrainguinal arteries. *Ann Vasc Surg*. 1990;4:85–93.
5. Veith FJ, Moss CM, Daly V, Fell SC, and Haimovici H. New approaches to limb salvage by extended extra-anatomic bypasses and prosthetic reconstructions to foot arteries. *Surgery*. 1978;84:764–74.
6. Parsons RE, Suggs WD, Veith FJ et al. Polytetrafluoroethylene bypasses to infrapopliteal arteries without cuffs or patches: A better option than amputation in patients without autologous vein. *J Vasc Surg*. 1996;23:347–456.

CHAPTER 27

Results of PREVENT III: A Multicenter, Randomized Trial of Edifoligide for the Prevention of Vein Graft Failure in Lower Extremity Bypass Surgery

Conte MS, Bandyk DF, Clowes AW, Moneta GL, Seely L, Lorenz TJ, Namini H, Hamdan AD, Roddy SP, Belkin M et al. PREVENT III Investigators. J Vasc Surg. 2006 Apr;43(4):742–51; discussion 751

ABSTRACT

Objective The PREVENT III study was a prospective, randomized, double-blinded, multicenter phase III trial of a novel molecular therapy (edifoligide; E2F decoy) for the prevention of vein graft failure in patients undergoing infra-inguinal revascularization for critical limb ischemia (CLI).

Methods From November 2001 through October 2003, 1,404 patients with CLI were randomized to a single intra-operative ex-vivo vein graft treatment with edifoligide or placebo. After surgery, patients underwent graft surveillance by duplex ultrasonography and were followed up for index graft and limb endpoints to 1 year. A blinded Clinical Events Classification committee reviewed all index graft endpoints. The primary study endpoint was the time to nontechnical index graft re-intervention or major amputation due to index graft failure. Secondary endpoints included all-cause graft failure, clinically significant graft stenosis (>70% by angiography or severe stenosis by ultrasonography), amputation/re-intervention-free survival, and nontechnical primary graft patency. Event rates were based on Kaplan-Meier estimates. Time-to-event endpoints were compared by using the log-rank test.

Results Demographics, comorbidities, and procedural details reflected a population with CLI and diffuse atherosclerosis. Tissue loss was the presenting symptom in 75% of patients. High-risk conduits were used in 24% of cases, including an alternative vein in 20% (15% spliced vein and 5% non-great saphenous vein) and 6% less than 3 mm in diameter; 14% of the cases were re-operative bypass grafts. Most (65%) grafts were placed to infra-popliteal targets. Perioperative (30-day) mortality occurred in 2.7% of patients. Major morbidity included myocardial infarction in 4.7% and early graft occlusion in 5.2% of patients. Ex-vivo treatment with edifoligide was well tolerated.

There was no significant difference between the treatment groups in the primary or secondary trial endpoints, primary graft patency, or limb salvage. A statistically significant improvement was observed in secondary graft patency (estimated Kaplan-Meier rates were 83% edifoligide and 78% placebo; P = 0.016) within 1 year. The reduction in secondary patency events was manifest within 30 days of surgery (the relative risk for a 30-day event for edifoligide was 0.45; 95% confidence interval, 0.27–0.76; P = 0.005). For the overall cohort at 1 year, the estimated Kaplan-Meier rate for survival was 84%, that for primary patency was 61%, that for primary assisted patency was 77%, that for secondary patency was 80%, and that for limb salvage was 88%.

Conclusions In this prospective, randomized, placebo-controlled clinical trial, ex vivo treatment of lower extremity vein grafts with edifoligide did not confer protection from re-intervention for graft failure.

AUTHOR COMMENTARY BY MICHAEL CONTE

Despite the continued evolution of endovascular technologies, infra-inguinal bypass surgery remains an important and effective treatment option for patients with advanced peripheral arterial disease (PAD). Recent data from the Vascular Quality Initiative demonstrate that open bypass was used as the initial revascularization in 37% of cases with CLI.[1] A recent multicenter German registry reported a 24% rate of initial bypass interventions.[2] While autogenous vein remains the conduit of choice for infra-inguinal bypass, durability and re-interventions remain an issue. Over 5 years, 30%–50% of lower extremity vein grafts will lose primary patency, largely as a result of de-novo stenoses occurring within the graft body or peri-anastomotic regions. A high percentage of these events occur within the first 2 years after implantation. Graft surveillance and prophylactic re-interventions can maintain assisted patency in many patients (typically 70% or greater at 5 years), but with added cost and attendant morbidity. While the use of evidence-based pharmacotherapies (anti-thrombotic, lipid-lowering) and lifestyle modification (e.g., smoking cessation) for PAD is critical to reduce long-term major adverse events, there is no specific treatment as yet proven to reduce the risk of vein graft failure.

Bypass grafts offer a unique opportunity for targeted drug or biologic interventions. The tissue is readily accessible for local delivery of agents prior to the initiation of the post-implantation response. Most vein grafts have minimal pre-existing pathology and thus treatment strategy can focus on modulation of the downstream healing process to reduce stenosis and occlusion. However, the mechanisms underlying vein graft disease are complex, involving inflammation, thrombosis, cell migration, proliferation, and matrix metabolism.[3–6] Surgical handling of the vein results in significant, yet highly variable, degrees of endothelial loss, cellular and biochemical injury. The prototypical mid-term vein graft lesion demonstrates profound intimal thickening comprised of both cells (actin (+) vascular smooth muscle cells [VSMC] and/or myofibroblasts) and matrix, with variable degrees of adventitial fibrosis. Animal studies have demonstrated a brisk early proliferative response in the vein graft wall following arterialization. This process resembles neointimal hyperplasia following arterial injury (e.g., angioplasty) but is longer in duration. Moreover, a certain degree of wall thickening is required for biomechanical stabilization of the venous graft within the arterial hemodynamic environment.

The Project of Ex-Vivo Vein Graft Engineering via Transfection III (PREVENT III) trial was a phase 3 multicenter, double-blind, placebo-controlled randomized clinical trial (RCT) that tested a novel molecular strategy to prevent vein graft failure in patients with CLI.[7] The study drug, edifoligide, is a double-stranded oligodeoxynucleotide designed as a competitive inhibitor ("decoy") to a key transcription factor (E2F) that regulates progression through the cell cycle. When administered to VSMC, edifoligide dramatically inhibits proliferation with no or minimal toxicity. It was effective at reducing neointimal hyperplasia in several animal models, including a rabbit carotid interposition vein graft.[8,9] The drug is readily delivered to grafts using non-distending pressure in a simple isolation chamber within minutes, and thus the intervention was easily translated to an intra-operative setting. Early human pilot studies in both lower extremity[10] and coronary[11] vein grafts suggested safety, feasibility, and signals of efficacy. Thus the sponsor, a biotechnology start-up company (Corgentech, South San Francisco, CA), developed a phase 3 clinical evaluation program consisting of parallel lower extremity (PREVENT III) and coronary bypass (PREVENT IV) RCTs. To complete this prodigious effort they subsequently partnered with a large pharmaceutical company (Bristol-Myers Squibb, New York, NY). The parallel phase 3 studies were designed to gain FDA approval for the drug to prevent vein bypass graft failure. If successful, they would establish a new paradigm of best practice in coronary and peripheral revascularization.

The PREVENT III (PIII) trial ultimately enrolled 1,404 CLI patients from 83 North American sites over a 2-year period.[12] It represented a collaborative effort from a broad range of academic and community surgeons. The inclusion criteria were broad and utilized the contemporary clinical definition of "critical limb ischemia" (tissue loss or rest pain with confirmative hemodynamic studies). Any type of autogenous vein graft, including spliced veins and arm veins, could be included. A single-segment great saphenous vein conduit was used in 80%, and re-do bypass grafts constituted 16% of the index procedures in the trial. Among the enrolled subjects, 75% presented with tissue loss, 64% were diabetic, and 12% had dialysis-dependent renal failure. Distal bypass targets included 53% tibial and 12% pedal arteries. Thus this study was quite representative of real-world contemporary practice of revascularization in CLI. The study protocol mandated intensive postoperative graft surveillance, with duplex ultrasonography at 1, 3, 6, and 12 months. The protocol also specified criteria for vein graft re-intervention, including recurrent clinical symptoms, angiographic and/or duplex evidence of severe (>70%) stenosis.

The primary study endpoint in PIII was time to "nontechnical" index graft failure within 12 months of enrollment. A blinded clinical events committee was chartered to review all cases of graft failure and major limb amputation in the trial. Prespecified criteria were used to determine technical failure, designed to eliminate graft events that were clearly unrelated to the development of intrinsic vein graft or anastomotic disease. Because of the underlying hypothesis, the study was intently focused on the identification of significant graft lesions and the impact of the study drug to reduce graft-related events.

The results of PIII demonstrated no difference in the incidence of the primary efficacy endpoint between placebo (25.5%) and edifoligide-treated (25.2%) grafts. There were also no differences in all-cause clinical failure (36% vs. 35%), freedom from clinically significant graft stenosis (46% vs. 44%), and amputation/re-intervention-free survival (49% vs. 50%). The overall cohort demonstrated primary (61%), primary assisted (77%), and secondary (81%) graft patency rates at 1 year. There was a significantly greater secondary patency (83% vs. 78%, $p = 0.016$) in the edifoligide-treated grafts (Figure 27.1). Other key outcomes included an overall 2.7% mortality and 5.2% incidence of early graft failure at 30 days. At 1 year, patient survival was 84% and freedom from major amputation was 88%. These results remain as a contemporary quality benchmark for infra-inguinal bypass surgery in CLI.

Similar to PREVENT III, the PREVENT IV trial demonstrated no difference in the primary efficacy endpoint among 3,000 randomized subjects who underwent coronary artery bypass surgery.[13] The disappointing results of these two large-scale clinical trials were convincing and clear. Edifoligide, when administered to vein grafts ex-vivo as a single treatment at the time of implantation, did not reduce graft failure. Yet these trials marked the potential arrival of intra-operative molecular therapy in cardiovascular surgery and yielded important data on the conduct and outcomes of these common procedures. As such they remain as benchmarks in their fields and predicates for future attempts using drugs, biologics, or hybrid technologies to improve bypass surgery.

Following the primary publication of the PIII study results, the investigators completed a series of pre-planned secondary analyses examining patient-level risk factors, technical determinants, quality of life (QOL), re-interventions and other postoperative outcomes.[14–23] The multicenter scale of the study, combined with the rigor of data collection for a regulatory trial, provided great opportunity to examine clinical outcomes of vein bypass surgery in this population. The importance of adequate quality great saphenous vein (Figure 27.2),[22] the influence of graft-related events on QOL,[19] the durability of surgical versus endovascular graft revisions,[14] and the associations between race, gender, and graft failure[17] were key findings. A model ("PIII Risk Score") to predict amputation-free survival at 1-year following revascularization in CLI was developed[23] and subsequently validated in other registries.[20] Finally, patient-level data from the placebo arm of PIII was used to help develop suggested objective performance goals for endovascular interventions in this population.[24]

In the end, the major limitation of the PIII trial was the inability to determine the mechanisms of vein graft failure and why the molecular intervention had failed to

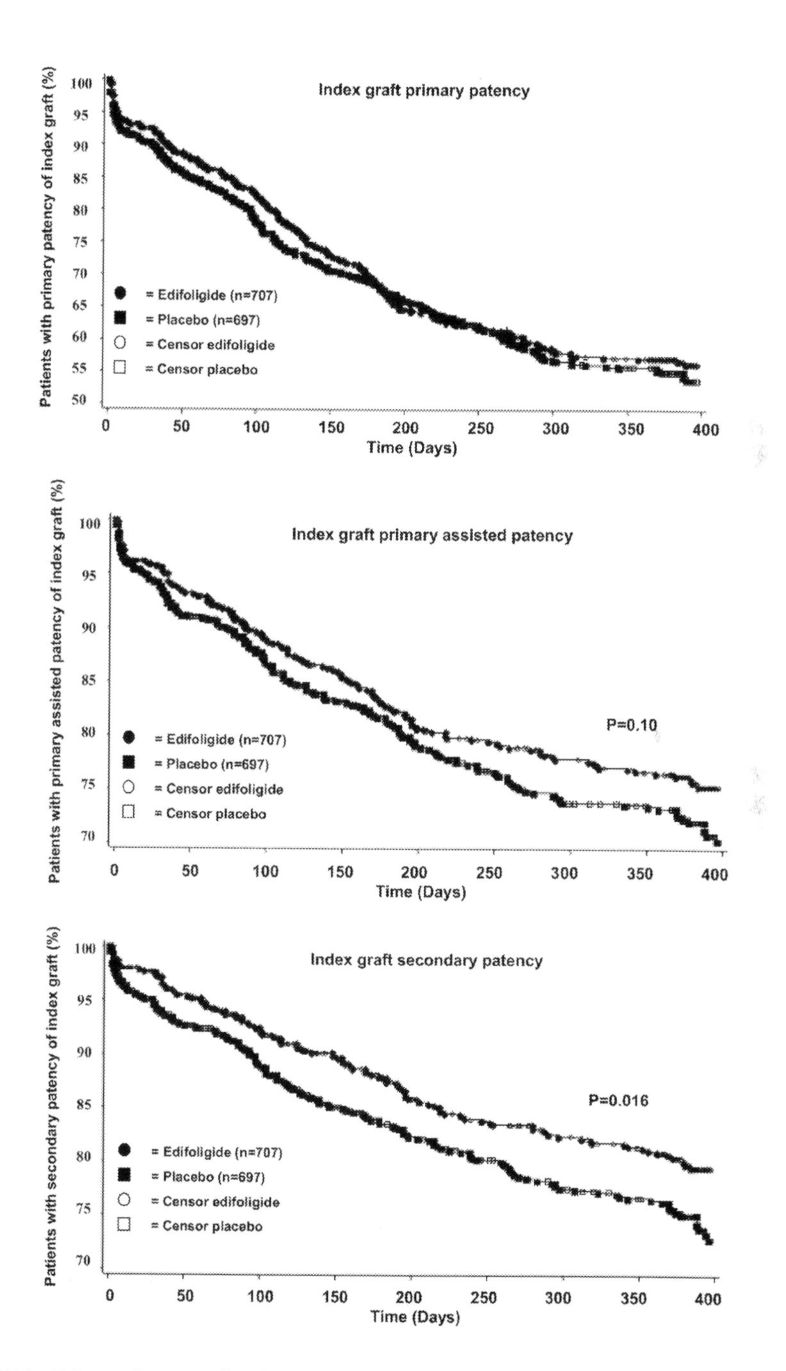

Figure 27.1 Primary (top panel), primary assisted (middle panel), and secondary (lower panel) patency of index vein bypass grafts performed for critical limb ischemia (N = 1,404) in the PREVENT III trial. The overall estimated rates for all subjects in the trial were 61%, 77%, and 80%, respectively at 1 year. Secondary graft patency was significantly higher in the edifoligide-treated group (p = 0.016).

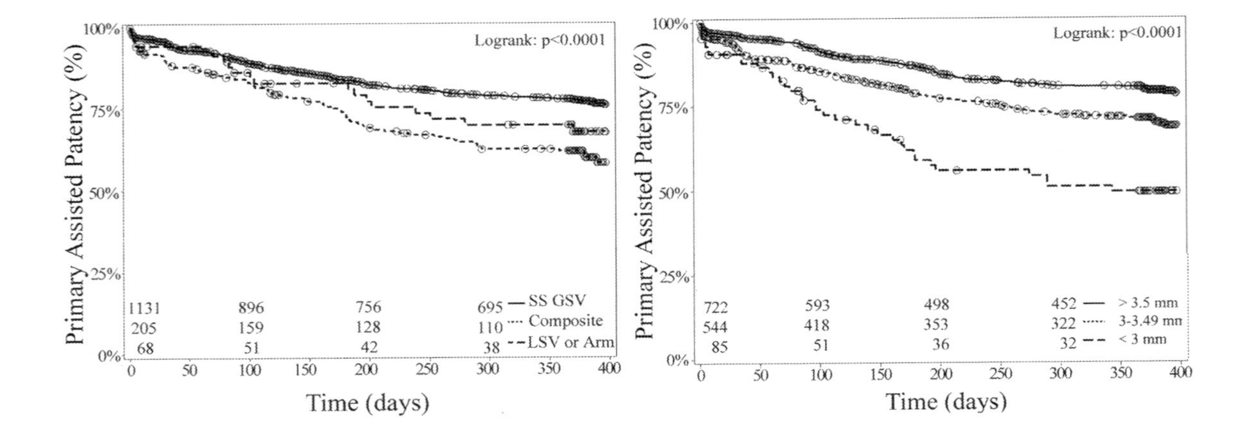

Figure 27.2 Impact of key technical factors on bypass outcomes in critical limb ischemia. Primary assisted patency of vein grafts in the PREVENT III trial based on conduit type (left panel; SSGSV = single segment great saphenous vein versus composite [spliced veins] versus lesser saphenous vein [LSV] or arm vein grafts) and estimated minimal graft diameter at implantation (right panel). In the trial, 43% of patients received an SSGSV graft with diameter >3.5 mm. These patients experienced 30-day graft failure rate of 1.7%, primary patency 72%, and secondary patency 87% at 1 year.

deliver. Clinical graft failure encompasses a broad range of patient factors, anatomic, technical, and biologic causes. High-resolution axial imaging studies, genomics, metabolomics, coagulation profiling and leukocyte phenotyping could have produced new insights into this challenging surgical problem. A well-executed vein bypass graft remains the most durable reconstruction for advanced PAD, yet graft disease is still a largely unsolved problem with significant impact on patients. The promise of the PIII trial, to re-engineer a better vein graft by a targeted molecular strategy, remains as relevant and tantalizing today as it was two decades ago.

REFERENCES

1. Simons JP, Schanzer A, Flahive JM et al. Survival prediction in patients with chronic limb-threatening ischemia who undergo infrainguinal revascularization. *J Vasc Surg: Off Publ, Soc Vasc Surg [and] Int Soc Cardiovasc Surg, North American Chapter.* 2019;69(6S):137S–51S e133.
2. Bisdas T, Borowski M, Torsello G. Current practice of first-line treatment strategies in patients with critical limb ischemia. *J Vasc Surg*. 2015;62(4):965–73. e963.
3. Conte MS, Mann MJ, Simosa HF, Rhynhart KK, and Mulligan RC. Genetic interventions for vein bypass graft disease: A review. *J Vasc Surg: Off Publ, Soc Vasc Surg [and] Int Soc Cardiovasc Surg, North American Chapter*. 2002;36(5):1040–52.
4. Owens CD, Ho KJ, and Conte MS. Lower extremity vein graft failure: A translational approach. *Vasc Med*. 2008;13(1):63–74.
5. de Vries MR, and Quax PHA. Inflammation in vein graft disease. *Front Cardiovasc Med.* 2018;5:3.
6. de Vries MR, Simons KH, Jukema JW, Braun J, and Quax PH. Vein graft failure: From pathophysiology to clinical outcomes. *Nature Rev Cardiol.* 2016;13(8):451–70.
7. Conte MS, Lorenz TJ, Bandyk DF, Clowes AW, Moneta GL, and Seely BL. Design and rationale of the PREVENT III clinical trial: Edifoligide for the prevention of infrainguinal vein graft failure. *Vasc Endovasc Surg*. 2005;39(1):15–23.
8. Mann MJ, Gibbons GH, Kernoff RS et al. Genetic engineering of vein grafts resistant to atherosclerosis. *Proc Natl Acad Sci U S A*. 1995;92(10):4502–6.
9. Mann MJ, Gibbons GH, Tsao PS et al. Cell cycle inhibition preserves endothelial function in genetically engineered rabbit vein grafts. *The J Clin Investigation*. 1997;99(6):1295–301.
10. Mann MJ, Whittemore AD, Donaldson MC et al. Ex-vivo gene therapy of human vascular bypass grafts with E2F decoy: The PREVENT single-centre, randomised, controlled trial. *Lancet*. 1999;354(9189):1493–8.
11. Grube E, Felderhoff T, Fitzgerald P et al. Phase II Trial of the E2F Decoy in Coronary Bypass Grafting. (Abstract). Paper presented at: American Heart Association Annual Meeting (Late Breaking Clinical Trials), 2001; Anaheim, CA.
12. Conte MS, Bandyk DF, Clowes AW et al. Results of PREVENT III: A multicenter, randomized trial of edifoligide for the prevention of vein graft failure in lower extremity bypass surgery. *J Vasc Surg: Off Publ, Soc Vasc Surg [and] Int Soc Cardiovasc Surg, North American Chapter*. 2006;43(4):742–51; discussion 751.
13. Alexander JH, Hafley G, Harrington RA et al. Efficacy and safety of edifoligide, an E2F transcription factor decoy, for prevention of vein graft failure following coronary artery bypass graft surgery: PREVENT IV: A randomized controlled trial. *JAMA: J Am Med Association*. 2005;294(19):2446–54.

14. Berceli SA, Hevelone ND, Lipsitz SR et al. Surgical and endovascular revision of infrainguinal vein bypass grafts: Analysis of midterm outcomes from the PREVENT III trial. *J Vasc Surg: Off Publ, Soc Vasc Surg [and] Int Soc Cardiovasc Surg, North American Chapter*. 2007;46(6):1173–9.
15. Conte MS, Bandyk DF, Clowes AW, Moneta GL, Namini H, and Seely L. Risk factors, medical therapies and perioperative events in limb salvage surgery: Observations from the PREVENT III multicenter trial. *J Vasc Surg: Off Publ, Soc Vasc Surg [and] Int Soc Cardiovasc Surg, North American Chapter*. 2005;42(3):456–64; discussion 464-455.
16. Nguyen LL, Brahmanandam S, Bandyk DF et al. Female gender and oral anticoagulants are associated with wound complications in lower extremity vein bypass: An analysis of 1,404 operations for critical limb ischemia. *J Vasc Surg: Off Publ, Soc Vasc Surg [and] Int Soc Cardiovasc Surg, North American Chapter*. 2007;46(6):1191–7.
17. Nguyen LL, Hevelone N, Rogers SO et al. Disparity in outcomes of surgical revascularization for limb salvage: Race and gender are synergistic determinants of vein graft failure and limb loss. *Circulation*. 2009;119(1):123–30.
18. Nguyen LL, Lipsitz SR, Bandyk DF et al. Resource utilization in the treatment of critical limb ischemia: The effect of tissue loss, comorbidities, and graft-related events. *J Vasc Surg: Off Publ, Soc Vasc Surg [and] Int Soc Cardiovasc Surg, North American Chapter*. 2006;44(5):971–5; discussion 975-976.
19. Nguyen LL, Moneta GL, Conte MS, Bandyk DF, Clowes AW, and Seely BL. Prospective multicenter study of quality of life before and after lower extremity vein bypass in 1,404 patients with critical limb ischemia. *J Vasc Surg: Off Publ, Soc Vasc Surg [and] Int Soc Cardiovasc Surg, North American Chapter*. 2006;44(5):977–83; discussion 983-974.
20. Schanzer A, Goodney PP, Li Y et al. Validation of the PIII CLI risk score for the prediction of amputation-free survival in patients undergoing infrainguinal autogenous vein bypass for critical limb ischemia. *J Vasc Surg*. 2009;50(4):769–75.
21. Schanzer A, Hevelone N, Owens CD, Beckman JA, Belkin M, and Conte MS. Statins are independently associated with reduced mortality in patients undergoing infrainguinal bypass graft surgery for critical limb ischemia. *J Vasc Surg: Off Publ, Soc Vasc Surg [and] Int Soc Cardiovasc Surg, North American Chapter*. 2008;47(4):774–81.
22. Schanzer A, Hevelone N, Owens CD et al. Technical factors affecting autogenous vein graft failure: Observations from a large multicenter trial. *J Vasc Surg: Off Publ, Soc Vasc Surg [and] Int Soc Cardiovasc Surg, North American Chapter*. 2007;46(6):1180–90; discussion 1190.
23. Schanzer A, Mega J, Meadows J, Samson RH, Bandyk DF, Conte MS. Risk stratification in critical limb ischemia: Derivation and validation of a model to predict amputation-free survival using multicenter surgical outcomes data. *J Vasc Surg: Off Publ, Soc Vasc Surg [and] Int Soc Cardiovasc Surg, North American Chapter*. 2008;48(6):1464–71.
24. Conte MS, Geraghty PJ, Bradbury AW et al. Suggested objective performance goals and clinical trial design for evaluating catheter-based treatment of critical limb ischemia. *J Vasc Surg: Off Publ, Soc Vasc Surg [and] Int Soc Cardiovasc Surg, North American Chapter*. 2009;50:1462–73.

CHAPTER 28

Statins Are Independently Associated with Reduced Mortality in Patients Undergoing Infrainguinal Bypass Graft Surgery for Critical Limb Ischemia

Schanzer A, Hevelone N, Owens CD, Beckman JA, Belkin M, Conte MS. J Vasc Surg. 2008 Apr;47(4):774–81

ABSTRACT

Objective Evidence suggesting a beneficial effect of cardioprotective medications in patients with lower extremity atherosclerosis derives largely from secondary prevention studies of heterogeneous populations. Patients with critical limb ischemia (CLI) have a large atherosclerotic burden with related high mortality. The effect of such therapies in this population is largely inferred and unproven.

Methods The Project of Ex-Vivo vein graft Engineering via Transfection III (PREVENT III) cohort comprised 1,404 patients with CLI who underwent lower extremity bypass grafting in a multicenter, randomized prospective trial testing the efficacy of edifoligide for the prevention of graft failure. Propensity scores were used to evaluate the influence of statins, beta-blockers, and antiplatelet agents on outcomes while adjusting for demographics, comorbidities, medications, and surgical variables that may influence drug use. Primary outcomes were major adverse cardiovascular events < or =30 days, vein graft patency, and 1-year survival assessed by Kaplan-Meier method. Potential determinants of 1-year survival were modeled using a multivariate Cox regression.

Results In this cohort, 636 patients (45%) were taking statins, 835 (59%) were taking beta-blockers, and 1,121 (80%) were taking antiplatelet drugs. Perioperative major adverse cardiovascular events (7.8%) and early mortality (2.7%) were not measurably affected by the use of any drug class. Statin use was associated with a significant survival advantage at 1 year of 86% vs. 81% (hazard ratio [HR], 0.71; 95% confidence interval [CI], 0.52–0.98; $P = 0.03$) by analysis of both unweighted and propensity score-weighted data. Use of beta-blockers and antiplatelet drugs had no appreciable impact on survival. None of the drug classes were associated with graft patency measures at 1 year. Significant predictors of 1-year mortality by Cox regression modeling were statin use (HR, 0.67; 95% CI, 0.51–0.90; $P = 0.001$), age >75 (HR, 2.1; 95% CI, 1.60–2.82; $P = 0.001$), coronary artery disease (HR, 1.5; 95% CI, 1.15–2.01; $P = 0.001$), chronic kidney disease stages 4 (HR, 2.0; 95% CI, 1.17–3.55; $P = 0.001$) and 5 (HR, 3.4; 95% CI, 2.39–4.73; $P < 0.001$), and tissue loss (HR, 1.9; 95% CI, 1.23–2.80; $P = 0.003$).

Conclusions Statin use is associated with improved survival in CLI patients 1 year after surgical revascularization. Further studies are indicated to determine optimal dosing in this population and to definitively address the question of relationship to graft patency. These data add to the growing literature supporting statin use in patients with advanced peripheral arterial disease.[1]

AUTHOR COMMENTARY BY ANDRES SCHANZER AND HAZEL MARECKI

Research Objective Establish evidence for a beneficial effect of cardioprotective medications, statins, antiplatelet agents, and beta-blockers in patients with peripheral vascular disease with critical limb-threatening ischemia (CLI).

Study Design A retrospective analysis was performed on the PREVENT III multicenter database using propensity score methodology to evaluate the association of statins, beta blockers, and antiplatelet agents, with survival, while adjusting for potential confounders. A multivariate Cox regression model was also used to further identify independent determinants of 1-year survival.

Sample Size The study cohort included 1,404 patients with critical limb-threatening ischemia who underwent infra-inguinal bypass with autogenous vein conduit at 83 hospitals in Canada and the United States between November 2001 and October 2003. Of this cohort, 636 (45%) were taking statins, 835 (59%) were taking beta-blockers, and 1,121 (80%) were taking antiplatelet agents.

Follow-Up PREVENT III patients were followed for 1 year post-infra-inguinal bypass surgery.[2]

Inclusion/Exclusion Criteria PREVENT III[3] inclusion criteria specified ≥18 years of age, infra-inguinal bypass graft with autogenous vein conduit for the indication of CLI defined as gangrene, nonhealing ischemic ulcer, or ischemic rest pain. Exclusion criteria were claudication as indication for lower extremity bypass and or use of nonautogenous conduit. All PREVENT III patients were included in reanalysis of cardioprotective medications.

Intervention or Treatment Received Not applicable.

Results None of the studied drug classes had a measurable effect on major adverse cardiovascular events (7.8%) or early perioperative mortality (2.7%). Statins were found to confer a survival benefit at one year (86% vs. 81%, HR 0.71%, 95% CI:

0.52–0.98; p = 0.03) by analysis of unweighted and propensity score-weighted data (Figure 28.1). Beta-blockers and antiplatelet agents had no measured impact on survival. None of the studied medications had an appreciable effect on 1-year patency. Beta-blockade improved 1-year primary patency in the unweighted data but was not significant in the propensity score-weighted analysis. Cox regression significant predictors of 1-year mortality were statin use (HR 0.67; CI 0.51–0.90, P = 0.001), age >75 (HR 2.1; 95% CI 1.60–2.82, p = 0.001), CAD (HR 1.5; CI: 1.15–2.01; p = 0.01), CKD stage IV (HR 2.0; CI: 1.17–3.55, p = 0.001) and stage V (HR 3.4; 95% CI 2.39–4.73, p < 0.001), and tissue loss (HR 1.9; CI 1.23–2.80, p = 0.003) (Table 28.1).

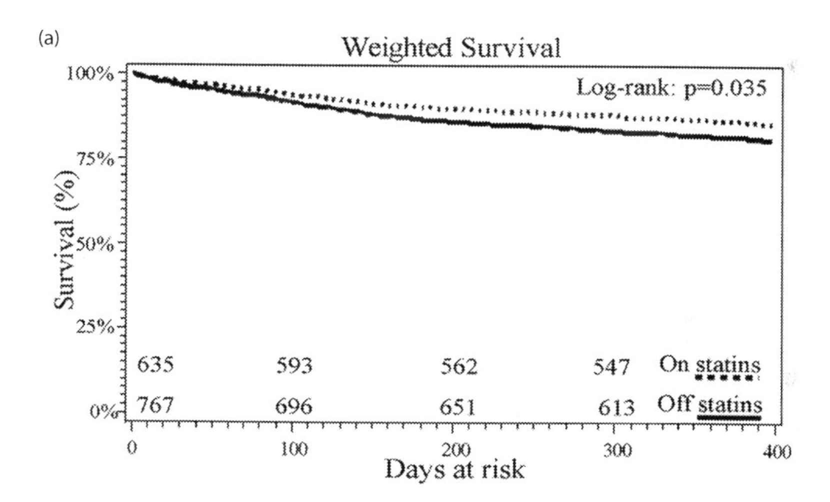

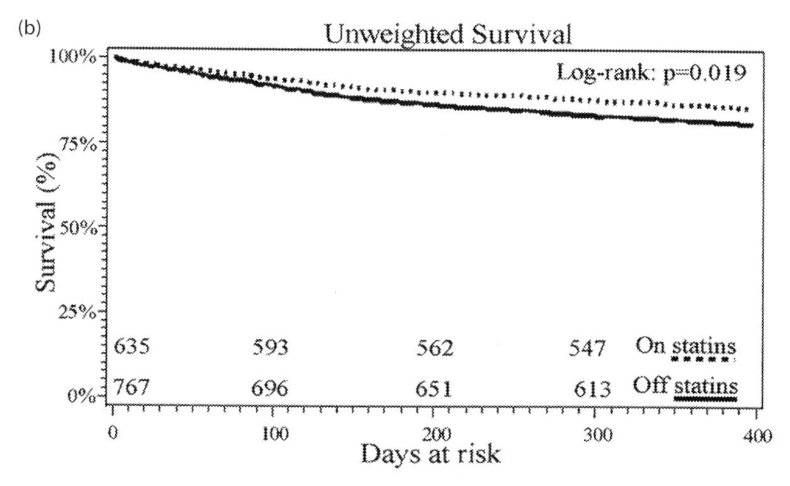

Figure 28.1 One-year survival by the Kaplan-Meier method in patients taking statins (dashed line) versus no (solid line). (a) Weighted propensity score (p = 0.03). (b) Unweighted propensity score (p = 0.02).

Table 28.1 Multivariate Analysis Identifying Impact of Risk Factor Predictors for 1-Year Mortality in the PREVENT III Cohort

Variable	Hazard Ratio (95% CI)	P
Age >75	2.13 (1.60–2.82)	<0.01
Female sex	1.09 (0.81–1.46)	0.58
Race/ethnicity		
White	1.0 (ref)	...
African American	0.82 (0.56–1.20)	0.3
Other	0.97 (0.63–1.50)	0.9
Risk factors for PAD		
Smoking	0.93 (0.68–1.28)	0.65
Diabetes mellitus	1.31 (0.96–1.79)	0.09
Hypertension	1.04 (0.70–1.54)	0.84
Coronary artery disease	1.52 (1.15–2.01)	<0.01
Prior IBG	0.84 (0.61–1.16)	0.3
Chronic kidney disease		
Stage 4	2.04 (1.17–3.55)	0.01
Stage 5	3.36 (2.39–4.73)	<.01
CLI criterion[a]		
Rest pain	1.0 (ref)	...
Tissue loss	1.86 (1.23–2.80)	<0.01
Medications		
Statin	0.68 (0.51–0.90)	<0.01
β-blocker	1.10 (0.82–1.46)	0.52
Aspirin	0.86 (0.63–1.19)	0.37
Surgical characteristics		
Proximal anastomosis		
CFA	1.0 (ref)	...
SFA	0.89 (0.64–1.23)	0.47
Popliteal	0.65 (0.42–1.00)	0.05
Distal anastomosis		
Popliteal, AK	1.0 (ref)	...
Popliteal, BK	1.22 (0.86–1.72)	0.26
Tibial	0.82 (0.48–1.40)	0.48
Pedal	0.86 (0.54–1.36)	0.52
Conduit diameter		
<3 mm	1.40 (0.85–2.30)	0.19
3–3.49 mm	0.83 (0.62–1.10)	0.21
>3.5 mm	1.0 (ref)	...
Institutional setting		
U.S., academic	0.90 (0.68–1.20)	0.48
U.S., private	1.0 (ref)	...
Canada	0.54 (0.27–1.09)	0.09

Abbreviation: *AK*, above knee; *BK*, below the knee; *CFA*, common femoral artery; *CLI*, critical limb ischemia; *IBG*, infrainguinal bypass graft; *PAD*, peripheral arterial disease; *PREVENT III*, Project of Ex-Vivo vein graft Engineering via Transfection; *SFA*, superficial femoral artery; *U.S.*, United States.

[a] Most severe.

Study Limitations Unlike a randomized controlled trial, propensity score weighting only adjusts for known confounders and does not adjust for unknown confounders. Cox regression modeling assumes a constant rate of underlying risk which is continuous over time in order to allow for variation in hazards of multiple variables.

Additionally, the relatively small study cohort had limited statistical power to detect differences, especially 30-day differences, in cardiovascular events or early mortality; this may represent a type-1 error. Finally, cohort homogeneity limited this study's generalizability to patients with aorto-iliac occlusive disease, aneurysmal disease, or who undergo bypass for an indication of intermittent claudication.

Relevant Studies

Heart Protection Study[4,5]: Statins demonstrated to confer 22% relative risk reduction in major vascular events in patients with peripheral arterial disease, broadly defined as "intermittent claudication, previous arterial revascularization, amputation, or aneurysm repair."

PREVENT III[2,3]: Multicenter randomized control trial designed to study the effects of edifoligide, a dsDNA molecule that inhibits cell-cycle progression hypothesized to reduce neointimal hyperplasia. All included patients had CLI defined as gangrene, non-healing ulceration, or ischemic rest pain. Study drug (e.g,. edifoligide) was found to confer no benefit on graft patency, cardiovascular events, or 1-year survival.[1]

CRITISCH Registry[6]: Prospective multicenter registry examined patients with critical limb ischemia treated with statin therapy versus without, with treatment crossovers and nonadherent patients excluded. Statin therapy was associated with increased amputation-free survival and lower rates of mortality and major adverse cardiovascular or cerebral events. However, statin therapy was not associated with lower amputation rates.

Suckow et al. (VSGNE)[7]: Patients with critical limb ischemia within the Vascular Study Group of New England Registry from 2003 to 2011 were examined retrospectively regarding use of statin medications for crude, adjusted, and propensity-matched rates of survival, 1-year amputation and graft occlusion. Statin therapy was associated with improved 5-year survival (63% vs. 54%, $p = 0.01$) but not associated with improved graft patency or decreased amputation.

Study Impact The identification of a quantifiable mortality benefit to the HMG Co-A reductase inhibitors, or statin medications, brought to light the importance of systemic treatment for the disease process of atherosclerosis. Patients with critical limb-threatening ischemia displayed the most severe form of atherosclerotic peripheral arterial disease and also experienced high rates of cardiovascular mortality, 50%–75% at 5 years.[8] It is difficult to conduct randomized control trials in patients with systemic vascular disease, but the statistical methods of using propensity score weights and Cox proportional hazards regression modeling to reanalyze the PREVENT III cohort provided a rigorous way in which to analyze a carefully collected cohort of vascular surgery patients.

With time, our understanding of the mechanism by which statins exert a mortality benefit in patients with atherosclerotic vascular disease has grown. Cholesterol has long been known to contribute to the development of atherosclerosis. From the late 1940s, Gofman and Donner at UC Berkeley identified differences in cholesterol lipoprotein content profiles which contributed to atherosclerosis. The science and treatment of hyperlipidemia was revolutionized by Goldstein and Brown's Nobel prize winning discovery of the genetic cause of familial hypercholesterolemia, an abnormally active form of 3-hydroxy-3-methylgluatamyl coenzyme A (HMG-CoA) reductase, the rate-limiting step in cholesterol synthesis. The resultant abnormal HMG-CoA reductase is no longer inhibited by high levels of high-density lipoprotein (HDL). Patient lipid profiles have traditionally been monitored for proof of successful treatment with statin medications, but a new understanding of the role of lipids in inflammatory processes has led to new markers. Lipid laden macrophages and lymphocytes produce IL-6, IL-1β, fibrinogen, and CRP, all of which had independently been shown to be associated with the development and progression of peripheral arterial disease. The PROVE_IT_TIMI trial showed that an hsCRP <2 is at least as important of a predictor as compared to LDL, and a better predictor of CV events in women.[9,10] The JUPITER trial additionally supports reduction of CRP <2 and LDL <13 with 44% risk reduction in MI, stroke, or unstable angina.[11] A new class of medications from the same inflammatory pathway includes the PCSK9 inhibitors, added to the U.S. market in 2015, with evidence showing decreased risk of arterial revascularization or cardiac death. The science of hyperlipidemia and inflammation is ever-evolving, and its importance for the vascular surgery population is becoming increasingly clear.

Throughout the study, between 2001 and 2003, only 45% of the PREVENT III cohort was treated with statin medications. Given that this cohort was diagnosed, meticulously followed, and treated for critical limb ischemia within the context of a large international trial, it is likely that the proportion of patients with critical limb ischemia on statins outside of the trial was even lower. This study suggested that vascular surgeons have a responsibility to become experts in medical management, not just surgical management. Medically treating systemic atherosclerotic disease in surgical patients influences their mortality. In the current era, guideline documents are clear that all patients with critical limb-threatening ischemia, as well as those with other atherosclerotic vascular disease, should be placed on high intensity statin medications to reduce cardiovascular mortality.[12] A growing literature has now demonstrated that statins are associated with decreased abdominal aortic aneurysm growth rates,[13] decreased stroke rates associated with carotid artery disease,[14] and improved amputation-free survival in patients with critical limb ischemia.[15] Taken in aggregate, all of these data have led to a global increase in the proportion of patients with vascular disease taking statin medications. Almost certainly, this increased use of statins has decreased cardiovascular events and prolonged life in patients with vascular disease.

REFERENCES

1. Schanzer A, Hevelone N, Owens CD, Beckman JA, Belkin M, and Conte MS. Statins are independently associated with reduced mortality in patients undergoing infrainguinal bypass graft surgery for critical limb ischemia. *J Vasc Surg*. 2008;47(4):774–81.e1.
2. Conte MS, Bandyk DF, Clowes AW et al. Results of PREVENT III: A multicenter, randomized trial of edifoligide for the prevention of vein graft failure in lower extremity bypass surgery. *J Vasc Surg*. 2006;43(4):742–51.e1.
3. Conte MS, Lorenz TJ, Bandyk DF, Clowes AW, Moneta GL, and Seely BL. Design and rationale of the PREVENT III Clinical Trial: Edifoligide for the prevention of Infrainguinal Vein Graft failure. *Vasc Endovascular Surg*. 2005;39(1):15–23.
4. MRC/BHF Heart Protection Study of cholesterol lowering with simvastatin in 20 536 high-risk individuals: A randomised placebocontrolled trial. *Lancet*. 2002;360(9326):7–22.
5. Randomized trial of the effects of cholesterol-lowering with simvastatin on peripheral vascular and other major vascular outcomes in 20,536 people with peripheral arterial disease and other high-risk conditions. *J Vasc Surg*. 2007;45(4):645–54.e1.
6. Stavroulakis K, Borowski M, Torsello G et al. Association between statin therapy and amputation-free survival in patients with critical limb ischemia in the CRITISCH registry. *J Vasc Surg*. 2017;66(5):1534–42.
7. Suckow BD, Kraiss LW, Schanzer A et al. Statin therapy after infrainguinal bypass surgery for critical limb ischemia is associated with improved 5-year survival. *J Vasc Surg*. 2015;61(1):126–33.e1.
8. Davies MG. Critical limb ischemia: Advanced medical therapy. *Methodist Debakey Cardiovasc J*. 2012;8(4):3–9. http://www.ncbi.nlm.nih.gov/pubmed/23342181. Accessed April 26, 2019.
9. Ridker PM, Cannon CP, Morrow D et al. C-Reactive protein levels and outcomes after statin therapy. *N Engl J Med*. 2005;352(1):20–8.
10. Morrow DA, de Lemos JA, Sabatine MS et al. Clinical relevance of c-reactive protein during follow-up of patients with acute coronary syndromes in the Aggrastat-to-Zocor Trial. *Circulation*. 2006;114(4):281–8.
11. Ridker PM, Danielson E, Fonseca FAH et al. Rosuvastatin to prevent vascular events in men and women with elevated C-Reactive protein. *N Engl J Med*. 2008;359(21):2195–207.
12. Conte MS, Bradbury AW, Kolh P et al. Global vascular guidelines on the management of chronic limb-threatening ischemia. *J Vasc Surg*. 2019;69(6S):3S–125S.e40.
13. Schouten O, van Laanen JHH, Boersma E et al. Statins are associated with a reduced infrarenal abdominal aortic aneurysm growth. *Eur J Vasc Endovasc Surg*. 2006;32(1):21–6.
14. Amarenco P, Labreuche J, Lavallée P, and Touboul P-J. Statins in stroke prevention and carotid atherosclerosis. *Stroke*. 2004;35(12):2902–9.
15. Westin GG, Armstrong EJ, Bang H et al. Association between statin medications and mortality, major adverse cardiovascular event, and amputation-free survival in patients with critical limb ischemia. *J Am Coll Cardiol*. 2014;63(7):682–90.

CHAPTER 29

Long-Term Results of In Situ Saphenous Vein Bypass: Analysis of 2058 Cases

Shah DM, Darling RC 3rd, Chang BB, Fitzgerald KM, Paty PS, Leather RP. *Ann Surg. 1995 Oct;222(4):438–46; discussion 446–8*

ABSTRACT

Purpose To evaluate the long-term patency and outcome of patients undergoing infra-inguinal reconstruction using the in situ saphenous vein.

Methods From 1957 to 1995, 3,148 autogenous vein bypasses were performed of which 2,058 used saphenous vein in situ for their reconstruction. The indications for operation were primarily limb threatening ischemia in 91% (1,875 out of 2,058). 88% of the patients with an intact ipsilateral greater saphenous vein had in situ saphenous vein bypasses completed successfully. Outflow consisted of 69% (1,023) bypasses performed to the infra-popliteal level, and 76% (1,562 of 2,058) were completed using the modified closed in situ technique. Follow-up was completed in 95% of the patients from 0 to 120 months. Groups were divided into long and short bypasses. Long bypasses were considered bypasses that were performed within 10 cm of the femoral bifurcation and 10 cm of the malleolus distally. Those with small veins under 4 mm versus larger veins, open versus closed in situ techniques, diabetics versus non-diabetics, and men versus women were analyzed.

Results 88% of patients with in situ with an intact ipsilateral saphenous vein could have an in situ bypass completed. Primary patency was 84% at 1 year, 72% at 5 years, and 55% at 10 years. Secondary- or primary-assisted patency was 91% at 1 year, 81% at 5 years, and 70% at 10 years. No statistically significant difference in patency was found in long versus short bypasses. There was no statistical difference in patency between larger versus smaller veins as well as no statistical difference in primary and secondary patency based on sex or diabetic status. Limb-salvage rates were 99% at 30 days, 97% at 1 year, 95% at 5 years, and 90% at 10 years.

Conclusions The infra-inguinal inflow source, length of bypass, specific outflow vessel, or vein diameter do not have a significant effect on immediate or long-term bypass performance. These data suggest the in situ saphenous vein is an excellent conduit for femoropopliteal and femoral to infra-geniculate bypasses for limb salvage.

AUTHOR COMMENTARY BY R. CLEMENT DARLING III, BENJAMIN B. CHANG, AND PAUL B. KREIENBERG

Research Question/Objective This was a study designed to evaluate the mid- and long-term results of in situ bypass. This was a technique that was evaluated by numerous surgeons including Karl Victor Hall of Norway. At our institution, Drs. Robert Leather and Alistair Karmody developed the first practical and successful method of in situ bypass. Our group has had extensive experience in distal bypasses and were interested to look at the long-term results of in situ reconstruction and compare them historically to the data on reverse vein bypasses.

Study Design From 1975 to 1995, 3,148 autogenous vein bypasses were performed of which 2,058 used saphenous vein in situ for their reconstruction. The indications for operation were primarily limb-threatening ischemia in 91% (1,875 out of 2,058). Eighty-eight percent of the patients with an intact ipsilateral greater saphenous vein had in situ saphenous vein bypasses completed successfully. Outflow consisted of 69% (1,023 out of 2,058) bypasses performed to the infrapopliteal level, and 76% (1,562 out of 2,058) were completed using the modified closed in situ technique.

Follow-Up In the postoperative period, bypass patency and limb salvage were determined at 2 weeks, 3 months, 6 months, 12 months, and every 6 months thereafter. This included physical exams, pulse volume recordings, segmental limb pressures, and duplex ultrasonography. Follow-up was completed in 95% of the patients from 0 to 120 months. Groups were divided into long and short bypasses. Long bypasses were considered bypasses that were performed within 10 cm of the femoral bifurcation and 10 cm of the malleolus distally. Those with small veins under 4 mm versus larger veins, open versus closed in situ techniques, diabetics versus nondiabetics, and men versus women were analyzed.

Results Eighty-eight percent of patients with in situ with an intact ipsilateral saphenous vein could have an in situ bypass completed. Primary patency was 84% at 1 year, 72% at 5 years, and 55% at 10 years. Secondary- or primary-assisted patency was 91% at 1 year, 81% at 5 years, and 70% at 10 years. No statistically significant difference in patency were found in long versus short bypasses. There was no statistical difference in patency between larger versus smaller veins as well as no statistical difference in primary and secondary patency based on sex or diabetic status. Limb-salvage rates were 99% at 30 days, 97% at 1 year, 95% at 5 years, and 90% at 10 years.

Study Limitations This was a single center series of patients undergoing in situ for inguinal reconstruction. Since the patients all had ipsilateral saphenous vein they were primarily de novo procedures that were not re-operative, thus creating a selection bias versus type of patient currently seen in most practices. This is also a retrospective analysis of prospectively collected surgery group's database.

Relevant Studies Drs. Linton and Darling in 1962 published their seminal paper on autogenous saphenous vein bypass in femoropopliteal obliterative arterial disease in *Surgery*. This was a landmark paper which demonstrated that infra-inguinal reconstruction could be performed safely and with a good long-term result. Since that time, there have been numerous papers from many institutions that performed large volumes of distal reconstructions in high-risk patients such as diabetics, patients with renal failure, patients with profound foot sepsis, with excellent results. One of the technical concerns of performing reverse vein reconstructions was the fact that one had to use the smaller portion of the vein for the proximal anastomosis on the large artery and the larger portion of vein on the smaller blood vessel distally which made some surgeons concerned about size mismatch, especially to the tibial vessels. In that year, it was not common to go below the knee until some of the subsequent data from Dr. Porter's group in Oregon, Campbell and Gibbons group at the Deaconess Hospital, and Drs. Mannick and Conte's group at The Brigham demonstrated that a more aggressive approach could save patients even with tibial occlusive disease. Dr. Leather and Dr. Karmody were the first to successfully employ in situ bypass techniques. There was a tremendous discussion, especially between Dr. Porter and Dr. Leather, of the benefits and the limitations of reverse vein versus in situ techniques. Those proponents for in situ felt that the warm ischemia time of the intima of the vein would be less leading to preservation of endothelial function and decreased ischemic injury to the vein, thereby decreasing short-term occlusion and long-term restenosis. Also, using the in situ technique one could use smaller veins which allowed one to aggressively treat more distal lesions and especially do long bypasses from the common femoral region down to the peri-malleolar tibial vessels using one piece of vein that was tapered in order to make both anastomoses easier. The most different aspect of the in situ technique was the ability to atraumatically disrupt the valves to allow flow from proximal to distal along the vein bypass.

Drs. Connolly and Charles Robb of London, as early as 1958, discussed the technical aspects, hemodynamic issues with saphenous vein bypass and thought the in situ vein reconstruction was too time consuming. They thought the fistula problem might outweigh the possible advantages. The development of instruments that could render the valves incompetent without causing undue vein injury in the process (the "valve incision" technique) was the primary reason that the in situ approach could become a practical and successful technique for distal bypass. Once the technical aspects of valve disruption were overcome, the next goal was to see how this affected patency. This was the thesis of the long-term results of in situ saphenous bypass by Dr. Shah et al. This was another long-term outcome paper which demonstrated that in situ bypass could be performed with remarkable longevity and limb salvage. The results seen by Dr. Shah, Dr. Leather, and our group demonstrated that they were considerably better than those from historic controls, and although many people adopted this technique there was still a bitter battle between those who preferred reverse vein reconstructions versus in situ.

Study Impacts This study was one of the first long-term results about a new distal reconstructive technique, the in situ saphenous vein bypass. Technical aspects had been worked out in the past but there was still a bitter discussion as to whether this technique could be taught and also whether the results would parallel or be better than those with reverse vein bypass. There were proponents on each side and although this paper was not to diminish the utility of reverse vein bypass, it was a way of showing not only that in situ bypasses work but distal reconstruction using long segments of single piece vein had excellent long-term patency and limb salvage. It also demonstrated that men and women have the same patency rates, which had been a concern in the past, and that diabetics did equally well as non-diabetics. This latter data was also corroborated by the numerous long-term studies from Frank Pomposelli, Gary Gibbons, David Campbell, and Franc Logerfo at the Deaconess Hospital in Boston. I strongly believe that the importance of this paper was not only on its technical aspects of distal reconstruction emphasizing the technical aspects of distal reconstruction for performing an in situ bypass, but more importantly it established that distal reconstruction to the lower third of the leg worked equally as well as those bypasses to the popliteal artery. Prior to this, these long bypasses were considered desperate, too complicated, and too time consuming for many surgeons and the main excuse was that they weren't going to work so why should one put in the effort. Again, this paper demonstrated that these long reconstructions technically could be performed with excellent short- and long-term results and the limb-salvage rate was equal if not better than prior reports. The database from this same group now documents the results of more than 6,000 in situ bypasses and 15,000 leg bypasses overall. An aggressive approach to limb salvage, endovascular and open, if performed in a balanced way can deliver extremely good limb-salvage results in patients with very difficult and extensive infra-inguinal occlusive disease.

SUGGESTED READING

Connolly JE. The history of the in situ saphenous vein bypass. *J Vasc Surg*. 2011;53:241–44.

Fogle MA, Whittemore AD, Couch NP, and Mannick JA. A comparison of in situ and reversed saphenous vein grafts for infrainguinal reconstruction. *J Vasc Surg*. 1987;5:46–52.

Hall KV. The great saphenous vein used in situ as an arterial shunt after extirpation of the vein valves. A preliminary report. *Surgery*. 1962;51:492–5.

Kunlin J. Le Traitement de l'arterite obtitrante par la greffe veineuse. *Arch Mal Coeur*. 1949;42:371.

Leather RP, and Karmody AM. In-situ saphenous vein arterial bypass for the treatment of limb ischemia. *Adv Surg*. 1986;19:175–219.

Leather RP, Powers SR, and Karmody AM. A reappraisal of the in situ saphenous vein arterial bypass: Its use in limb salvage. *Surger*. 1979;86:453–61.

Leather RP, and Shah DM. Experiences with in situ lower extremity saphenous vein bypass procedures. *Surg Annu*. 1988;20:257–71.

Leather RP, Shah DM, Chang BB, and Kaufman JL. Resurrection of the in situ saphenous vein bypass. 1,000 cases later. *Ann Surg*. 1988 Oct;208(4):435–42.

Leather RP, Shah DM, and Karmody AM. Infrapopliteal arterial bypass for limb salvage-increased patency and utilization of the saphenous vein used in-situ. *Surgery*. 1981;90:1000–1008.

Linton R, and Darling RC. Autogenous saphenous vein bypass grafts in femoropopliteal obliterative arterial disease. *Surgery*. 1962;51:62–72.

Pomposelli FB, Kansal N, Hamdan AD et al. A decade of experience with dorsalis pedis artery bypass: Analysis of outcome in more than 1,000 cases. *J Vasc Surg*. 2003 Feb;37(2):307–15.

Porter JM. In situ versus reversed vein graft: Is one superior? *J Vasc Surg*. 1987;5:779–80.

Shah DM, Darling RC 3rd, Chang BB, Fitztgerald KM, Paty PS, and Leather RP. Long-term results of in situ saphenous vein bypass. Analysis of 2,058 cases. *Ann Surg*. 1995 Oct;222(4):438–46; discussion 446–8.

Suggs WD, Sanchez LA, Woo D, Lipsitz EC, Ohki T, and Veith FJ. Endoscopically assisted in situ lower extremity bypass graft: A preliminary report of a new minimally invasive technique. *J Vasc Surg*. 2001 Oct;34(4):668–72.

Taylor LM Jr, Edwards JM, and Porter JM. Present status of reversed vein bypass grafting: Five-year results of a modern series. *J Vasc Surg*. 1990 Feb;11(2):193–205.

CHAPTER 30

Contemporary Management of Acute Mesenteric Ischemia: Factors Associated with Survival

Park WM, Gloviczki P, Cherry KJ Jr, Hallett JW Jr, Bower TC, Panneton JM, Schleck C, Ilstrup D, Harmsen WS, Noel AA. J Vasc Surg. 2002 Mar;35(3):445–52

ABSTRACT

Purpose Acute mesenteric ischemia (AMI) is a morbid condition with a difficult diagnosis and a high rate of complications, which is associated with a high mortality rate. For the evaluation of the results of current management and the examination of factors associated with survival, we reviewed our experience.

Methods The clinical data of all the patients who underwent operation for AMI between January 1, 1990, and December 31, 1999, were retrospectively reviewed, clinical outcome was recorded, and factors associated with survival rate were analyzed.

Results Fifty-eight patients (22 men and 36 women; mean age, 67 years; age range, 35 to 96 years) underwent the study. The cause of AMI was embolism in 16 patients (28%), thrombosis in 37 patients (64%), and nonocclusive mesenteric ischemia (NMI) in five patients (8.6%). Abdominal pain was the most frequent presenting symptom (95%). Twenty-five patients (43%) had previous symptoms of chronic mesenteric ischemia. All of the patients underwent abdominal exploration, preceded with arteriography in 47 (81%) and with endovascular treatment in eight. Open mesenteric revascularization was performed in 43 patients (bypass grafting, n = 22; thromboembolectomy, n = 19; patch angioplasty, n = 11; endarterectomy, n = 5; reimplantation, n = 2). Thirty-one patients (53%) needed bowel resection at the first operation. Twenty-three patients underwent second-look procedures, 11 patients underwent bowel resections (repeat resection, n = 9), and three patients underwent exploration only. The 30-day mortality rate was 32%. The rate was 31% in patients with embolism, 32% in patients with thrombosis, and 80% in patients with NMI. Multiorgan failure (n = 18 patients) was the most frequent cause of death. The cumulative survival rates at 90 days, at 1 year, and at 3 years were 59%, 43%, and 32%, respectively, which was lower than the rate of a Midwestern white control population ($P < 0.001$). Six of the 16 late deaths (38%) occurred because of complications of mesenteric ischemia. Age less than 60 years ($P < 0.003$) and bowel resection ($P = 0.03$) were associated with improved survival rates.

Conclusions The contemporary management of AMI with revascularization with open surgical techniques, resection of nonviable bowel, and liberal use of second-look procedures results in the early survival of two thirds of the patients with embolism and thrombosis. Older patients, those who did not undergo bowel resection, and those with NMI have the highest mortality rates. The long-term survival rate remains dismal. Timely revascularization in patients who are symptomatic with chronic mesenteric ischemia should be considered to decrease the high mortality rate of AMI.

AUTHOR COMMENTARY BY WOOSUP M. PARK AND PETER GLOVICZKI

Research Question/Objective Acute mesenteric ischemia is a morbid condition with a high mortality rate.[1] The objective of this study was to evaluate what patient and treatment factors were associated with survival in the short- and mid-term.

Study Design Single-center retrospective case series.

Sample Size 58 patients.

Follow-Up 3 years.

Inclusion/Exclusion Criteria Patients presenting with acute mesenteric ischemia presenting to the vascular surgery service and undergoing laparotomy from January 1, 1990 to December 31, 1999 were included for study.

Intervention or Treatment Received All patients underwent initial exploratory laparotomy with treatment guided by intra-operative findings including revascularization in 43 patients and bowel resection in 31. Second look procedures were performed in 23 patients, of whom 11 underwent bowel resection (further resection in 9). The 47 patients underwent preoperative contrast arteriography and eight of these had an initial endovascular procedure.

Results Fifty-eight patients with acute mesenteric ischemia (1990–1999), 22 men and 37 women, ages ranging from 35 to 96 years, underwent exploratory laparotomy. Pre-operative contrast arteriography was performed on 47 patients (81%) and eight of these had initial endovascular intervention. The cause of acute mesenteric ischemia was embolism in 28%, thrombosis in 64%, and nonocclusive mesenteric ischemia in 8.6%. Open revascularization was performed on 43 patients, consisting of bypass grafting in 22 patients, thromboembolectomy in 19, patch angioplasty in 11, endarterectomy in five, and mesenteric reimplantation in two. Bowel resection was required in 31 patients (53%) during the first laparotomy. Of the 23 patients undergoing second look laparotomy, an additional 11 patients had bowel resection, of whom nine had repeat bowel resection. The 30-day mortality rate was 32% (embolism

31%, thrombosis 32%, and nonocclusive mesenteric ischemia 81%), with multiorgan failure representing the most frequent cause of death. Overall survival at 90 days, 1 year, and 3 years was 59%, 43%, and 32%; 38% of the late deaths (6 of 16) were due to complications of mesenteric ischemia. Factors associated with improved survival included age less than 60 years ($P < 0.003$) and bowel resection ($P = 0.03$). The study concluded that revascularization with open surgical techniques, resection of the nonviable bowel, and a liberal use of second look procedure improves survival of these patients. Older patients, those not undergoing resection of dead bowel, and those with nonocclusive mesenteric ischemia had the highest mortality rates and where long-term overall survival was poor, and elective revascularization of chronic mesenteric ischemia should be pursued more aggressively.

Study Limitations This was a single institution retrospective study that only included patients who had an open laparotomy for acute mesenteric ischemia. The selection of these patients skews the mortality results. Overall, mortality of acute mesenteric ischemia is far greater than the 32% presented as this study, since there were many excluded patients too moribund for operation and those who died before diagnosis of acute mesenteric ischemia could be made. The small number of five patients with nonocclusive mesenteric ischemia limits any major conclusion but it emphasizes the high mortality of this subset of patients. A significant limitation was the lack of endovascular therapy in the 1990s that certainly changed contemporary management of these patients. It is noteworthy that those who underwent bowel resection had a better overall survival than those who did not. In addition, those who underwent successful surgical revascularization did better if they had embolism or thrombosis.

Relevant Studies This paper provided an analysis of a large operative series of patients undergoing surgical treatment of acute mesenteric ischemia. Since its publication, Ryer et al.[2] updated this Mayo Clinic series, comparing a subsequent decade of patients (1990s vs. 2000s), excluding nonocclusive mesenteric ischemia, and found that while the patients were older, no difference in mortality was found between eras (27% vs. 17%, $P = 0.28$). This was despite an increase in the utilization of endovascular therapies. No difference in outcomes could be discerned between patients treated with endovascular versus open surgical revascularization. A contemporary publication of acute mesenteric ischemia from Kougias et al.[3] from Baylor College of Medicine found a similarly high rate of 30-day mortality (31%) in 72 patients from 1993 to 2005. Scali et al.[4] compared antegrade versus retrograde bypass configurations for revascularization in acute mesenteric ischemia found an overall mortality rate of 26% with no difference in outcomes between configurations.

Arthurs et al.[5] studied 78 consecutive patients with acute mesenteric ischemia treated between 1999 and 2008 in a retrospective case series from the Cleveland Clinic. Endovascular therapy was the preferred treatment in 81% versus operative revascularization in 18%. Successful endovascular revascularization was achieved in 87% and resulted in a lower mortality rate than with open revascularization (36% vs. 50%, $P < 0.05$). Endovascular therapy was associated with a lower rate of acute renal failure and respiratory failure. Beaulieu et al.[6] looked at the data from the National Inpatient Sample Database and found 514 patients undergoing open surgery and 165 patients undergoing endovascular treatment with a greater mortality in open surgery (open 39.3% vs. endo 24.9%, P = 0.01). This paper demonstrated the increasing use of endovascular techniques over open surgery during the study period of 2005–2009.

While open revascularization is performed simultaneously with exploratory laparotomy and bowel resection, endovascular revascularization typically is performed before laparotomy. The rapid dissemination of endovascular techniques and accumulation of experience has resulted in the adoption of hybrid techniques involving direct access to the diseased vessel and performing retrograde open mesenteric stenting (ROMS). It is particularly helpful in revascularizing flush occlusions of the superior mesenteric artery in cases where the transfemoral endovascular approach may be difficult or not possible. Oderich et al[7] reported from a multicenter study of ROMS in acute and subacute on chronic mesenteric ischemia and found an acceptable primary patency rate of 76% at 2 years, with a 45% 30-day mortality for acute mesenteric ischemia. Comparably, Roussel et al. reported a 1-year primary patency of 92% with a 30-day mortality of 25% in 25 patients with acute mesenteric ischemia treated with ROMS.

As in ST segment myocardial infarctions (STEMI) and strokes, the successful treatment of acute mesenteric ischemia is also time dependent. Since the publication of our paper, all series on acute mesenteric ischemia demonstrated a similarly high rate of mortality and need for bowel resection, indicating that for many patients, the diagnosis and treatment come too late to successfully treat this deadly disease. Using an approach similar to STEMI and stroke, Roussel et al.[8] created an intestinal stroke center with multidisciplinary treatment protocols and processes. From 2009–2014, 83 patients were treated for acute mesenteric ischemia in a dedicated intestinal stroke center with focus on early diagnosis, revascularization, and exploration. 30-day mortality was 6.9% with a 2-year survival of 89.2%. While these excellent results represent a selected subpopulation of patients, it cannot be argued that creating protocols and pathways that favor early diagnosis and trigger early intervention and operation is not a great use of resources. Establishing a dedicated acute intestinal ischemia team and management protocol may not just be helpful, but critical in driving down the mortality rate of acute mesenteric ischemia.

REFERENCES

1. Park WM, Gloviczki P, Cherry KJ Jr, Hallett JW Jr, Bower TC, Panneton JM, Schleck C, Ilstrup D, Harmsen WS, and Noel AA. Contemporary management of acute mesenteric ischemia: Factors associated with survival. *J Vasc Surg*. 2002 Mar;35(3):445–52.
2. Ryer EJ, Kalra M, Oderich GS, Duncan AA, Gloviczki P, Cha S, and Bower TC. Revascularization for acute mesenteric ischemia. *J Vasc Surg*. 2012;55:1682–9.

3. Kougias P, Lau D, El Sayed AF, Zhou W, Huynh TT, and Lin PH. Determinants of mortality and treatment outcome following surgical interventions for acute mesenteric ischemia. *J Vasc Surg*. 2007;46:467–74.
4. Scali ST, Ayo D, Giles KA et al. Outcomes of antegrade and retrograde open mesenteric bypass for acute mesenteric ischemia. *J Vasc Surg*. 2019;69:129–40.
5. Arthurs ZM, Titus J, Bannazadeh M, Eagleton MJ, Srivastava S, Sarac TP, and Clair DG. A comparison of endovascular revascularization with traditional therapy for the treatment of acute mesenteric ischemia. *J Vasc Surg*. 2011;53:698–704.
6. Beaulieu RJ, Arnaoutakis KD, Abularrage CH, Efron DT, Schneider E, and Black JH. Comparison of open and endovascular treatment of acute mesenteric ischemia. *J Vasc Surg*. 2014;59:159–64.
7. Oderich GS, Macedo R, Stone DH et al. on behalf of the Low Frequency Vascular Disease Research Consortium Investigators. Multicenter study of retrograde open mesenteric artery stenting through laparotomy for treatment of acute and chronic mesenteric ischemia. *J Vasc Surg*. 2018;68:470–80.
8. Roussel A, Castier Y, Nuzzo A, Pellenc Q, Sibert A, Panis Y, Bouhnik Y, and Corcos O. Revascularization of acute mesenteric ischemia after creation of a dedicated multidisciplinary center. *J Vasc Surg*. 2015;62:1251–6.

CHAPTER 31

Contemporary Outcomes of Intact and Ruptured Visceral Artery Aneurysms

Shukla AJ, Eid R, Fish L, Avgerinos E, Marone L, Makaroun M, Chaer RA. J Vasc Surg. 2015 Jun;61(6):1442–8

ABSTRACT

Objective The treatment outcomes of ruptured visceral artery aneurysms (rVAAs) have been sparsely characterized, with no clear comparison between different treatment modalities. The purpose of this paper was to review the perioperative and long-term outcomes of open and endovascular interventions for intact visceral artery aneurysms (iVAAs) and rVAAs.

Methods This was a retrospective review of all treated VAAs at one institution from 2003 to 2013. Patient demographics, aneurysm characteristics, management, and subsequent outcomes (technical success, mortality, re-intervention), and complications were recorded.

Results The study identified 261 patients; 181 patients were repaired (77 ruptured, 104 intact). Pseudoaneurysms were more common in rVAAs (81.8% vs. 35.3% for iVAAs; $P < 0.001$). The rVAAs were smaller than the iVAAs (20.7 mm vs. 27.5 mm; $P = 0.018$), and their most common presentation was abdominal pain; 29.7% were hemodynamically unstable. Endovascular intervention was the initial treatment modality for 67.4% (75.3% for rVAAs, 61.5% for iVAAs). The perioperative complication rate was higher for rVAAs (13.7% vs. 1% for iVAAs; $P = 0.003$), as was mortality at 30 days (13% vs. 0% for iVAAs; $P = 0.001$), 1 year (32.5% for rVAAs vs. 4.1% for iVAAs; $P < 0.001$), and 3 years (36.4% for rVAAs vs. 8.3% for iVAAs; $P < 0.001$). Lower 30-day mortality was noted with endovascular repair for rVAAs (7.4% vs. 28.6% open; $P = 0.025$). Predictors of mortality for rVAAs included age (odds ratio, 1.04; $P = 0.002$), whereas endovascular repair was protective (odds ratio, 0.43; $P = 0.037$). Mean follow-up was 26.2 months, and Kaplan-Meier estimates of survival were higher for iVAAs at 3 years (88% vs. 62% for rVAAs; $P = 0.045$). The 30-day re-intervention rate was higher for rVAAs (7.7% vs. 19.5% for iVAAs; $P = 0.019$) but was similar between open and endovascular repair (8.2% vs. 15%; P = NS).

Conclusions rVAAs have significant mortality. Open and endovascular interventions are equally durable for elective repair of VAAs, but endovascular interventions for rVAAs result in lower morbidity and mortality. Aggressive treatment of pseudoaneurysms is electively recommended at diagnosis regardless of size.

AUTHOR COMMENTARY BY RABIH CHAER

This paper was inspired by a middle-aged man I cared for while on call over Christmas, with a ruptured pancreaticoduodenal arcade (PDA) aneurysm and upper GI bleeding. A multidisciplinary evaluation including vascular surgery and hepatobiliary surgery was done, and it was clear that while there is no standardized approach to treat those patients, surgical resection is highly morbid. After successful initial coil embolization via a superior mesenteric artery branch, the patient bled again a few days later, requiring additional coiling to seal aneurysm perfusion from the gastroduodenal artery. He fully recovered, but this case sparked our interest into investigating visceral artery aneurysms (VAAs), particularly in the setting of rupture, with the hypothesis that endovascular treatment is equally effective and durable as surgical resection, but much less morbid.

Ruptured VAAs carry a high risk of mortality. Although open and endovascular treatment of intact nonruptured visceral aneurysms is safe and durable, endovascular repair of ruptured aneurysms results in lower morbidity and mortality.

Our published series is the largest to date on ruptured VAAs and shows a significant mortality of 11.9% at 30 days and all-cause mortality of 41.3% at 2 years. The significant mortality observed in our series with ruptures can be explained by the high prevalence of pseudoaneurysms, which typically result from underlying hepatobiliary disease, and the significant number of PDA aneurysms, which are difficult to diagnose and treat. PDA aneurysms and all visceral pseudoaneurysms carry a high risk for rupture, and we recommend that they should be repaired early on regardless of size.

Endovascular treatment of ruptures resulted in lower morbidity and mortality compared with open repair (28.6% vs. 7.4%). The low 30-day mortality as well as the low major complication rate of 8.9% sits in sharp contrast to the open group (28.6% major complication and mortality at 30 days). The benefit of endovascular repair may be derived from the combination of lower morbidity compared with open repair as well as the ability to more accurately diagnose and treat the source of the bleed. The latter is enhanced further when a contrasted CT scan is available as it often becomes difficult to find a small pseudoaneurysm in the peripancreatic region.

It is our hope that this work will lead to increased awareness of the importance of a standardized, multidisciplinary approach to visceral aneurysms and early endovascular intervention for PDA aneurysms and visceral pseudoaneurysms regardless of size, and that this be reflected in future societal clinical practice guidelines.

CHAPTER 32

Clinical Importance and Management of Splanchnic Artery Aneurysms

Stanley JC, Wakefield TW, Graham LM, Whitehouse WM Jr, Zelenock GB, Lindenauer SM. J Vasc Surg. 1986 May;3(5):836–40

ABSTRACT

Splanchnic artery aneurysms are unusual but important vascular lesions. Nearly 22% of all reported splanchnic artery aneurysms present as clinical emergencies, including 8.5% that result in death. More than 2,000 of these aneurysms have been documented in the literature. The most commonly involved vessels, in decreasing order of frequency, include the history and treatment must be individualized.

EXPERT COMMENTARY BY DAWN MARIE COLEMAN

Research Question/Objective This study was undertaken to characterize the clinical importance and management of splanchnic artery aneurysms.

Study Design Review.

Sample Size Not applicable, although the authors cite "more than 2,000 splanchnic artery aneurysms have been documented in the literature."

Follow-up Not applicable.

Inclusion/Exclusion Criteria Not applicable.

Intervention or Treatment Received Not applicable.

Results This narrative clinical review summarizes the clinical importance and management of splanchnic artery aneurysms. The authors reference that nearly 22% of all reported splanchnic artery aneurysms present as clinical emergencies, including 8.5% that result in death. The most commonly involved vessels, in decreasing order of frequency include: splenic > hepatic > superior mesenteric > celiac > gastric-gastroepiploic > jejunal-ileal-colic > pancreaticoduodenal-pancreatic > gastroduodenal.

Splenic artery aneurysms are associated with arterial fibrodysplasia, portal hypertension, and multiparity, with up to 20% reported as symptomatic. Rupture rates are estimated as 95% during pregnancy, resulting in severe mortality rates for mother (70%) and fetus (95%). Aneurysm size >2.5 cm, pregnancy, child-bearing age and symptoms were referenced as indication for surgical therapy. The authors further report a mortality rate for ruptured aneurysms in non-pregnant patients is 25%, suggesting that on the basis of a 2% incidence of rupture with associated 25% mortality rate, operative mortality rates must be <0.5% to justify elective surgical repair.

Hepatic artery aneurysms are attributed to atherosclerosis, acquired medial degeneration, trauma, infection associated with illicit drug use, and other arteriopathies. The majority (80%) are extrahepatic, while 20% are intrahepatic with site involvement well defined: 63% located in the common hepatic artery, 28% in the right hepatic artery, 5% in the left hepatic artery, and 4% affecting bilateral hepatic arteries. Rupture into the biliary tract and peritoneal are reported with equal frequency and the authors further recommend operative therapy for most aneurysms as the frequency of hepatic artery aneurysm rupture is less than 20% and the mortality rate associated with such approximates 35%.

Superior mesenteric artery aneurysms are attributed primarily to infection (60%), and specifically to the fact that mycotic aneurysms occurring as a result of nonhemolytic streptococci in left-sided bacterial endocarditis involve this vessel more frequently than any other muscular artery. The authors propose that while the exact rupture rate for these aneurysms is unknown, it is "relatively high" and most lesions should be treated operatively with aneurysmectomy and formal arterial reconstruction, the preferred modality over ligation.

Celiac artery aneurysms are associated with rupture rates of 13% and associated mortality rates of 50%. Approximately half will be associated with concomitant aortic or visceral aneurysm. Aneurysmectomy and arterial reconstruction with saphenous vein is proposed for treatment. Gastric and gastroepiploic artery aneurysms are described as mainly "acquired," either as a result of medial degeneration or a consequence of peri-arterial inflammation, with secondary atherosclerosis common. These aneurysms often present ruptured (90% of cases), without antecedent symptoms. Rupture results in GI bleeding (70%) > intraperitoneal hemorrhage (30%). Treatment with ligation is recommended or extragastric lesions, while intramural aneurysms are best excised with the involved portion of the stomach (partial gastrectomy). Pancreaticoduodenal, pancreatic, and gastroduodenal artery aneurysms are commonly cited to result from periarterial inflammation, typically as a consequence of pancreatitis with vascular necrosis or erosion by adjacent pseudocysts. These aneurysms commonly are associated with epigastric pain and rupture is common (up to 75%), especially in cases of inflammation with rupture-associated mortality rates that approach 50%. The authors propose a role for transcatheter embolization to control acute bleeding, with a high complication rate, and acknowledge the difficulties of simple ligation secondary to anatomic challenges.

Conclusions Splanchnic artery aneurysms are unusual but important vascular lesions. Each splanchnic aneurysm has a unique natural history for which treatment must be individualized.

Study Limitations Clinical review (narrative); without methodology to support systematic review or meta-analysis.

Relevant Studies Because of the increased use of sophisticated forms of intra-abdominal imaging, including magnetic resonance imaging and angiography (MRI, MRA) and computerized tomographic scans and angiography (CT, CTA), occult visceral artery aneurysms are being diagnosed with increased frequency and at smaller sizes.[1] Improvements in endovascular therapies have also allowed an enhanced ability for treatment of these often anatomically complex lesions with a large variety of individualized and precise catheter-based therapies. The natural history of splanchnic aneurysms and their potential for rupture is poorly defined due to their overall low frequency, and while larger institutional case series have been reported, they may be biased toward a representation of unusual presentations and successful outcomes. Regardless, it is clear even from case reports and institutional series that a significant proportion of visceral artery aneurysms present with rupture supporting a careful approach toward their diagnosis and management.

A recent systematic review and meta-analysis of the management of visceral artery aneurysms included 80 observational studies that were mostly noncomparative, encompassing 2,845 aneurysms, of which 775 were splenic, 359 were hepatic, 226 were pancreaticoduodenal and gastroduodenal, 95 were superior mesenteric, 87 were celiac, 15 were jejunal, ileal, or colic, and 9 gastric or gastroepiploic.[2] This review cites importantly the natural history of slow growth, with a tendency toward nonrupture when small.[3] It also considers the role for endovascular techniques (i.e., embolization, coiling, and covered stents), which have been widely adapted to treat splanchnic artery aneurysm because of the minimally invasive nature, anticipated shorter recovery time, and generally lower risk of morbidity and death. Across all aneurysms, differences in mortality between open and endovascular approaches were not statistically significant. The endovascular approach was used more often and associated with shorter hospital stay and lower rates of cardiovascular complications but higher rates of re-intervention. Postembolization syndrome rates ranged from 9% (renal) to 38% (splenic) and coil migration ranged from 8% (splenic) to 29% (renal). Access site complications were low (<5%).

The Society for Vascular Surgery proposed Clinical Practice Guidelines on the management of visceral artery aneurysm in 2020.[1] This document summarizes that, because of their potential for rupture, most visceral artery pseudoaneurysms, mycotic aneurysms, and many larger and asymptomatic true aneurysms warrant intervention. Treatment can generally be accomplished by either open surgical or endovascular approaches, with the goal of preventing aneurysm expansion and potential rupture by exclusion from the arterial circulation while maintaining necessary distal or collateral bed perfusion. In areas of the visceral circulation with an abundance of collateral flow, for example in the splenic artery, proximal and distal ligation of the aneurysm segment is a viable surgical option. This can also be accomplished with endovascular isolation of the aneurysmal segment, either by placement of a stent graft or by coil embolization of the proximal and distal arterial segment. The preferred treatment for each patient and aneurysm must be individualized to account for vascular anatomy and comorbidities.

Study Impact This historic review nicely emphasizes the unique etiology and end-stage natural history of splanchnic artery aneurysms, with an emphasis on early and open surgical treatment to obviate high rupture-related mortality.

REFERENCES

1. Chaer RA, Abularrage CJ, Coleman DM, Eslami MH, Kashyap VS, Rockman C, and Murad H. The society for vascular surgery clinical practice guidelines on the management of visceral aneurysms. *J Vasc Surg*. 2020;pii:S0741-5214(20)30156–7. doi: 10.1016/j.jvs.2020.01.039.
2. Barrionuevo P, Malas MB, Nejim B et al. A systematic review and meta-analysis of the management of visceral artery aneurysms. *J Vasc Surg*. 2019;70(5):1694–9.
3. Abbas MA, Stone WM, Fowl RJ et al. Splenic artery aneurysms: Two decades experience at Mayo clinic. *Ann Vasc Surg*. 2002;16(4):442–9.

CHAPTER 33

Popliteal Artery Aneurysms: A 25-Year Surgical Experience

Shortell CK, DeWeese JA, Ouriel K, Green RM. J Vasc Surg. 1991;14(6):771–9

ABSTRACT

Operative repair was undertaken for 51 popliteal aneurysms in 39 patients between 1958 and 1990. Operation was performed on an emergency basis in 19 extremities with limb-threatening ischemia and as an elective procedure in 32 extremities. Cumulative limb salvage (94%) rates and patency rates (67%) became significantly different at 6 years ($p < 0.05$). Graft patency was affected by clinical presentation and runoff. After 1 year, cumulative patency for extremities with limb-threatening ischemia was significantly lower than for those having an elective operation (69% vs. 100%, $p < 0.05$). Runoff did not influence graft patency until 3 years, at which time cumulative patency was better in extremities with good runoff than in extremities with poor runoff (89% vs. 30%, $p < 0.05$). Limb salvage was affected only by presentation. All limb loss (three patients) occurred within the first month in extremities with graft occlusion after operation for limb-threatening ischemia. Runoff did not influence patency rates for extremities with limb-threatening ischemia, since no difference was observed in runoff between the two groups. We conclude that elective repair is indicated in all patients with popliteal aneurysms. It is associated with little risk to the patient, and prevents the need for operation in the setting of limb-threatening ischemia with its poorer overall results and definite incidence of amputation.

AUTHOR COMMENTARY BY E. HOPE WEISSLER AND CYNTHIA K. SHORTELL

Research Question/Objective What factors affect operative results following popliteal artery aneurysm repair?

Study Design Retrospective review.

Sample Size 39 patients, 51 aneurysms.

Follow-Up 10 years for overall patency and salvage analyses.

Inclusion/Exclusion Criteria Excluded patients presenting with irreversible ischemia requiring amputation.

Intervention or Treatment Received

Operative repair: 32 short-segment distal superficial femoral artery to popliteal artery bypasses, 10 standard femoropopliteal bypasses, and nine femorotibial bypasses. Forty-nine were done with saphenous vein, two with prosthetic conduit.

Results

Morbidity and mortality: 30-day mortality was 6%, 30-day patency was 94%, 30-day amputation was 6%. Eleven additional patients died over the course of follow-up due to unrelated causes.

Patency versus salvage: 94% patency and limb-salvage rates at both 1- and 6-month follow-up (all three early graft failures led to limb loss). Patency declined to 67% at 6 years but limb salvage remained unchanged at 94%. From 3 years up to 10 years, patency was significantly better in patients with good runoff (two or more vessel run-off versus one or none), but there was no difference up until 3 years.

Elective procedure versus limb-threatening ischemia: All three patients with limb loss presented initially with limb-threatening ischemia. No elective patients required amputation. Limb salvage was therefore 84% in the ischemic presentation population and 100% in the elective population.

Postoperative aneurysmal enlargement: Four patients developed massive enlargement of the excluded popliteal aneurysm at least 5 years after operation. All patients had saccular aneurysms, were symptomatic, and underwent resection of the enlarged arterial segments. No feeding collaterals could be found during any of the operations, but one was encased in a venous network and densely adherent to the popliteal vein.

Study Limitations This study was retrospective and aneurysm size was not able to be included as a covariate because angiographic data was lacking in 20 of 51 extremities. It was not entirely clear if and when patients were lost to follow-up or censored due to death.

Relevant Studies

1. *Gifford, 1953*: 100 popliteal aneurysms with a 26% complication rate among asymptomatic patients and 20% amputation rate overall.
2. *Reilly, 1983*: 244 popliteal aneurysms with a 2.8% complication rate among asymptomatic patients, 16.2% complication rate among chronically symptomatic patients, and 29.3% complication rate among acutely symptomatic patients.
3. *Whitehouse, 1983*: Nine amputations among patients who presented with thrombosed aneurysms versus no amputations among asymptomatic patients. 18% limb loss rate among 32 aneurysms treated nonsurgically.

4. *Anton, 1986*: 10-year limb-salvage rates of 93% among 55 asymptomatic patients and 79% among 68 patients who presented with complications of aneurysms.
5. *Greenberg, 1998*: Presented the results of catheter-directed lysis in five patients with acutely thrombosed popliteal aneurysms and absent infrapopliteal runoff followed by surgical bypass. There were no amputations, though two patients' bypasses thrombosed (one thrombosed twice), and two patients suffered residual neurologic deficits.
6. *Huang, 2014*: Compared results of 42 endovascular repairs (10 emergent) and 107 open repairs (14 emergent), demonstrating equivalent 30-day outcomes between the two modalities stratified by urgency. There was a trend toward decreased freedom from major adverse events among elective endovascular repairs, decreased primary patency rates for emergent endovascular repairs, and increased re-interventions for elective endovascular repairs.

Study Impact Discussion of which popliteal arterial aneurysms to repair and which to watch did not begin with this paper, but this paper did alter the landscape of the debate due to its finding that elective repair of popliteal aneurysms was associated with no amputation or mortality. Worse limb-related outcomes were seen among patients presenting with ischemic symptoms. This was in contrast to prior reports of significant complications following operative repair among asymptomatic patients and suggested that observation of asymptomatic popliteal aneurysms carried a higher risk of limb loss than did operative repair.[1,2,4,7] Management of asymptomatic popliteal aneurysms therefore shifted toward intervention. Indeed, multiple groups have subsequently confirmed that patients presenting with symptomatic aneurysms do significantly worse than asymptomatic patients following repair.[8–10]

Finally, the change in approach to repairing asymptomatic popliteal aneurysms catalyzed by our paper appears to have carried over to the use of endovascular modalities, which have been adopted for use in this area as well.

Over the last 20 years, discussion has focused not on *whether* asymptomatic aneurysms should be repaired, but on whether there are any asymptomatic aneurysms that *don't* need to be fixed. What our paper suggested, and what the lack of consensus regarding observation of aneurysms shows, is that the natural history of popliteal aneurysmal disease is not predictable enough to design a reliable surveillance regimen for. In this way, management of popliteal aneurysms is similar to other disease processes (such as shaggy aorta or arterial thoracic outlet) in which the risks of observation include atheroembolic events, rather than disease processes in which the major event of concern is rupture (such as aortic aneurysms) or stepwise progression of disease (such as peripheral arterial disease).

In our paper, size was not assessed as a covariate, largely because changing diagnostic techniques over the study period did not provide comparable size measurements. As cross-sectional CT or MR angiography has become more ubiquitous, interest has grown in using size as an indication of which asymptomatic aneurysms can safely be observed. Most studies (including our paper) use 2 centimeters as a cutoff for intervention of asymptomatic aneurysms, but this remains controversial given mixed reports about the likelihood of aneurysm thrombosis and thromboembolic events in smaller aneurysms.[9,11] Presence of mural thrombus has also been proposed as an indication for intervention on asymptomatic aneurysms.

The growing popularity and availability of two techniques have in recent years exerted increasing influence on the risk benefit analysis surrounding repair of asymptomatic popliteal aneurysms. Endovascular options allowing popliteal aneurysm repair with less physiologic stress have continued the shift toward intervention.[12–16] In addition, more sophisticated endovascular clot removal strategies have allowed some patients presenting with acute limb ischemia to be emergently managed with delayed elective definitive repairs. This strategy has been reported to result in limb-related outcomes similar to patients who did not present with acute limb ischemia,[16,17] potentially mitigating the risks of observation of asymptomatic aneurysms.

As with many other areas of modern surgical practice, increased complexity and sophistication of available data has led not to more detailed and reliable treatment algorithms, but instead to a renewed focus on individual patients' treatment goals, overall health status, anatomy, and tolerance for risk. Since the publication of our paper in 1991, when recommendations were usually strictly adhered to regardless of individual patient factors, we have gradually changed our approach to the selection of patients for whom elective repair, be it open or endovascular, is offered. It is therefore our practice when considering treatment of asymptomatic popliteal aneurysms to consider not just the size and presence of mural thrombus but also the patient's age, activity level, and operative risk. Factors such as comorbidities, BMI, venous conduit, runoff, evidence of prior embolic events from the aneurysm, and patient preference all play an important role in the decision.

REFERENCES

1. Gifford RW JR, Hines EA, and Janes JM. An analysis and follow-up study of one hundred popliteal aneurysms. *Surgery*. 1953;33:284–93.
2. Reilly MK, Abbott WM, and Darling RC. Aggressive surgical management of popliteal aneurysms. *Am J Surg*. 1983;145:498–502.
3. Whitehouse WM JR, Wakefield TW et al. Limb-threatening potential of arteriosclerotic popliteal artery aneurysms. *Surgery*. 1983;93:694–9.
4. Anton GE, Hertzer NR, Beven EG et al. Surgical management of popliteal aneurysms: Trends in presentation, treatment, and results from 1952–1984. *J Vasc Surg*. 1986;3:125–34.
5. Greenberg R, Wellander E, Nyman U et al. Aggressive treatment of acute limb ischemia due to thrombosed popliteal aneurysms. *Eur J Rad*. 1998;28:211–8.
6. Huang Y, Gloviczki P, Oderich GS et al. Outcomes of endovascular and contemporary open surgical repairs of popliteal artery aneurysm. *J Vasc Surg*. 2014;50:631–8.
7. Lowell RC, Gloviczki P, Hallett JW et al. Popliteal artery aneurysms: The risk of nonoperative management. *Ann Vasc Surg*. 1994;8:14–23.

8. Mahmood A, Salaman R, Sintler M et al. Surgery of popliteal artery aneurysms: A 12-year experience. *J Vasc Surg*. 2003;37:586–93.
9. Dawson I, Sie R, van Baalen JM et al. Asymptomatic popliteal aneurysm: Elective operation versus conservative follow-up. *Br J Surg*. 1994;81:1504–7.
10. Pulli R, Dorigo W, Troisi N et al. Surgical management of popliteal artery aneurysms: Which factors affect outcomes? *J Vasc Surg*. 2006;43:481–7.
11. Ascher E, Markevich N, Schutzer RW et al. Small popliteal artery aneurysms: Are they clinically significant? *J Vasc Surg*. 2003;37:755–60.
12. Marin ML, Veith FJ, Panetta TF et al. Transfemoral endoluminal stented graft repair of a popliteal artery aneurysm. *J Vasc Surg*. 1994;19:754–7.
13. Idelchik GM, Dougherty KG, Hernandez E et al. Endovascular exclusion of popliteal artery aneurysms with stent-grafts: A prospective single-center experience. *J Endovasc Ther*. 2009;16:215–23.
14. Rajasinghe HA, Tzilinis A, Keller T et al. Endovascular exclusion of popliteal artery aneurysms with expanded polytetrafluorethylene stent-grafts: Early results. *Vasc Endovasc Surg*. 2007;40:460–6.
15. Golchehr B, Zeebregts CJ, Reijnen MMPJ et al. Long-term outcome of endovascular popliteal artery aneurysm repair. *J Vasc Surg*. 2018;67:1797–804.
16. Tielliu IFJ, Verhoeven ELG, Zeebregts CJ et al. Endovascular treatment of popliteal artery aneurysms: Results of a prospective cohort study. *J Vasc Surg*. 2005;41:561–7.
17. Carpenter JP, Barker CF, Robert B et al. Popliteal artery aneurysms: Current management and outcome. *J Vasc Surg*. 1994;19:65–73.

Chapter 34

A Prospective Double-Blind Randomized Controlled Trial of Radiofrequency versus Laser Treatment of the Great Saphenous Vein in Patients with Varicose Veins

Nordon IM, Hinchliffe RJ, Brar R, Moxey P, Black SA, Thompson MM, Loftus IM. Ann Surg. 2011 Dec;254(6):876–81

ABSTRACT

Background Endovenous ablation of varicose veins using radiofrequency ablation (RFA) and endovenous laser therapy (EVLT) has reported advantages over traditional open surgical treatment. There is little evidence comparing the efficacy and patient-reported outcomes between the two endovenous solutions. This study compares the RFA and EVLT strategies in a prospective double-blind clinical trial.

Methods Consecutive patients with primary unilateral great saphenous vein (GSV) reflux undergoing endovenous treatment were randomized to RFA (VNUS ClosureFAST) or EVLT (810-nm diode laser). The primary outcome measure was GSV occlusion at 3 months after treatment. Secondary outcome measures were occlusion at 7 days, postoperative pain, analgesic requirement, and bruising, assessed at day 7 after surgery. Quality of life (QoL) was assessed preoperatively and 3 months after surgery using the Aberdeen Varicose Vein Questionnaire (AVVQ) and EQ-5D.

Results A total of 159 patients were randomized to RFA (79 patients) or EVLT (80 patients). Groups were well matched for demographics, disease extent, severity, and preoperative QoL. Duplex scanning confirmed 100% vein occlusion at 1 week in both groups. At 3 months, occlusion was 97% for RFA and 96% for EVLT; P = 0.67. Median (interquartile range) percentage above-knee bruise area was greater after EVLT 3.85% (6.1) than after RFA 0.6% (2); P = 0.0001. Postoperative pain assessed at each of the first 7 postoperative days was less after RFA (P = 0.001). Changes in the AVVQ (P = 0.12) and EQ-5D (P = 0.66) at 3 months were similar in both groups.

Conclusions RFA and EVLT offer comparable venous occlusion rates at 3 months after treatment of primary GSV varices; with neither modality proving superior. RFA is associated with less periprocedural pain, analgesic requirement, and bruising.

AUTHOR COMMENTARY BY THAKSHYANEE BHUVANAKRISHNA AND IAN NORDON

Research Question/Objective The objective of this study was to compare radiofrequency ablation (RFA) and endovenous laser therapy (EVLT) of the great saphenous vein (GSV) in patients with varicose veins.

Study Design Prospective double-blind randomized controlled trial.

Sample Size 159 patients.

Follow-Up 3 months.

Inclusion Criteria Age (18–80 yrs), primary varicose veins, GSV territory, symptomatic varicose veins [>CEAP 2].

Exclusion Criteria Pregnancy, age <18 or >80 yrs, excessive tortuosity of GSV—not amenable to endovenous treatment, recurrent varicose veins, recent deep vein thrombosis/pulmonary embolus, anticoagulant medication, intolerant of nonsteroidal anti-inflammatory drugs, small saphenous vein reflux, deep venous incompetence.

Intervention Received All patients received a general anesthetic (GA), and standardized perioperative analgesia and anesthetic agents were administered after a protocol specific to the study. No thromboprophylaxis or antibiotics were used.

The GSV was cannulated percutaneously at the level of the knee using a Seldinger technique and duplex ultrasound guidance. Standard tumescent anesthesia was used. In both groups, phlebectomy hooks were used for simultaneous avulsion of infragenicular varicosities that had been marked before surgery.

Endovenous laser therapy was performed using a Vari-Lase Bright tip laser fiber (Vascular Solutions Inc. USA). The fiber was withdrawn continuously at 2 mm/sec (12 W power) with a target 80 J/cm energy utilization. For those undergoing radiofrequency ablation, VNUS ClosureFAST catheters (Medtronic, USA) were used for segmental RFA. Double treatment of the most proximal segment was performed. External compression of the treated segment was applied with target power less than 20 W at 120°C.

Results 465 patients referred with varicose veins to our vascular surgery service were screened, 159 were randomized, 87 to EVLT and 79 to RFA treatment strategies. There was no crossover of patients between the treatment arms after randomization or before treatment and patients were well matched. The GSV diameter, CEAP grade, and QOL scores were similar between groups. Median length of vein treated, procedural time, volume of tumescence, and number of avulsions were all well matched. All patients underwent phlebectomies.

The primary outcome measured was GSV occlusion at 3 months assessed by an independent vascular scientist blinded to the treatment modality. At 1 week after surgery, 100% (n = 154) of cases demonstrated GSV occlusion at the treated segment on duplex scanning. At 3 months, five of 138 treated veins were patent—three of 68 EVLT treated veins were patent (96% success), and two of 70 RFA treated veins were patent (97% success); there was no statistical significance between groups (P = 0.67).

Secondary outcome measures included pain assessed using a visual analog score, analgesia consumption, bruising volume measured using digital analysis software, complications, return to work, and quality of life. Postoperative pain was considerably less after RFA. Median pain scores for EVLT versus RFA at day 1, day 3, and day 7 were 28 versus 9.5 (P = 0.001), 23.5 versus 6 (P = 0.001), and 13.5 versus 0 (P = 0.001), respectively.

EVLT led to a greater area of leg bruising than RFA; median area 3.85% (range, 0%–27.4%) versus 0.6% (range, 0%–11.5%); (P = 0.0001) at 1 week after surgery.

Complications were rare in both groups. The incidence of burns, paresthesia, and thrombophlebitis was 2% for each independent complication in the entire cohort. No patients sustained a deep vein thrombosis or pulmonary embolus.

The median (range) time of return to work was 7 days (1–60) in the EVLT group, compared to 9 days (0–28) after RFA, which was not statistically significant (P = 0.76).

Groups were well matched for preoperative QOL measured by both AVVQ score and EQ-5D. There was no difference in improvement in QOL as measured by either tool at 3-months postsurgery.

Study Limitations The primary limitation of this study was the number of patients lost to follow-up. However, this was expected, accounting for the primary endpoint being chosen as 3 months. The pre-study power calculation took this number into account and an appropriate number of patients attended. 87% of patients randomized were available for a duplex scan at 3-month follow-up. This rate of lost-to-follow-up appears standard for this genre of trial; another recent varicose vein trial lost 12% of patients at 6 weeks. Younger patients are less likely to attend follow-up unless they have experienced adverse outcomes or require further treatments.

Second, this study utilized a general anesthetic protocol to ensure standardization of the perioperative patient experience and allow for phlebectomies to be performed. This is not current practice as the majority of endovenous cases are now performed in an ambulatory setting under local anesthesia.

Finally, while this study only compares two techniques in practice, it is important to acknowledge that there are other treatment options available, for example, foam sclerotherapy, and mechanochemical endovenous ablation (MOCA) which are well tolerated and allow for complete treatment of varicosities.

This study showed both EVLT and RFA were equally successful with excellent reliable vein occlusion rates; RFA had better outcomes when evaluating perioperative pain and bruising. Nevertheless, both techniques are continually being improved and any advancements that would provide for better patient experience should be compared against these outcomes.

Relevant Studies Since publication, RCTs continue to be delivered exploring the most effective and most cost-efficient methods to treat varicose veins. The CLASS trial confirmed that EVLT was preferred to surgery and foam sclerotherapy for both clinical effectiveness and cost-efficiency.[1] EVLT and RFA continue to be proven to be more clinically effective than the novel MOCA at 1 year,[2] while the clinical benefit of early endovenous ablation of superficial venous reflux, in addition to compression therapy and wound dressings, reduces the time to healing of venous leg ulcers, increases ulcer-free time, and is likely to be cost effective (EVRA RCT).[3]

The evidence from this paper and others published since continues to demonstrate that treatment of varicose veins improves quality of life and is cost effective.

Study Impact At the time of publication of this article, it was the first study in its field to demonstrate clinically important endpoints within a prospective double-blinded RCT independent of industry support or oversight. The key difference between RFA and EVLT is in perioperative bruising and pain. Radiofrequency ablation is associated with significantly less pain and bruising than EVLT when measured 1 week after treatment. This is a relevant endpoint for patients who need to return to work and normal activities quickly.

This study was conceived when endovenous vein treatments were in their infancy. Laser ablation and radiofrequency ablation had their advocates. As is often the situation with evolving technologies, both modalities were heavily promoted by their industry backers.

While both RFA and EVLT offered comparable venous occlusion rates at 3 months after treatment of primary GSV varices, neither modality was superior.

These techniques are now generally available to patients in an office-based practice, under local anesthetic. This has almost completely negated the need for what now seems barbaric open GSV ligation, stripping, and avulsions.

Since its introduction into practice, EVLT has evolved. While initially being pioneered as a technique using the 810 nm laser fiber wavelength in the United States, the current practice utilizes 910 nm laser fiber wavelength, with the aim of advancements being to maximize local damage to the varicose vein while minimizing damage to adjacent tissues. A 1470 nm diode laser may be demonstrating superiority to RFA, yet given the efficacy of both treatments superiority will be difficult to prove.

RFA has had its own advancements since the original catheter was introduced. The technique utilizes bipolar radiofrequency to cause heating of tissue. Over the years, unlike its previous generations, the latest RFA technology avoids overheating resulting in burning of the tissue by reducing the radiofrequency flow when the coating of the electrode gets warm. The VNUS Closure system has been replaced by Venefit™ providing a more precise heating of the 7 cm vein segments while maintaining excellent results.

Overall, current outcomes from endovenous technologies are predictable and reliable. In modern practice with advancements in both EVLT and RFA it is hard to determine superiority. The early trials certainly stimulated industry to develop their product and provide better outcomes and treatment options to our patients.

REFERENCES

1. Brittenden J, Cotton SC, Elders A et al. Clinical effectiveness and cost-effectiveness of foam sclerotherapy, endovenous laser ablation and surgery for varicose veins: results from the Comparison of LAser, Surgery and foam Sclerotherapy (CLASS) randomised controlled trial. *Health Technol Assess*. 2015;19(27):1–342.
2. Vahaaho S, Mahmoud O, Halmesmaki K et al. Randomized clinical trial of mechanochemical and endovenous thermal ablation of great saphenous varicose veins. *Br J Surg*. 2019;106(5):548–54.
3. Gohel MS, Heatley F, Liu X et al. Early versus deferred endovenous ablation of superficial venous reflux in patients with venous ulceration: The EVRA RCT. *Health Technol Assess*. 2019;23(24)1–96.

CHAPTER 35

Contemporary Outcomes after Venography-Guided Treatment of Patients with May-Thurner Syndrome

Rollo JC, Farley SM, Oskowitz AZ, Woo K, DeRubertis BG. J Vasc Surg Venous Lymphat Disord. 2017 Sep;5(5):667–76

ABSTRACT

Objective Patients with May-Thurner syndrome (MTS) present with a spectrum of findings ranging from mild left leg edema to extensive iliofemoral deep venous thrombosis (DVT). Whereas asymptomatic left common iliac vein (LCIV) compression can be seen in a high proportion of normal individuals on axial imaging, the percentage of these persons with symptomatic compression is small, and debate exists about the optimal clinical and diagnostic criteria to treat these lesions in patients with symptomatic venous disease. We evaluated our approach to venography-guided therapy for individuals with symptomatic LCIV compression and report the outcomes.

Methods All patients with suspected May-Thurner compression of the LCIV between 2008 and 2015 were analyzed retrospectively. Patients with chronic iliocaval lesions not associated with compression of the LCIV were excluded from analysis. Criteria for intervention included LCIV compression in the setting of (1) leg edema/venous claudication with associated venographic findings (collateralization, iliac contrast stagnation, and contralateral cross-filling), or (2) left leg deep venous thrombosis. Outcome measures included presenting Clinical, Etiology, Anatomy, Pathophysiology (CEAP) score, postintervention CEAP score, primary patency, and secondary patency. Technical success was defined as successful stent implantation without intra-operative device complications, establishment of in-line central venous flow, and less than 30% residual LCIV stenosis.

Results Of the 63 patients evaluated, 32 (51%) had nonthrombotic MTS and presented with leg edema (100%) or venous claudication (47%). Thirty-one patients (49%) had thrombotic MTS and presented with acute (26%) or chronic (71%) DVT, leg edema (100%), or venous claudication (74%). The mean presenting CEAP score was 3.06 and 3.23 for nonthrombotic and thrombotic MTS, respectively. Forty-four patients (70%) underwent successful intervention with primary stenting (70%) or thrombolysis and stenting (30%); 14 nonthrombotic MTS patients were treated conservatively with compression therapy alone, and five thrombotic MTS patients were treated with lysis or angioplasty alone. Clinical improvement and decrease in CEAP score occurred in 95% and 77% of stented patients compared with 58% and 32% of nonstented patients. Complete symptom resolution was achieved in 48% of patients overall, or 64% of stented patients and only 21% of nonstented patients. Complications included two early re-occlusions. Primary and secondary 2-year patency rates were 93% and 97% (mean follow-up, 20.3 months) for stented patients.

Conclusions Venography-guided treatment of MTS is associated with excellent 1-year patency rates and a significant reduction in symptoms and CEAP score. Treating symptomatic MTS patients on the basis of physiologically relevant venographic findings rather than by intravascular ultrasound imaging alone results in excellent long-term patency and clinical outcomes but may result in undertreatment of some patients who could benefit from stent implantation.

AUTHOR COMMENTARY BY BRIAN DERUBERTIS AND RAMEEN MORIDZADEH

In our seminal publication "Contemporary outcomes after venography-guided treatment of patients with May-Thurner syndrome," we believe we significantly added to the existing literature regarding the diagnosis and management of patients with May-Thurner syndrome (MTS). This syndrome typically presents with either chronic mild to moderate leg swelling or acute deep vein thrombosis (DVT), and while the latter group has already shown a propensity for life-threatening complications and thus requires aggressive treatment with thrombus removal and iliac vein stenting, the non-thrombotic May-Thurner patients may only be mildly symptomatic and often present at a very young age. It is currently unknown whether iliac vein stenting, the results of which are not clear 20–40 years postprocedure, is appropriate for all of these patients, many of whom are below the age of 40 years. Among our aims of this manuscript, therefore, was to describe our algorithm for diagnosis and treatment of patients with thrombotic and nonthrombotic May-Thurner syndrome, determine if we could help identify those nonthrombotic May-Thurner patients that were most likely to benefit from iliac vein stenting, and evaluate the effectiveness of percutaneous intervention for May-Thurner syndrome in a contemporary series of patients.

Our manuscript included a retrospective analysis of a prospectively maintained single-center database of 102 patients with left-sided venous occlusive disease between 2008 and 2015, selecting only patients with compression of the left common iliac vein by the right common iliac artery (n = 70 patients). Excluded were other nonthrombotic iliac vein lesions such as retroperitoneal fibrosis, pelvic tumors, or other compressive syndromes.

Indications for iliac vein stenting required all of the following to be present: failed trial of compression therapy, sufficiently severe symptoms affecting quality of life, and radiographic contrast venography findings that suggested that there was a truly physiologic perturbation in venous flow patterns. These findings included contrast stagnation in the common and external iliac vein on venography, evidence of collateralization to the pelvic, lumbar or other retroperitoneal collateral veins, or cross-filling to the contralateral right iliac venous system through the hypogastric veins. Once these findings were confirmed by venography, patients who had failed conservative therapy were treated with intravascular ultrasound (IVUS)-guided stent implantation, with IVUS used not for determining whether to proceed with stent implantation but instead for proper sizing and placement of stents. Patients with thrombotic MTS and acute DVT underwent thrombolysis prior to iliac vein stenting. Outcomes were assessed clinically with improvement in the CEAP class 1–6 and patency was documented with duplex ultrasound examination.

In this study, 63 patients demonstrated clear MTS and had available follow-up, with 31 presenting with acute DVT, representing the thrombotic MTS group, and 32 presenting with chronic leg swelling without concomitant DVT, representing the nonthrombotic MTS group. The mean age was 46 years, and 76% of patients were female. Forty-six percent of patients in the thrombotic MTS group had a hypercoagulable condition. For nonthrombotic MTS, all patients presented with left leg edema, and venous claudication was present in 47%. In contrast, thrombotic MTS patients presented with sudden onset left leg swelling and were diagnosed with acute DVT or had a prior diagnosis of left leg DVT and presented with postthrombotic syndrome symptoms. The mean CEAP score for the entire series was 3.14.

All patients in the thrombotic MTS group were treated with iliac vein stenting with or without thrombus removal strategies of lysis or pharmacomechanical thrombectomy. In the nonthrombotic group, 18 of the 32 patients were treated with iliac vein stenting and 14 were treated with conservative management (compression therapy, venous-lymphatic massage, life-style modifications). There was a 100% technical success rate for those patients undergoing attempt at iliac venous stenting, and one of the key findings of this study was the difference in clinical improvement between stented versus nonstented patients. Comparing all patients who underwent stenting versus those who did not, stented patients had better clinical outcomes after intervention (95% vs. 58%, respectively; $p < 0.001$), were more likely to have a decrease in CEAP score (77% vs. 32%, respectively; $p < 0.001$), and were more likely to have complete clinical resolution of venous symptoms (64% vs. 21%, respectively; $p < 0.001$). At 24 months, primary and secondary patency rates in the stented patients were 87% and 93%, respectively. Importantly, however, disease progression was rare for patients managed conservatively in the nonstented group and none of these patients developed left iliofemoral DVT during the study period.

While some publications appear to advocate for use of IVUS findings as a major driver of the determinate for stent indication in nonthrombotic patients, the diagnostic and treatment algorithm that evolved at our center over the study period of this paper included reliance on contrast venography findings as the primary determinate to guide intra-procedural decision-making regarding treatment.[1] Intravascular ultrasound was then used to guide the technical aspects of the implantation procedure and aided in both stent sizing as well as placement. This combination of the use of contrast venography and clinical presentation for determining the appropriateness of stent implantation as well as the use of IVUS for guiding technical aspects of the intervention contributes to the significance of this article relative to the existing literature on the treatment of patients with May-Thurner syndrome.

While IVUS is a sensitive measure of iliac vein compression and cross-sectional area assessment, axial imaging in normal individuals has demonstrated some degree of iliac vein compression and narrowing in over 50%.[2] This would suggest IVUS may be an overly sensitive test for the indication of stent implantation, and while stent implantation is generally associated with good outcomes, potential complications can include stent fracture, migration, restenosis, and occlusion. These complications have been shown to be uncommon in the short and intermediate term, but no data exists to describe the likelihood of these complications decades after implantation. This is an important factor in the risk-benefit analysis for these interventions considering the young age of many of these nonthrombotic MTS patients.

In addition to the diagnostic and technical points discussed in this paper, another important distinction between this manuscript and others detailing the treatment of patients with venous lesions was the inclusion of only those patients with documented iliac vein compression syndromes. In reviewing the existing literature on venous stenting, many manuscripts include a heterogenous collection of patients with May-Thurner syndrome, chronic postthrombotic venous occlusive lesions, and malignant obstruction.[3–5] While the treatment of these patients may be similar and involve identical implants, outcomes can vary considerably based on treatment indication, and thus this manuscript excluded many patients treated at our institution for lesions not caused by iliac vein compression syndromes, and these excluded patients were reported on in a subsequent manuscript focused entirely on these postthrombotic lesions.[6]

With respect to findings, this manuscript demonstrates that excellent outcomes are attained with the use of iliac vein stents for the treatment of MTS, thus adding to the growing body of literature demonstrating favorable results with the endovascular management of these patients.[7,8] However, in this manuscript we also examined and reported upon those patients with nonthrombotic treated conservatively, thus providing further insight into the natural history of patients diagnosed with MTS who are not managed with iliac vein stenting. One of the critical findings in this study included the fact that stented patients proved to have better clinical outcomes and reduction in CEAP scores than nonstented patients, perhaps suggesting that a more aggressive approach than we normally employ would be an acceptable (or possibly even more favorable) strategy for these nonthrombotic patients. However, it is important to note that none of the nonthrombotic patients treated conservatively without stenting suffered progression of their venous symptoms or acute DVT during the study period, suggesting the safety of this approach in these patients, and that initial management with conservative measures of compression and patient education does not preclude stenting at a later time.

Limitations included the retrospective nature of the study. In addition, clinical assessment of venous symptom improvement was nonstandardized and did not include quality-of-life measures.

Ultimately, this manuscript serves as a landmark study for the care of patients with thrombotic and nonthrombotic May-Thurner syndrome. The authors emphasize a selective stenting strategy that requires both precise evaluation of clinical presentation and venographic findings for the decision to proceed with stent implantation, which is then carried out with IVUS imaging for technical guidance. This selective strategy may allow for a more thoughtful approach to iliac vein stenting, thus obviating unwarranted iliac stents in some patients while maintaining excellent clinical outcomes.

REFERENCES

1. Montminy ML, Thomasson JD, Tanaka GJ, Lamanilao LM, Crim W, and Raju S. A comparison between intravascular ultrasound and venography in identifying key parameters essential for iliac vein stenting. *J Vasc Surg Venous Lymphat Disord*. 2019 Nov;7(6):801–7.
2. Kibbe MR, Ujiki M, Goodwin AL, Eskandari M, and Matsumura J. Iliac vein compression in an asymptomatic patient population. *J Vasc Surg* 2004;39:937–43.
3. Juhan C, Hartung O, Alimi Y, Barthélemy P, Valerio N, and Portier F. Treatment of nonmalignant obstructive iliocaval lesions by stent placement: Mid-term results. *Ann Vasc Surg*. 2001 Mar;15(2):227–32.
4. Williams ZF, and Dillavou ED. A systematic review of venous stents for iliac and venacaval occlusive disease. *J Vasc Surg Venous Lymphat Disord*. 2020 Jan;8(1):145–53.
5. Devcic Z, Techasith T, Banerjee A, Rosenberg JK, and Sze DY. Technical and anatomic factors influencing the success of inferior vena caval stent placement for malignant obstruction. *J Vasc Interv Radiol*. 2016 Sep;27(9):1350–60.
6. Rollo JC, Farley SM, Jimenez JC, Woo K, Lawrence PF, and DeRubertis BG. Contemporary outcomes of elective iliocaval and infrainguinal venous intervention for post-thrombotic chronic venous occlusive disease. *J Vasc Surg Venous Lymphat Disord*. 2017 Nov;5(6):789–99.
7. Hager ES, Yuo T, Tahara R, Dillavou E, Al-Khoury G, Marone L, Makaroun M, and Chaer RA. Outcomes of endovascular intervention for May-Thurner syndrome. *J Vasc Surg Venous Lymphat Disord*. 2013 Jul;1(3):270–5.
8. Raju S. Long-term outcomes of stent placement for symptomatic nonthrombotic iliac vein compression lesions in chronic venous disease. *J Vasc Interv Radiol*. 2012 Apr;23(4):502–3.

CHAPTER 36

The VANISH-2 Study: A Randomized, Blinded, Multicenter Study to Evaluate the Efficacy and Safety of Polidocanol Endovenous Microfoam 0.5% and 1.0% Compared with Placebo for the Treatment of Saphenofemoral Junction Incompetence

Todd KL 3rd, Wright DI. VANISH-2 Investigator Group. Phlebology. 2014 Oct;29(9):608–18. doi: 10.1177/0268355513497709. Epub 2013 Jul 17

ABSTRACT

Objective To determine efficacy and safety of polidocanol endovenous microfoam in treatment of symptoms and appearance in patients with saphenofemoral junction (SFJ) incompetence due to reflux of the great saphenous vein or major accessory veins.

Method Patients were randomized equally to receive polidocanol endovenous microfoam 0.5%, polidocanol endovenous microfoam 1.0%, or placebo. The primary efficacy endpoint was patient-reported improvement in symptoms, as measured by the change from baseline to week 8 in the 7-day average electronic daily diary VVSymQ™ score. The co-secondary endpoints were the improvement in appearance of visible varicosities from baseline to week 8, as measured by patients and by an independent physician review panel.

Results In 232 treated patients, polidocanol endovenous microfoam 0.5% and polidocanol endovenous microfoam 1.0% were superior to placebo, with a larger improvement in symptoms (VVSymQ [6.01 and −5.06, respectively, versus −2.00; $P < 0.0001$]) and greater improvements in physician and patient assessments of appearance ($P < 0.0001$). These findings were supported by the results of duplex ultrasound and other clinical measures. Of the 230 polidocanol endovenous microfoam-treated patients (including open-label patients), 60% had an adverse event compared with 39% of placebo; 95% were mild or moderate. No pulmonary emboli were detected, and no clinically important neurologic or visual adverse events were reported. The most common adverse events in patients treated with polidocanol endovenous microfoam were retained coagulum, leg pain, and superficial thrombophlebitis; most were related to treatment and resolved without sequelae.

Conclusion Polidocanol endovenous microfoam provided clinically meaningful benefit in treating symptoms and appearance in patients with varicose veins. Polidocanol endovenous microfoam was an effective and comprehensive minimally invasive treatment for patients with a broad spectrum of vein disease (clinical, etiology, anatomy, pathophysiology clinical class C2 to C6) and great saphenous vein diameters ranging from 3.1 to 19.4 mm. Treatment with polidocanol endovenous microfoam was associated with mild or moderate manageable side effects. VVSymQ is an important new, validated instrument for symptom assessment in patients with varicose veins.

EXPERT COMMENTARY BY JUAN CARLOS JIMENEZ

Research Question The question meant to be answered by this study was:

> "Is commercially manufactured polidocanol endovenous microfoam (PEM) sclerosant safe and effective for the treatment of patients with symptomatic, incompetent superficial axial and tributary veins?"

Study Design This was a 5-year, randomized, multicenter, parallel-group study using two different concentrations of PEM (0.5% and 1.0%) compared with placebo. These were administered in blinded fashion. The patients were followed to week 8 for this particular paper and a subsequent publication reported results to 1 year.[1]

Sample Size The study population consisted of patients aged 18–75 years who had SFJ reflux (>0.5 seconds) due to reflux of the great saphenous vein (GSV) or major accessory veins by preoperative duplex ultrasound. The total number of patients randomized was 235 and 230 patients completed week 8 follow-up. CEAP clinical class 2–6 patients were included in the study. CEAP clinical class distribution was 31.9% C2, 40.1% C3, 22.8% C4, and 5.2% C5/C6.

Follow-Up After the initial treatment, patients had a 1-week follow-up visit with duplex ultrasound. Patients without thrombotic postoperative complications were then seen at 4 and 8 weeks post-treatment. If deep venous thrombosis (DVT) was present on the initial 1-week duplex scan (DVT, or common femoral thrombus extension; CFVTE), then patients underwent additional duplex scans 1 and 2 weeks later and then monthly until the thrombi stabilized or resolved. The primary endpoint was patient-reported improvement in symptoms as measured by VVSymQ. The co-secondary endpoints of the study were the improvement in appearance of visible varicose veins from baseline to week 8 as measured by IPR-V^3 and PA-V^3 scores. Clinically meaningful change was evaluated by patients and independent panelists using PGIC and CGIC questionnaires. Tertiary endpoints were response to treatment by duplex ultrasound, improvement in venous clinical severity score (VCSS), and improvements in VEINES-QOL scores.

Exclusion Criteria (1) Patients with DVT or pulmonary embolism, (2) inability to comply with post-treatment compression due to severe peripheral arterial disease or leg obesity, (3) incompetence of the small saphenous vein, deep venous reflux, or reduced mobility, and (4) major surgery, pregnancy, or prolonged hospitalization within 3 months.

Intervention or Treatment Received Patients received a maximum 15 mL of either: (1) PEM 0.5%, (2) PEM 1.0%, (3) PEM 0.125% control, or (4) placebo.

Results There were statistically significant improvements for both the 0.5% and 1.0% treatments groups compared with placebo. Overall, there was a 64% reduction in symptoms in the treatment groups compared with 22% in the placebo group ($p < 0.0001$). Statistically significant improvement in appearance was also noted in the 0.5% and 1.0% treatment groups. Elimination of SFJ reflux and/or complete occlusion of the GSV was achieved in 83% and 86% of patients who received PEM 0.5% and PEM 1.0%, respectively. No cerebrovascular events or anaphylactic shock occurred. Thrombotic adverse events occurred in 10.4% of patients. Thrombus extension into the common femoral vein occurred in nine patients (3.9%). None were occlusive. There were six proximal deep vein thromboses (2.6%), seven distal deep vein thromboses (3%), and two patients had gastrocnemius thrombi. Half of the patients received anticoagulation and the remainder were managed with nonsteroidal anti-inflammatory medications and/or compression and observation. There were no differences in the outcome between patients who were treated or not treated with anticoagulation. All patients were followed until their thrombi resolved or stabilized (median 29 days). No pulmonary emboli were noted.

Relevant Studies Included in reference list.

Study Impact The VANISH-2 trial was a pivotal phase 3 study which helped gain Food and Drug Administration (FDA) approval for Varithena® (Smith and Nephew, Andover, MA, USA). This trial demonstrated an excellent safety profile for this novel, commercially manufactured chemical formulation for polidocanol for treating larger superficial varicose veins. Prior to the availability of Varithena, endovenous liquid sclerosants (i.e., polidocanol, sodium tetradecyl sulfate, etc.) were mixed with room air using the Tessari method.[2] This is commonly referred to as "physician compounded foam" (PCF) and served to treat a larger luminal surface area for varicose veins. FDA-approved usage of polidocanol is limited to spider and reticular veins, thus PCF sclerotherapy of larger varicose veins ($\geq$3 mm) is not a formally approved indication. This method results in sclerosant foam with inconsistent bubble size and high nitrogen content. Transient ischemic symptoms and stroke have been reported following administration of physician compounded foam sclerotherapy likely due to patients with patent foramen ovale.[3] The incidence of patent foramen ovale in the general population has been reported as high as 26%–59%.[4,5] The commercial processing of Varithena results in a 1% polidocanol foam with a 65:35 O_2 to CO_2 ratio with a nitrogen content less than 0.8%. The more rapidly absorbed bubbles in Varithena result in less risk of clinically significant systemic embolization and this was demonstrated by Regan and Gibson in a recent study.[6]

This trial also demonstrated excellent symptom relief and appearance following this nonthermal, nontumescent method for treating patients with incompetent, symptomatic varicose veins. Several instruments for measuring patient satisfaction and symptomatic improvement were utilized and all demonstrated a statistically and clinically significant improvement in patients with chemical ablation compared with placebo. Although already considered a "noninvasive" technique, thermal (radiofrequency and laser) ablation requires injection with a spinal of tumescent solution to the subcutaneous tissue surrounding the GSV. Chemical ablation not only eliminates the risk of thermal spread to the surrounding tissues, it does not require injection of tumescent fluid which may significantly increase the discomfort to patients undergoing radiofrequency or laser ablation.

A disadvantage of chemical (compared with thermal) ablation appears to be the increased technical heterogeneity of the procedures which may be performed. With radiofrequency and laser ablation, the treatment catheter is directed into the primary axial vein and specific areas within the vein are targeted for treatment. Polidocanol endovenous microfoam can be injected into superficial veins both proximal and distal to access sites and refluxed into communicating tributary and perforator veins, theoretically increasing the surface area of the vein lumen coming into direct contact with the sclerosant. Injection of sclerosant foam systemically into the superficial venous system is a less directed technique than thermal ablation, allowing a higher theoretical risk of deep venous thrombosis. A limitation of this study is that it did not report which patients underwent chemical ablation of axial veins alone compared with patients who underwent concomitant treatment of axial and tributary veins.

There was an increased incidence of post-treatment thrombotic events (10.4%) and common femoral vein thrombus extension (3.9%) in the VANISH-2 trial compared with many studies reporting outcomes following thermal ablation (radiofrequency and laser).[7,8] Another randomized trial by Gibson and colleagues demonstrated similar outcomes.[9] Albeit, the post-treatment ultrasound monitoring protocol in the VANISH-2 trial required detailed surveillance and none of the patients experienced any serious adverse events (i.e., pulmonary embolus, stroke) as a result. Whether chemical ablation has a truly higher risk of DVT is a question which can be answered with randomized trials directly comparing thermal and Varithena treatments. At our institution, we have reported excellent results with RFA of both the great and small saphenous veins with a common femoral extension risk of 1.8%.[10,11] Anecdotally, our early clinical experience with Varithena has been excellent although these results have not yet been formally reported. We have added it to our armamentarium of treatment options for these patients.

The VANISH-2 trial was one of the initial, pivotal trials setting the wheels in motion for FDA approval of Varithena. It is likely that investigators in the coming decade will provide additional information regarding newer nonthermal and nontumescent techniques for treating patients with symptomatic varicose veins. It is important for vascular surgeons to be aware of this particular study and determine whether this novel, nonthermal, nontumescent technique is inferior, equivalent, or superior to an already clinically safe and effective treatment: thermal saphenous ablation.

REFERENCES

1. Todd KL 3rd, Wright D, Orfe E. The durability of treatment effect with polidocanol endovenous microfoam on varicose vein symptoms and appearance (VANISH-2). *J Vasc Surg Venous Lymphat Disord*. 2015;3:258–264.
2. Xu J, Wang YF, Chen AW et al. A modified Tessari method for producing more foam. *Springerplus*. 2016;5:129.
3. Forlee MV, Grouden M, Moore DJ et al. Stroke after varicose vein foam injection sclerotherapy. *J Vasc Surg*. 2006;43:162–4.
4. Hagen PT, Scholz DG, Edwards WD. Incidence and size of patent foramen ovale during the first 10 decades of life. *Mayo Clin Proc*. 1984;59(1):17–20.
5. Wright DD, Gibson KD, Barclay J et al. High prevalence of right-to-left shunt in patients with symptomatic great saphenous vein incompetence and varicose veins. *J Vasc Surg*. 2010;51:104–7.
6. Regan JD, Gibson KS, Rush JE et al. Clinical significance of cerebrovascular gas emboli during polidocanol endovenous ultra-low nitrogen microfoam ablation and correlation with magnetic resonance imaging in patients with right-to-left shunt. *J Vasc Surg*. 2011;53:131–7.
7. Nordon IM, Hinchliffe RJ, Brar R et al. A prospective double-blind randomized controlled trial of radiofrequency versus laser treatment of the great saphenous vein in patients with varicose veins. *Ann Surg*. 2011;254:876–71.
8. Healy DA, Kimura S, Power D et al. A systematic review and meta-analysis of thrombotic events following endovenous thermal ablation of the great saphenous vein. *Eur J Vasc Endovasc Surg*. 2018;56:94–100.
9. Gibson K, Kabnick L, Varithena® 013 Investigator group. A multicenter, randomized, placebo-controlled study to evaluate the efficacy and safety of Varithena® (Polidocanol endovenous microfoam 1%) for symptomatic, visible varicose veins with saphenofemoral junction incompetence. *Phlebology*. 2017;32:185–93.
10. Harlander-Locke M, Jimenez JC, Lawrence PF et al. Management of endovenous heat-induced thrombus using a classification system and treatment algorithm following segmental thermal ablation of the small saphenous vein. *J Vasc Surg*. 2013;58:427–31.
11. Harlander-Locke M, Jimenez JC, Lawrence PF et al. Endovenous ablation with concomitant phlebectomy is a safe and effective method of treatment for symptomatic patients with axial reflux and large incompetent tributaries. *J Vasc Surg*. 2013;58:166–72.

CHAPTER 37

Rosuvastatin to Prevent Vascular Events in Men and Women with Elevated C-Reactive Protein

Ridker PM, Danielson E, Fonseca FAH, Genest J, Gotto AM, Kastelein JP et al. *N Engl J Med 2008;359:2195–207*

ABSTRACT

Background Increased levels of the inflammatory biomarker high-sensitivity C-reactive protein predict cardiovascular events. Since statins lower levels of high-sensitivity C-reactive protein as well as cholesterol, we hypothesized that people with elevated high-sensitivity C-reactive protein levels but without hyperlipidemia might benefit from statin treatment.

Methods We randomly assigned 17,802 apparently healthy men and women with low-density lipoprotein (LDL) cholesterol levels of less than 130 mg per deciliter (3.4 mmol per liter) and high-sensitivity C-reactive protein levels of 2.0 mg per liter or higher to rosuvastatin, 20 mg daily, or placebo and followed them for the occurrence of the combined primary endpoint of myocardial infarction, stroke, arterial revascularization, hospitalization for unstable angina, or death from cardiovascular causes.

Results The trial was stopped after a median follow-up of 1.9 years (maximum, 5.0). Rosuvastatin reduced LDL cholesterol levels by 50% and high-sensitivity C-reactive protein levels by 37%. The rates of the primary endpoint were 0.77 and 1.36 per 100 person-years of follow-up in the rosuvastatin and placebo groups, respectively (hazard ratio for rosuvastatin, 0.56; 95% confidence interval [CI], 0.46 to 0.69; $P < 0.00001$), with corresponding rates of 0.17 and 0.37 for myocardial infarction (hazard ratio, 0.46; 95% CI, 0.30 to 0.70; $P = 0.0002$), 0.18 and 0.34 for stroke (hazard ratio, 0.52; 95% CI, 0.34 to 0.79; $P = 0.002$), 0.41 and 0.77 for revascularization or unstable angina (hazard ratio, 0.53; 95% CI, 0.40 to 0.70; $P < 0.00001$), 0.45 and 0.85 for the combined endpoint of myocardial infarction, stroke, or death from cardiovascular causes (hazard ratio, 0.53; 95% CI, 0.40 to 0.69; $P < 0.00001$), and 1.00 and 1.25 for death from any cause (hazard ratio, 0.80; 95% CI, 0.67 to 0.97; $P = 0.02$). Consistent effects were observed in all subgroups evaluated. The rosuvastatin group did not have a significant increase in myopathy or cancer but did have a higher incidence of physician-reported diabetes.

Conclusions In this trial of apparently healthy persons without hyperlipidemia but with elevated high-sensitivity C-reactive protein levels, rosuvastatin significantly reduced the incidence of major cardiovascular events. (ClinicalTrials.gov number, NCT00239681.)

EXPERT COMMENTARY BY JUAN CARLOS JIMENEZ

Research Question Does administration of rosuvastatin 20 mg to patients with low LDL levels and elevated high-sensitivity C-reactive protein (hsCRP) levels decrease the rate of first major cardiovascular events?

Study Design The JUPITER study (Justification for the Use of Statins in Prevention: an Intervention Trial Evaluating Rosuvastatin) was a randomized, double-blind, placebo-controlled trial. It was a multicenter trial conducted at 1,315 sites in 26 countries.

Sample Size The study population consisted of 17,802 participants.

Follow-Up Follow-up visits were scheduled at 13 weeks post-randomization. Then follow-up occurred at 6, 12, 18, 24, 30, 36, 42, 48, 54, and 60 months after randomization.

Inclusion Criteria Men (>50 years) and women (>60 years) were eligible if they had no history of cardiovascular disease, their serum LDL levels were less than 130 mg/dL and their hsCRP level was greater than 2.0 mg/L.

Intervention or Treatment Received Patients were randomized to either a treatment group (rosuvastatin 20 mg daily) or a placebo group.

Results The study was terminated after a median follow-up of 1.9 years. At the 12-month visit, the rosuvastatin group, as compared with the placebo group, had a 50% lower median LDL cholesterol level (mean difference, 47 mg per dL [1.2 mmol per liter]), a 37% lower median hsCRP level, and a 17% lower median triglyceride level ($P < 0.001$ for all three comparisons). There were 142 first major cardiovascular events in the rosuvastatin group compared with 251 in the placebo group. The rates of the primary endpoint were 0.77 and 1.36 per 100 person-years of follow-up in the rosuvastatin and placebo groups, respectively (hazard ratio for rosuvastatin, 0.56; 95% confidence interval [CI], 0.46 to 0.69; $P < 0.00001$). Rosuvastatin was also associated with statistically significant reductions in fatal or nonfatal MI, fatal or nonfatal stroke, arterial revascularization, unstable angina, deep venous thrombosis, pulmonary embolism, and rates of death from any cause. There were no differences reported adverse events in both groups. Physician-reported diabetes was higher in the rosuvastatin group ($p = 0.01$).

Relevant Studies Included in reference list.

Study Impact The JUPITER trial was one of the first to demonstrate the beneficial effects of statins on decreasing first cardiovascular events independent of lipid-lowering effects. The study was stopped early after only 1.9 years by its Independent Data and Safety Monitoring Board due to the significant improved outcomes noted in the rosuvastatin group. Patients in the treatment group demonstrated a relative risk reduction (RRR) for all vascular events of 44%, 48% RRR for stroke, and a 20% RRR for all-cause mortality. Relative risk for myocardial infarction was decreased by 54% and deep venous thrombosis/pulmonary embolism were reduced by 43%. This occurred in patients who all began the study with LDL levels <130 mg/dL. Important to vascular surgeons, rosuvastatin also resulted in a 46% RRR in arterial revascularization procedures in this trial.

The hypothesis that systemic inflammation leads to the development of atherosclerotic plaque had been described prior to the JUPITER trial, however this study cemented its clinical relevance.[1] The researchers demonstrated that elevated hsCRP levels were predictive of vascular events in seemingly "healthy" patients with low LDL levels and no history of prior cardiovascular morbidity. In fact, the greatest absolute risk and the greatest absolute risk reduction for major vascular events were noted among those patients with the highest elevation in hsCRP. In addition, the outcomes in the JUPITER study were the first to demonstrate clear benefits for women and also for black and Hispanic patients.

Critics of the trial argue that the rate of the primary endpoint (a composite five different cardiovascular events) was low in both groups (0.77% per year in the rosuvastatin group and 1.36% in the placebo group).[2] Thus, the absolute risk reduction was only 0.59% per year or 1.2% over the trial's 2-year duration. This outcome is less profound than the 44% relative risk reduction demonstrated, leading to the potential conclusion that the positive effects of statins were overestimated in JUPITER. Additionally, the number of patients needed to be treated (NNT) to prevent one combination of the vascular events represented by the primary endpoint was relatively high at 169 persons for 1 year. These limitations have prompted concerns regarding expanding the clinical indications of statin therapy as recommended by the authors.

Nevertheless, the clinical benefits in JUPITER relate directly to the patient population treated by vascular and endovascular surgeons. A recent meta-analysis suggests that statin therapy reduces abdominal aortic aneurysm progression, rupture, and leads to lower rates of perioperative mortality following elective AAA repair.[3] Statins are also associated with improved outcomes following peripheral endovascular revascularization,[4] infra-inguinal bypass surgery,[5] carotid endarterectomy,[6] carotid stenting,[7] aorto-femoral bypass,[8] coronary artery bypass grafting,[9] and thoracic endovascular aortic repair for aortic dissection.[10] Higher amputation-free survival has also been demonstrated in patients taking statins with critical limb ischemia although improved limb-salvage rates have not been definitively shown.[11] As not only vascular "surgeons" but also comprehensive vascular "specialists," we are responsible for ensuring that our patients are receiving optimal medical therapy for their atherosclerotic risk factors prior to, during, and after intervention. The implications and lessons learned from the JUPITER trial are essential knowledge for the 21st century vascular and endovascular surgeon to ensure the best-practice clinical patient outcomes.

REFERENCES

1. Hansson GK, and Libby P. The immune response in atherosclerosis: A double-edged sword. *Nat Rev Immunology*. 2006;6: 508–19.
2. Vaccarino V, Bremner JD, and Kelley ME. JUPITER: A few words of caution. *Circ Cardiovasc Qual Outcomes*. 2009;2:286–88.
3. Salata K, Syed M, Hussain MA et al. Statins reduce abdominal aortic aneurysm growth, rupture and perioperative mortality: A systematic review and meta-analysis. *J Am Heart Assoc*. 2018;7:e008657
4. De Grijs D, Teixeira P, and Katz S. The association of statin therapy with the primary patency of femoral and popliteal artery stents. *J Vasc Surg*. 2017;67:1472–79.
5. Suckow BD, Kraiss LW, Schanzer A et al. Statin therapy after infrainguinal bypass surgery for critical limb ischemia is associated with improved 5-year survival. *J Vasc Surg*. 2015;61:126–33.
6. Arinze N, Farber A, Sachs T et al. The effect of statin use and intensity on stroke and myocardial infarction after carotid endarterectomy. *J Vasc Surg*. 2018;68:1398–1405.
7. Rizwan M, Faateh M, Dakour-Aridi H et al. Statins reduce mortality and failure to rescue after carotid artery stenting. *J Vasc Surg*. 2018;69:112–19.
8. Abdelkarim AH, Dakour-Aridi H, Gurakar M et al. Association between statin use and perioperative mortality after aortobifemoral bypass in patients with aortoiliac occlusive disease. *J Vasc Surg*. 2019;70:508–515.
9. Liakopoulos OJ, Kuhn EW, Slottosch I et al. Statin therapy in patients undergoing coronary artery bypass grafting for acute coronary syndrome. *Thorac Cardiovasc Surg*. 2018;66:434–441.
10. Rizwan M, Faateh M, Locham S et al. Effects of statin use on endovascular repair of thoracic aortic aneurysm and dissection. *J Vasc Surg*. 2018;67:e111–e112.
11. Stavroulakis K, Borowski M, Torsello G et al. Statin therapy is associated with increased amputation-free survival among patients with critical limb ischemia. *J Vasc Surg*. 2017;65:34S.

CHAPTER 38

Statin Use Improves Limb Salvage after Intervention for Peripheral Arterial Disease

Parmar GM, Novak Z, Spangler E, Patterson M, Passman MA, Beck AW, Pearce BJ. J Vasc Surg. 2019 Aug;70(2):539–46. doi: 10.1016/j.jvs.2018.07.089. Epub 2019 Feb 2

ABSTRACT

Background Statin use is recommended in all patients with peripheral arterial disease (PAD), owing to its morbidity and mortality benefits. However, the effect of statin use on limb salvage in patients with PAD after intervention is unclear. We examined the effect of statin use on limb salvage and survival among patients with PAD undergoing surgical or endovascular intervention.

Methods A total of 488 patients with PAD were identified who underwent surgical ($n = 297$) or endovascular ($n = 191$) intervention between 2009 and 2010. Information was collected from electronic medical records and the Social Security Death Index. Predictors of ongoing statin use were identified first by univariate analysis and then via multivariable logistic regression. Survival and freedom from amputation were identified using Kaplan-Meier plots and adjusted hazard ratios by Cox regression.

Results Of the 488 patients with PAD with intervention, 39% were non-whites, 44% were females, 41% received statins, 56% received antiplatelets, 26% received oral anticoagulants, 9% required a major amputation, and 11% died during follow-up of up to 88 months. Statin users were more often male ($P = 0.03$), white ($P = 0.03$), smokers ($P < 0.01$), and had higher comorbidities such as coronary artery disease ($P < 0.01$), hypertension ($P < 0.01$), and diabetes ($P < 0.01$). Antiplatelet use was not associated with limb salvage ($P = 0.13$), but did improve survival ($P < 0.01$). Dual antiplatelet therapy did not show any benefit over monotherapy for limb salvage ($P = 0.4$) or survival ($P = 0.3$). Statin use was associated with improved survival ($P = 0.04$), and improved limb salvage (hazard ratio, 0.3; 95% confidence interval, 0.1–0.7) after adjusting for severity of disease, traditional risk factors, and concurrent antiplatelet use.

Conclusions Statin use in patients with PAD with interventions was associated with improved limb salvage and survival. Despite existing guidelines, statin therapy was low in our PAD population, and efforts are ongoing to increase their use across the health care system.

AUTHOR COMMENTARY BY GAURAV M. PARMAR AND ADAM W. BECK

Research Question/Objective To examine the effect of statin use on limb salvage and overall survival among patients with PAD undergoing surgical or endovascular intervention.

Study Design Retrospective observational study of a prospectively maintained registry.

Sample Size 488 PAD patients.

Follow-Up Up to 88 months.

Inclusion Criteria PAD patients who underwent index surgical or endovascular intervention between 2009 and 2010 at an academic medical center.

Intervention or Treatment Received Statin therapy.

Results See abstract.

Study Limitations We did not have information regarding the effectiveness of statin therapy in controlling lipid levels. However, recent studies have shown benefits of statin therapy even in patients with normal lipid levels. We also did not have information regarding medication compliance, nor the exact initiation/duration of statin therapy. Although the benefits of statin therapy are greatest in patients who are on a longer duration of treatment, there are also notable advantages in patients recently initiated on statin therapy.

Relevant Studies Not applicable.

Study Impact Our study demonstrates that statin therapy not only improves overall survival as previously described in literature, but it is also independently associated with reduced need of amputation in patients undergoing surgical or endovascular intervention for PAD. There are very few high-quality studies available showing significant improvement in limb-related outcomes from statin therapy. Due to various recent guidelines recommending statin therapy in all patients with PAD for its mortality and cardiovascular benefits (Table 38.1),[1,2] a randomized clinical trial to answer this question is unlikely to be possible.

Vascular surgeons are the primary care takers for patients with PAD. Surgeons performed approximately 51% of the revascularization procedures (surgical or endovascular or hybrid) between 2006 and 2011 in the Medicare beneficiaries above 65 years of age, with the remaining 49% of the revascularization procedures (mostly endovascular) performed by cardiologists, radiologists, and others.[3] The existing literature shows that the

Table 38.1 Summary of 2016 American Heart Association (AHA)/American College of Cardiology Foundation (ACCF) Guideline-Directed Medical Therapy in Patients with Lower Extremity Peripheral Artery Disease

	Asymptomatic PAD	Symptomatic PAD	CLI/CLTI/SLTI
To Reduce Cardiovascular Mortality (Risk Factor Modification)			
Tobacco cessation	Yes (I)	Yes (I)	Yes (I)
Antiplatelet therapy	Reasonable (IIa)	Yes (I)[a]	Yes (I)[a]
Statin therapy	Yes (I)	High intensity if tolerated (I)	High intensity if tolerated (I)
Antihypertensive therapy	Yes (I)	Yes (I)	Yes (I)
ACEI/ARB	ACEI (IIa)	ACEI or ARB (IIa)	ACEI or ARB (IIa)
Glycemic control	Good practice medicine – expert consensus (I)	Good practice medicine – expert consensus (I)	Good practice medicine – expert consensus (I)
Oral anticoagulation	HARM (III)	HARM (III)	HARM (III)
DAPT		Benefits not well established (IIb)	Benefits not well established (IIb)
Vorapaxar		Benefits not well established (IIb)	Benefits not well established (IIb)
Aspirin plus low-dose rivaroxaban		Consider in young patients with polyvascular disease and low bleeding risk[b]	Consider in young patients with polyvascular disease and low bleeding risk[b]
To Improve/Maintain Functional Status (Quality of Life)			
Cilostazol		Yes (I)[c]	Yes (I)[c]
Pentoxifylline		No benefit (III)	No benefit (III)
Chelation therapy		No benefit (III)	No benefit (III)
Supervised exercise therapy		Yes (I)	Yes (I)
Structured community- or home-based exercise program with behavioral change techniques		Can be beneficial (IIa)	Can be beneficial (IIa)
Alternative strategies of exercise therapy, including upper-body ergometry, cycling, and pain-free or low-intensity walking		Can be beneficial (IIa)	Can be beneficial (IIa)
Referral to interdisciplinary foot care team		Can be beneficial (IIa)	Can be beneficial (IIa)
To Prevent/Minimize Tissue Loss (Amputation)			
Referral to interdisciplinary foot care team			Yes (I)
DAPT			Reasonable after revasc (IIb)
Oral anticoagulation			Uncertain benefit after vein/prosthetic bypass (IIb)
Optimum glycemic control			Can be beneficial (IIa)
Pneumatic compression (arterial pump) devices			May be considered (IIb)
Hyperbaric oxygen therapy			Effectiveness unknown (IIb)

Note: Strength (Class) of Recommendation, (I): Benefit $\ggg$ Risk, (IIa): Benefit $\gg$ Risk, (IIb): Benefit $\geq$ Risk, (III): Benefit = Risk, (III)-HARM: Benefit < Risk.

Abbreviation: PAD: Peripheral Artery Disease, CLI: Critical Limb Ischemia, CLTI: Critical Limb-Threatening Ischemia, SLTI: Severe Limb Threatening Ischemia, DAPT: Dual Anti-Platelet Therapy, ACEI: Angiotensin Converting Enzyme Inhibitor, ARB: Angiotensin Receptor Blocker.

[a] 2017 European Society of Cardiology (ESC)/European Society for Vascular Surgery (ESVS) PAD management guidelines prefer clopidogrel to aspirin.

[b] Not incorporated in any guidelines yet.

[c] 2017 ESC/ESVS PAD management guidelines do not recommend cilostazol.

patients with PAD receive suboptimal medical therapy compared to patients with cardiovascular disease (CVD), despite similar mortality risks. Particularly, the utilization of statin therapy in PAD patients is disappointingly low (~40%), and this is even worse when it comes to surgical patients. The REduction of Atherothrombosis for Continued Health (REACH) registry showed that the statin prescription rate was significantly lower among vascular surgeons (33%) compared to cardiologists (79%).[4] This is not surprising because traditionally either primary care physicians or cardiologists have assumed the responsibility of cholesterol management. We hope one of the major impacts of this study is to help bridge this gap for PAD patients treated by vascular surgeons.

What are the reasons for suboptimal medical therapy in PAD patients? The PAD Awareness, Risk, and Treatment: New Resources for Survival (PARTNERS) program revealed poor physician awareness of PAD diagnosis as well as poor awareness of guideline-directed medical therapy in PAD patients.[5] Moreover, the primary focus on limb-related outcomes rather than the cardiovascular outcomes also drives this underutilization.[5] Patients prescribed with antiplatelet therapy are more likely to receive statin therapy in our study. We think that the physician guideline awareness for medical management drives this correlation between statin and antiplatelet use. We hope that our study will be useful in raising awareness by showing that the statin therapy not only improved cardiovascular outcomes in patients with PAD, but also improved limb-related outcomes (tissue loss). This should help mitigate the previously mentioned barriers and help in increasing the use of statin therapy in PAD patients.

Hoeks et al. showed that the PAD patients receiving guideline directed medical therapy (aspirin, statin, and beta-blockers) at the time of their vascular intervention had better survival at 3-year follow up.[6] They also showed that the utilization of these medications was significantly lower at baseline as well as 3 years after their initial intervention.[6] PAD patients requiring surgical or endovascular intervention are also sicker and would receive greater benefit from optimal medical therapy. Therefore, the time of vascular intervention can serve as a great point of contact to ensure that these patients are receiving appropriate medical therapy. We have noticed great improvement in the awareness about guideline-directed medical therapy among vascular surgeons in our division and are seeing increasing awareness among other surgeons in part due to large and targeted readership of the *Journal of Vascular Surgery*, and participation in the Society for Vascular Surgery Vascular Quality Initiative, where proper statin and antiplatelet therapy is a major focus.[7]

REFERENCES

1. Gerhard-Herman MD, Gornik HL, Barrett C et al. 2016 AHA/ACC Guideline on the Management of Patients with Lower Extremity Peripheral Artery Disease: Executive Summary. *Vasc Med (United Kingdom)*. 2017. doi:10.1177/1358863X17701592
2. Aboyans V, Ricco JB, Bartelink MLEL et al. 2017 ESC guidelines on the diagnosis and treatment of peripheral arterial diseases, in collaboration with the European society for vascular surgery (ESVS). *Russ J Cardiol*. 2018. doi:10.15829/1560-4071-2018-8-164-221

3. Jones WS, Mi X, Qualls LG et al. Trends in settings for peripheral vascular intervention and the effect of changes in the outpatient prospective payment system. *J Am Coll Cardiol*. 2015. doi:10.1016/j.jacc.2014.12.048
4. Kumbhani DJ, Steg G, Cannon CP et al. Statin therapy and long-term adverse limb outcomes in patients with peripheral artery disease: Insights from the REACH registry. *Eur Heart J*. 2014. doi:10.1093/eurheartj/ehu080
5. Hirsch AT, Murphy TP, Lovell MB et al. Gaps in public knowledge of peripheral arterial disease: The first national PAD public awareness survey. *Circulation*. 2007. doi:10.1161/CIRCULATIONAHA.107.725101
6. Hoeks SE, Scholte op Reimer WJM, Van Gestel YRBM et al. Medication underuse during long-term follow-up in patients with peripheral arterial disease. *Circ Cardiovasc Qual Outcomes*. 2009. doi:10.1161/CIRCOUTCOMES.109.868505
7. De Martino RR, Hoel AW, Beck AW et al. Participation in the vascular quality initiative is associated with improved perioperative medication use, which is associated with longer patient survival. *J Vasc Surg*. 2015. doi:10.1016/j.jvs.2014.11.073

CHAPTER 39

Major Adverse Limb Events and Mortality in Patients with Peripheral Artery Disease: The COMPASS Trial

Anand SS, Caron F, Eikelboom JW, Bosch J, Dyal L, Aboyans V, Abola MT, Branch KRH, Keltai K, Bhatt DL et al. J Am Coll Cardiol. 2018 May 22;71(20):2306–15

ABSTRACT

Background Patients with lower extremity peripheral artery disease (PAD) are at increased risk of major adverse cardiovascular events (MACE) and major adverse limb events (MALE). There is limited information on the prognosis of patients who experience MALE.

Objectives Among participants with lower extremity PAD, this study investigated: (1) if hospitalizations, MACE, amputations, and deaths are higher after the first episode of MALE compared with patients with PAD who do not experience MALE; and (2) the impact of treatment with low-dose rivaroxaban and aspirin compared with aspirin alone on the incidence of MALE, peripheral vascular interventions, and all peripheral vascular outcomes over a median follow-up of 21 months.

Methods We analyzed outcomes in 6,391 patients with lower extremity PAD who were enrolled in the COMPASS (Cardiovascular Outcomes for People Using Anticoagulation Strategies) trial. COMPASS was a randomized, double-blind placebo-controlled study of low-dose rivaroxaban and aspirin combination or rivaroxaban alone compared with aspirin alone. MALE was defined as severe limb ischemia leading to an intervention or major vascular amputation.

Results A total of 128 patients experienced an incident of MALE. After MALE, the 1-year cumulative risk of a subsequent hospitalization was 61.5%; for vascular amputations, it was 20.5%; for death, it was 8.3%; and for MACE, it was 3.7%. The MALE index event significantly increased the risk of experiencing subsequent hospitalizations (hazard ratio [HR]: 7.21; $p < 0.0001$), subsequent amputations (HR: 197.5; $p < 0.0001$), and death (HR: 3.23; $p < 0.001$). Compared with aspirin alone, the combination of rivaroxaban 2.5 mg twice daily and aspirin lowered the incidence of MALE by 43% ($p = 0.01$), total vascular amputations by 58% ($p = 0.01$), peripheral vascular interventions by 24% ($p = 0.03$), and all peripheral vascular outcomes by 24% ($p = 0.02$).

Conclusions Among individuals with lower extremity PAD, the development of MALE is associated with a poor prognosis, making prevention of this condition of utmost importance. The combination of rivaroxaban 2.5 mg twice daily and aspirin significantly lowered the incidence of MALE and the related complications, and this combination should be considered as an important therapy for patients with PAD. (Cardiovascular Outcomes for People Using Anticoagulation Strategies [COMPASS]; NCT01776424.)

EXPERT COMMENTARY BY JOE PANTOJA AND KAREN WOO

The paper "Major Adverse Limb Events and Mortality in Patients with Peripheral Artery Disease: The COMPASS Trial" by Anand et al. contributes two important findings to the care of patients with peripheral arterial disease (PAD): (1) it provides updated outcomes for patients who experience a major adverse limb event, and (2) it presents strong evidence for an antithrombotic regimen that may reduce complications of PAD.[1] Using a subset of patients enrolled in the Cardiovascular Outcomes for People Using Anticoagulation Strategies (COMPASS) trial, this study leveraged the strength of a randomized controlled trial to examine controversies in management of patients with PAD.[2]

The research objective of this study was two-fold: (1) to determine the outcomes of PAD patients after experiencing a major adverse limb event (MALE), and (2) to determine the impact of rivaroxaban in combination with aspirin on these outcomes. MALE was defined as a major limb amputation secondary to vascular insufficiency, acute limb ischemia requiring vascular interventions, or chronic limb ischemia requiring hospitalization and intervention. To accomplish these goals, a subgroup analysis was conducted for patients with PAD in the COMPASS trial. Briefly, the COMPASS trial was an industry sponsored, double-blinded, international, multicenter, randomized controlled trial that compared three antithrombotic regimens in reducing the risk of major adverse cardiac events in patients with stable coronary artery disease or PAD. The treatment arms were monotherapy aspirin 100 mg daily, monotherapy rivaroxaban 5 mg twice daily, and rivaroxaban 2.5 mg twice daily in combination with aspirin 100 mg daily. The PAD subgroup analysis study included COMPASS trial participants with a history of lower extremity PAD, defined as history of previous aorto-femoral bypass surgery, limb bypass surgery, percutaneous transluminal angioplasty revascularization of the iliac or infra-inguinal arteries, limb or foot amputation for arterial vascular disease, intermittent claudication confirmed by objective measures, and those with coronary artery disease and an ankle-brachial index of <0.9.

The COMPASS trial criteria for participation largely determined the population included in the present study. The COMPASS trial inclusion criteria included patients that were 65 years or older and those younger than 65 with documented atherosclerosis in at least two vascular beds or with at least two risk factors including current smoking, diabetes mellitus, stage 3 chronic kidney disease, heart failure, or a nonischemic stroke older than 1 month. Notable COMPASS trial exclusion criteria included patients who had an elevated bleeding risk including those with a history of stroke within a month, severe heart failure with ejection fraction <30%, stage 5 chronic kidney disease, a need for dual antiplatelet therapy or oral anticoagulant therapy, or liver disease with coagulopathy.[3]

For the subgroup analysis, the PAD patients were divided into two groups: those with MALE and those without. They were followed for 23 months. The two groups were compared to determine predictors of MALE. The cardiovascular outcomes after the development of MALE were also described. Last, the PAD population was divided into groups based on their antithrombotic regimen, and cardiovascular, limb, and death outcomes were compared between them.

Study Results This study included 6,391 patients with PAD of which 128 experienced a MALE. In patients with a previous history of vascular interventions, the incidence of MALE was 3.8% compared to 1.4% in those with claudication or no intervention. After experiencing the first limb event, the risk of hospitalization, amputation, and death increased substantially to 7-fold, 197-fold, and 3-fold, respectively, compared to the patients that did not experience MALE. The combination of rivaroxaban and aspirin reduced the rates of peripheral vascular outcomes including MALE and amputation compared to aspirin alone but increased the likelihood of bleeding. When comparing treatment groups, those receiving aspirin alone were twice as likely to experience MALE (2.5% vs. 1.5%) and vascular amputation (1.2% vs. 0.5%). However, those on combination therapy experienced major bleeding events at a higher rate compared to aspirin alone (3.2% vs. 2.0%). A significant benefit of combination antithrombotic therapy was seen in outcomes after a limb event. After patients experienced an initial MALE, those taking aspirin alone had a six-fold increase risk in death and a 10-fold increase risk in major adverse cardiovascular events or amputation compared to those taking combination therapy.

Study Limitations Although this study included a large number of PAD patients, there were several limitations. This was a subgroup analysis with a limited number of patients who experienced MALE. The original COMPASS study was not powered to answer the research questions posed by this study. It is unclear whether a greater number of patients with MALE would have changed the conclusions of this paper. However, the limitations of the small sample size are evident. For example, in this study's predictive univariate model, known risk factors for the development of MALE including smoking and diabetes were not predictive of MALE. The small sample size may have prevented further stratification of patients limiting the capacity to identify those that benefit from combination therapy while minimizing the risk of harm. Specifically, younger patients may be predisposed to fewer bleeding complications than older patients which may inform the risk-benefit ratio of combination therapy, yet an age analysis was not undertaken. Readers must also keep in mind that the COMPASS study was sponsored by manufacturers of the study drugs and a number of the investigators disclosed financial relationships with those manufacturers.

Study Impact Prior to the COMPASS trial, the data on medical therapy for the prevention of adverse cardiovascular events in PAD patients was ambiguous. Currently, the standard antithrombotic regimen includes antiplatelet therapy typically with a single agent. There have been a variety of trials comparing single and dual antiplatelet therapy with a variety of agents including aspirin, clopidogrel, ticagrelor, and vorapaxar. Results from these trials have shown modest risk reduction with single antiplatelet therapy and no net benefit in reduction of adverse cardiovascular event rate or death with dual antiplatelet therapy in PAD subgroup analysis.[4–7] Combination antiplatelet and anticoagulants have also shown no net benefit in PAD patients. Combination anticoagulant therapy has shown an increase in major bleeding events with a small to no difference in risk reduction.[8,9] However, the COMPASS trial proposed an antithrombotic regimen that combined low-dose anticoagulant (rivaroxaban 2.5 mg twice daily) and antiplatelet (aspirin 100 mg daily) and found such a profound risk reduction benefit that the trial was prematurely concluded. It is the first trial that has shown a substantial net benefit in preventing MALE, adverse cardiac events, and death in PAD patients.

The COMPASS trial findings are being recognized as practice changing advancements in the treatment of PAD patients but continue to have clinical applicability concerns. The COMPASS trial group has advocated for clinical implementation of their findings for patients meeting inclusion criteria, namely patients who have a high risk of developing an adverse cardiovascular event with symptomatic PAD or coronary arterial disease and asymptomatic PAD.[10] Despite this somewhat narrowed inclusion criteria, the risk of bleeding remains a clinical concern and an important factor when initiating this combination antithrombotic therapy. Given the risk of bleeding and the inclusion of patients with symptomatic and asymptomatic PAD, a stratified analysis of the effect of combined therapy on different subpopulations of patients with PAD would be helpful to determine if the combined therapy results in equally impressive outcomes in symptomatic and asymptomatic patients. However, it is unlikely that this analysis can be meaningfully performed due to the sample size.

The trial implemented restrictive exclusion criteria that are frequently comorbidities in the PAD population including atrial fibrillation. Furthermore, the additional atherosclerotic risk factors required of patients younger than 65 (part of the aforementioned inclusion criteria) may have selected a population that is less likely to have a major bleeding event and more likely to benefit from combination therapy. A recent analysis of the COMPASS trial data that calculated the number needed to treat for benefit (NNT-B) and harm (NNT-H) found that younger patients benefitted more and had a lower risk of harm than older patients (NNT-B: 48 vs. 91, NNT-H: 500 vs. 63, respectively).[11] Although this suggests that younger patients with high cardiovascular risk may be the targeted population, further age-based subgroup analysis is needed to assess the role of age in determining antithrombotic therapy. Last, the application of this regimen in the post-revascularization PAD patient is unknown. This is currently being assessed in the VOYAGER PAD (Vascular Outcomes Study of ASA Along with Rivaroxaban in Endovascular or Surgical Limb Revascularization for Peripheral

Arterial Disease) trial, an international randomized controlled trial that aims to assess the combination antithrombotic regimen in PAD patients after revascularization.[12]

REFERENCES

1. Anand SS, Caron F, Eikelboom JW et al. Major adverse limb events and mortality in patients with peripheral artery disease: The COMPASS trial. *J Am Coll Cardiol.* 2018 22;71(20):2306–15.
2. Eikelboom JW, Connolly SJ, Bosch J et al. Rivaroxaban with or without aspirin in stable cardiovascular disease. *N Engl J Med.* 2017 Oct 5;377(14):1319–30.
3. Bosch J, Eikelboom JW, Connolly SJ et al. Rationale, design and baseline characteristics of participants in the Cardiovascular Outcomes for People Using Anticoagulation Strategies (COMPASS) trial. *Can J Cardiol.* 2017 Aug 1;33(8):1027–35.
4. Cacoub PP, Bhatt DL, Steg PG, Topol EJ, Creager MA, CHARISMA Investigators. Patients with peripheral arterial disease in the CHARISMA trial. *Eur Heart J.* 2009 Jan;30(2):192–201.
5. Patel MR, Becker RC, Wojdyla DM et al. Cardiovascular events in acute coronary syndrome patients with peripheral arterial disease treated with ticagrelor compared with clopidogrel: Data from the PLATO Trial. *Eur J Prev Cardiol.* 2015 Jun;22(6):734–42.
6. Wiviott SD, Braunwald E, McCabe CH et al. Prasugrel versus clopidogrel in patients with acute coronary syndromes. *N Engl J Med.* 2007 Nov 15;357(20):2001–15.
7. Bonaca MP, Bhatt DL, Cohen M et al. Long-term use of ticagrelor in patients with prior myocardial infarction. *N Engl J Med.* 2015 May 7;372(19):1791–800.
8. Warfarin Antiplatelet Vascular Evaluation Trial Investigators, Anand S, Yusuf S, Xie C, et al. Oral anticoagulant and antiplatelet therapy and peripheral arterial disease. *N Engl J Med.* 2007 Jul 19;357(3):217–27.
9. Alexander JH, Lopes RD, James S et al. Apixaban with antiplatelet therapy after acute coronary syndrome. *N Engl J Med.* 2011 Aug 25;365(8):699–708.
10. Hussain MA, Wheatcroft M, Nault P et al. COMPASS for vascular surgeons: Practical considerations. *Curr Opin Cardiol.* 2019;34(2):178–84.
11. Kerkar P, Bose D, Nishandar T et al. A critical analysis of the COMPASS trial with respect to benefit-risk assessment using the numbers needed to treat: Applicability and relevance in Indian patients with stable cardiovascular disease. *Indian Heart J.* 2018 Dec;70(6):911–4.
12. Capell WH, Bonaca MP, Nehler MR et al. Rationale and design for the Vascular Outcomes Study of ASA along with rivaroxaban in endovascular or surgical limb revascularization for peripheral artery disease (VOYAGER PAD). *Am Heart J.* 2018;199:83–91.

CHAPTER 40

A Randomised, Blinded, Trial of Clopidogrel versus Aspirin in Patients at Risk of Ischaemic Events (CAPRIE)

CAPRIE Steering Committee. Lancet. 1996 Nov 16;348(9038):1329–39

EXPERT COMMENTARY BY RHUSHEET PATEL AND JESSICA BETH O'CONNELL

Antiplatelet therapy's role in reducing cardiovascular risk has been long established, first by the Antiplatelet Trialists' Collaboration meta-analysis study in 1994 and expounded upon by the Antithrombotic Trialists' Collaboration group's 2002 systemic review—both showing an approximately 20% odds reduction in vascular events in patients on antiplatelet therapy compared to controls.[1,2] However, prior to clopidogrel, no safe alternative to aspirin had been approved for the prevention of cardiovascular morbidity. Previously, ticlopidine, an alternate thienopyridine derivative to clopidogrel, had shown a significant decrease in the risk of adverse cardiovascular events compared to placebo but with an unfavorable side effect profile.

Published in 1996, the CAPRIE trial sought to assess the potential benefit and safety of clopidogrel compared with aspirin in reducing atherosclerotic risk, eventually leading to FDA approval of clopidogrel for this indication in 1997. Specifically, the CAPRIE trial looked to compare the risk of ischemic stroke, myocardial infarction (MI), and vascular death in patients with vascular disease on aspirin versus clopidogrel. In a multicenter, randomized trial, a total of 19,185 patients across 384 centers and 16 countries were enrolled among three subgroups, recent stroke (6,431 patients), recent MI (6,302), and peripheral arterial disease (PAD) (6,452). Patients were subsequently randomized to a 75 mg dose of clopidogrel or a 325 mg dose of aspirin by center and subgroup. The mean follow-up was 1.63 years for a total of 36,731 patient-years at risk. Patients with any early, permanent discontinuation of study drug for any reason other than the occurrence of an outcome event, approximately 4,059 (21.2%), were censored in analysis.[3]

Among all randomized patients, there was an 8.7% relative risk reduction in favor of clopidogrel over aspirin for the primary endpoint of ischemic stroke, MI, or vascular death. The corresponding on-treatment analysis (while on study drug or within

28 days of early permanent discontinuation) yielded a slightly higher, 9.4% relative risk reduction. Notably for vascular surgeons, intention-to-treat analysis also showed a 7.6% relative risk reduction favoring clopidogrel for the composite endpoint of ischemic stroke, MI, amputation, or vascular death. Although not powered to detect a treatment effect in the entire study cohort, subgroup analysis did reveal a 7.3% relative risk reduction in favor of clopidogrel for the primary endpoint in patients with recent stroke and a 23.8% risk reduction in patients with PAD. There was, however, a 3.7% relative risk *increase* in patients with recent MI. Given this finding, further analysis of all patients with *any* prior history of MI, including those previously categorized into the recent stroke and MI subgroups, showed a 7.4% relative risk reduction in favor of clopidogrel for the composite primary endpoint.

Posthoc analysis of the CAPRIE database by Bhatt et al. revealed that high-risk patients, identified as those with a history of coronary artery bypass grafting (CABG), more than one ischemic event, involvement of multiple vascular beds, diabetes, and those with hypercholesterolemia, all showed an amplified absolute and relative risk reduction of 14.9% with clopidogrel treatment.[4–7] Bhatt further showed a significant reduction in rehospitalizations for ischemic events (unstable angina, transient ischemic attack, and peripheral limb ischemia) or bleeding events in patients treated with clopidogrel over aspirin.[8]

There were no worrying findings of adverse events in either the clopidogrel of aspirin group. The frequency of rash was significantly higher in the clopidogrel group; however, this was reported as severe or requiring discontinuation of drug in only 1.2% of patients. Gastrointestinal hemorrhage and severe upper gastrointestinal discomfort were both more common in the aspirin group. There was no treatment effect upon liver function and no excessive neutropenia in the clopidogrel group, which had been a concern in the use of prior thienopyridine derivatives.

Finding an arguably only modest cardiovascular benefit for clopidogrel versus aspirin, especially in the context of clopidogrel's almost 20-fold higher cost at the time, the CAPRIE trial did not replace aspirin with clopidogrel, but importantly paved the way for a series of clinical trials that established clopidogrel's use alongside aspirin in dual antiplatelet therapy (DAPT). Multiple randomized clinical trials in the early 2000s first established the role of DAPT, with aspirin and clopidogrel, in improving outcomes for symptomatic cardiac patients. The Clopidogrel in Unstable Angina to Prevent Recurrent Events (CURE) trial in 2000 first showed a reduced rate of cardiovascular death/MI/stroke in the DAPT group versus aspirin therapy alone. Secondary outcome analysis also showed a reduced rate of recurrent ischemia in the DAPT group.[9] These results were bolstered further by the COMMIT trial: metoprolol and clopidogrel in patients with acute MI, which concluded that adding clopidogrel to aspirin resulted in a 9% relative risk reduction in the combined risk of death, reinfarction, or stroke after an MI, without increasing the risk of major bleeding.[10] Clopidogrel's role in post-cardiac percutaneous coronary interventions (PCI) patients was also established by the PCI-CURE subset and the early and sustained dual oral antiplatelet therapy following percutaneous coronary intervention (CREDO) trials. Both showed significantly lower rates of cardiovascular death/MI with the use of prolonged, up to 1-year, dual antiplatelet therapy following PCI.[11,12]

The aforementioned conclusions were hypothesized to extended to peripheral interventions and in 2012 the European MIRROR (management of peripheral arterial interventions with mono or dual antiplatelet) trial showed a significant reduction in target lesion revascularization and mortality in patients treated with DAPT for 6 months versus aspirin alone. Notably, at 12 months the reduction in rate of target lesion revascularization became nonsignificant although the mortality benefit of DAPT remained.[13] In 2010, the CASPAR (clopidogrel and acetylsalicylic acid in bypass surgery for peripheral arterial disease randomized) control trial pointed to a possible role of DAPT in reducing major adverse limb events in patients with prosthetic bypass grafts, however, showed no benefit in vein grafts.[14]

While no multi-specialty consensus guidelines for the use of antiplatelet therapy in PAD patients currently exists, the most recent Society for Vascular Surgery (SVS) clinical practice guidelines recommend, cardiac disease notwithstanding, at least single antiplatelet therapy with aspirin or clopidogrel for symptomatic patients; and consideration of DAPT for high-risk patients with acceptable bleeding risk to reduce the risk of cardiovascular events.[15] While no randomized trial data exists, DAPT is also generally recommended for at least 1 month post-infra-inguinal stent intervention in PAD patients.[16] In the case of visceral artery stenting, DAPT with aspirin and clopidogrel is similarly widely used to prevent thrombosis complications, although no level one evidence is currently available.

Since CAPRIE, clopidogrel has similarly found a place in thromboembolic stroke prevention secondary to extracranial carotid disease. The benefit of DAPT over single antiplatelet therapy in asymptomatic patients remains unclear, but multiple randomized trials have shown a benefit of combination of aspirin and clopidogrel in secondary stroke prevention in the months following a cerebrovascular event. The fast assessment of stroke and transient ischemic attack to prevent early recurrence (FASTER) trial was stopped early, but did show a trend toward fewer ischemic events in the DAPT versus aspirin alone group.[17] The clopidogrel in high-risk patients with acute nondisabling cerebrovascular events (CHANCE) trial was a multicenter RCT from China that showed a significant reduction, from 11.7% to 8.2%, in the rate of stroke with DAPT treatment in the first 90 days following an index stroke/TIA. Hemorrhagic complications were similar between both the DAPT and aspirin-alone groups.[18] Based on this data and the previously established role of clopidogrel in safely reducing all cause cardiovascular risk, the current American Heart and American Stroke Association guidelines recommend consideration of clopidogrel monotherapy in place of aspirin for secondary stroke prevention as well as consideration of DAPT in the first month following and ischemic stroke or TIA, but to not continue this therapy long term.[19] Based on two randomized control trials from Italy and the UK, dual antiplatelet therapy with aspirin and clopidogrel during the perioperative period of carotid stenting has also become the standard of care to reduce thromboembolic risk.[20,21] The ideal length of DAPT therapy in these cases remains unknown, however, most agree upon continuing aspirin and clopidogrel for at least 4 weeks postprocedure, as was done in the Carotid Revascularization Endarterectomy versus STenting (CREST) trial protocol.[22]

CAPRIE marked clopidogrel's coronation as a safe and efficacious antiplatelet agent that has since expanded its role in a growing environment of endovascular neurologic, cardiac, visceral, and peripheral interventions. As both an aspirin alternative and part of dual antiplatelet therapy, clopidogrel is already a mainstay of vascular medicine and as essential as surgical intervention. Now, as a recently approved generic, it will continue to be a part of the acute and chronic treatment of almost all vascular patients.

REFERENCES

1. Collins R, Peto R, Baigent C, Sandercock P, Dunbabin D, and Warlow C. Collaborative overview of randomised trials of antiplatelet therapy Prevention of death, myocardial infarction, and stroke by prolonged antiplatelet therapy in various categories of patients. *BMJ.* 1994;308(6921):81–106.
2. Baigent C, Sudlow C, Collins R, and Peto R. Collaborative meta-analysis of randomised trials of antiplatelet therapy for prevention of death, myocardial infarction, and stroke in high risk patients. *BMJ.* 2002;324(7329):71–86.
3. Gent M, Beaumont D, Blanchard J et al. A randomised, blinded, trial of clopidogrel versus aspirin in patients at risk of ischaemic events (CAPRIE). CAPRIE Steering Committee. *Lancet.* 1996;348(9038):1329–39.
4. Ringleb PA, Bhatt DL, Hirsch AT, Topol EJ, and Hacke W. Benefit of clopidogrel over aspirin is amplified in patients with a history of ischemic events. *Stroke.* 2004;35(2):528–32.
5. Bhatt DL, Chew DP, Hirsch AT, Ringleb PA, Hacke W, and Topol EJ. Superiority of clopidogrel versus aspirin in patients with prior cardiac surgery. *Circulation.* 2001;103(3):363–8.
6. Bhatt DL, Foody J, Hirsch AT, Ringleb P, Hacke W, Topol EJ. Complementary, additive benefit of clopidogrel and lipid-lowering therapy in patients with atherosclerosis. *J Am Coll Cardiol* 2000;35(suppl A):326.
7. Bhatt DL, Marso SP, Hirsch AT, Ringleb PA, Hacke W, Topol EJ. Amplified benefit of clopidogrel versus aspirin in patients with diabetes mellitus. *Am J Cardiol.* 2002;90(6):625–628. doi:10.1016/s0002-9149(02)02567-5
8. Bhatt DL, Hirsch AT, Ringleb PA, Hacke W, Topol EJ. Reduction in the need for hospitalization for recurrent ischemic events and bleeding with clopidogrel instead of aspirin. CAPRIE investigators. *Am Heart J.* 2000;140(1):67–73.
9. Yusuf S, Zhao F, Mehta SR, Chrolavicius S, Tognoni G, and Fox KK. Effects of clopidogrel in addition to aspirin in patients with acute coronary syndromes without ST-segment elevation. *N Engl J Med.* 2001;345(7):494–502.
10. Chen ZM, Jiang LX, Chen YP et al. Addition of clopidogrel to aspirin in 45,852 patients with acute myocardial infarction: Randomised placebo-controlled trial. *Lancet.* 2005;366(9497):1607–21.
11. Mehta SR, Yusuf S, Peters RJ et al. Effects of pretreatment with clopidogrel and aspirin followed by long-term therapy in patients undergoing percutaneous coronary intervention: The PCI-CURE study. *Lancet.* 2001;358(9281):527–33.

12. Steinhubl SR, Berger PB, Mann JT, 3rd et al. Early and sustained dual oral antiplatelet therapy following percutaneous coronary intervention: A randomized controlled trial. *JAMA*. 2002;288(19):2411–20.
13. Tepe G, Bantleon R, Brechtel K et al. Management of peripheral arterial interventions with mono or dual antiplatelet therapy--the MIRROR study: A randomised and double-blinded clinical trial. *Eur Radiol*. 2012;22(9):1998–2006.
14. Belch JJ, Dormandy J, Biasi GM et al. Results of the randomized, placebo-controlled clopidogrel and acetylsalicylic acid in bypass surgery for peripheral arterial disease (CASPAR) trial. *J Vasc Surg*. 2010;52(4):825–33, 833.e821–822.
15. Rooke TW, Hirsch AT, Misra S et al. 2011 ACCF/AHA Focused Update of the Guideline for the Management of Patients With Peripheral Artery Disease (updating the 2005 guideline): A report of the American College of Cardiology Foundation/American Heart Association Task Force on Practice Guidelines. *J Am Coll Cardiol*. 2011;58(19):2020–45.
16. Olinic D-M, Tataru DA, Homorodean C, Spinu M, and Olinic M. Antithrombotic treatment in peripheral artery disease. *Vasa*. 2018;47(2):99–108.
17. Kennedy J, Hill MD, Ryckborst KJ, Eliasziw M, Demchuk AM, and Buchan AM. Fast assessment of stroke and transient ischaemic attack to prevent early recurrence (FASTER): A randomised controlled pilot trial. *Lancet Neurol*. 2007;6(11):961–9.
18. Wang Y, Zhao X, Liu L et al. Clopidogrel with aspirin in acute minor stroke or transient ischemic attack. *N Engl J Med*. 2013;369(1):11–9.
19. Kernan WN, Ovbiagele B, Black HR et al. Guidelines for the prevention of stroke in patients with stroke and transient ischemic attack: A guideline for healthcare professionals from the American Heart Association/American Stroke Association. *Stroke*. 2014;45(7):2160–236.
20. McKevitt FM, Randall MS, Cleveland TJ, Gaines PA, Tan KT, and Venables GS. The benefits of combined anti-platelet treatment in carotid artery stenting. *Eur J Vasc Endovasc Surg*. 2005;29(5):522–7.
21. Dalainas I, Nano G, Bianchi P, Stegher S, Malacrida G, and Tealdi DG. Dual antiplatelet regime versus acetyl-acetic acid for carotid artery stenting. *Cardiovasc Intervent Radiol*. 2006;29(4):519–21.
22. Brott TG, Howard G, Roubin GS et al. Long-term results of stenting versus endarterectomy for carotid-artery stenosis. *N Engl J Med*. 2016;374(11):1021–31.

Chapter 41

Multidisciplinary Care Improves Amputation-Free Survival in Patients with Chronic Critical Limb Ischemia[1]

Chung J, Modrall JG, Ahn C, Lavery LA, Valentine RJ. J Vasc Surg. 2015 Jan;61(1):162–9[1]

AUTHOR COMMENTARY BY JAYER CHUNG

Research Question/Objective Compare the effect of multi-disciplinary care team versus standard wound care upon amputation-free survival (AFS) among chronic critical limb ischemia patients.

Study Design Single-center retrospective cohort.

Sample Size 146 patients.

Follow-Up Median 539 (IQR 314, 679) days.

Inclusion/Exclusion Criteria *Inclusion*: Adults ≥18 years of age with chronic critical limb ischemia (CLI) as defined by the following: >2 weeks of ischemic ulceration/gangrene in conjunction with objective evidence of hemodynamic insufficiency. Patients with prior partial foot amputations to the index limb were permitted. *Exclusion*: Patients presenting with nonatherosclerotic disease (Buerger's, history of antecedent acute limb ischemia). Patients with intermittent claudication only and patients with a major amputation to the index limb were also excluded.

Intervention or Treatment Received *Intervention*: Patients were defined as receiving multi-disciplinary care from the time of their initial consultation at the hospital. Multidisciplinary care (MDC) was defined by care that was directed in concert between the vascular surgery, podiatric surgery, and plastic surgery services from their initial presentation to the hospital/clinic. This is in contrast to standard wound care (SWC), where the general surgery service initially provided the directed care. Subsequent care was provided by a non-regimented, heterogeneous combination of general surgeons, wound care nurses, primary care physicians, mid-level providers, patient care providers, and/or the patients themselves.

Results Ischemic tissue loss was present in 85 patients (38 at Rutherford category 5, and 47 at Rutherford category 6). Within this cohort, 51 (60%) had MDC, and 34 (40%) had SWC. Fifty-eight patients (68%) underwent revascularization (open in 17, endovascular in 35, and hybrid in 6), 14 (8%) were managed with primary major amputation, and 13 (15%) declined revascularization. AFS was superior for patients in the MDC arm versus the SWC arm (593.3 ± 53.5 days vs. 281.0 ± 38.2 days; log-rank, P = 0.02). Wound-healing times favored the MDC arm over the SWC arm (444.5 ± 33.2 days vs. 625.2 ± 126.5 days), although this was not statistically significant (log-rank, P = 0.74). Multivariate modeling revealed that independent predictors of major amputation or death, or both, were nonrevascularized patients (hazard ratio [HR], 3.76; 95% confidence interval [CI], 1.78–8.02; P < 0.01), treatment by SWC (HR, 2.664; 95% CI, 1.23–5.77; P = 0.01), and baseline nonambulatory status (HR, 1.89; 95% CI, 1.17–2.85; P < 0.01).

Study Limitations Our cohort remains a relatively small single-center cohort drawn from the inner-city population of Dallas, Texas. This precluded our ability to perform a propensity score analysis. This would have been ideal to mitigate selection bias, which is likely present in our cohort due to the referral tendencies of the physicians seeking limb-salvage expertise. We could not clarify the role of diabetes (insulin-dependent vs. noninsulin dependent) and the role of glycemic control on AFS. Moreover, the study is observational, with no laboratory evaluations, imaging, or procedures performed outside of those deemed necessary by the physicians caring for the patient; hence, data are missing for some of the covariates. Cost analyses were not performed and warrant future study, especially in light of passage of the ACA. We also could not determine the optimal membership required of a multidisciplinary limb-salvage team.

Relevant Studies Prior to this publication, practice patterns had begun to evolve such that several centers were beginning to utilize a multidisciplinary team to care for the diabetic foot. The leaders of the American Podiatric Medical Association (APMA) and the Society for Vascular Surgery (SVS) had released guidelines recommending multidisciplinary care of limb-threatening ischemia.[2] However, there was little data that confirmed that multidisciplinary care truly improved outcomes. Since the publication, the manuscript has been cited 44 times, each ratifying the salubrious effect of multidisciplinary care teams. Most notably, the manuscript was cited in the most recent American Heart Association/American College of Cardiology Guidelines regarding the management of lower extremity peripheral arterial disease.[3]

Study Impact Multidisciplinary care teams had become standard practice for other disease states, such as coronary artery disease, and transcatheter aortic valve replacement, due to robust evidence showing the superiority of multidisciplinary care. The same theoretical benefits exist for the management of CLTI. These include shared decision-making, improved logistical organization and timeliness of care, and improved access to necessary resources, specialized procedures, and research studies. While multidisciplinary care has been popularized for chronic limb-threatening ischemia (CLTI), data supporting this practice had been sparse.[2] This data provided the seminal data that proved the benefit of MDC, which had been, prior to this publication, a theoretical benefit only. Multidisciplinary care halved the major amputation rate compared to the prior standard of care. After publication of the manuscript, multiple other publications have demonstrated similar magnitude salubrious effects of multidisciplinary care for CLTI. Because of the publication of our manuscript and others, multidisciplinary care has become the recommended standard of care for CLTI.[3]

Our data has enabled practicing vascular surgeons to have improved informed discussions regarding expected outcomes with and without a multidisciplinary care team. This data can also be utilized to aid hospital administrators to justify the value of creating a multidisciplinary limb-salvage team. In particular, the paper highlights the durability of amputation-free survival with a multidisciplinary approach. Unfortunately, CLTI patients tend to return with recurrent ischemic ulcerations and vascular insufficiency. This shows that the benefit imparted by multidisciplinary care teams is durable over a 2-year period. Given that there is an approximately 50% mortality of limb-threatening ischemia patients at 5 years, the 2-year outcome data is particularly valuable.

Finally, the authors showed that further marginal improvements in amputation-free survival may be achieved through improved wound care, instead of iterative improvements in revascularization techniques. The data showed that the marginal improvements in limb salvage were not due to improved revascularization specific outcomes, such as patency, the performance of endovascular-first approaches, or the performance of open surgical bypass. Instead, the improved amputation-free survival emanated from improved outcomes after partial foot amputations.

The paper also highlighted several areas of future research. Namely, the optimal complement of specialties remains debated. Some authors argue that a team with a vascular surgeon and a podiatrist are sufficient for a multidisciplinary approach. Certainly, our data endorses the value of this. However, other authors support the concept of more complex multidisciplinary teams, consisting of specialists in revascularization, atherosclerotic risk factor modification, wound care, prostheses and orthotics, diabetes management, infection control, and social work. The marginal benefit of each specialty input remains unknown for every patient with limb-threatening ischemia.

Hence, the costs associated with multidisciplinary care require further investigation. While our population benefited as a whole, not all patients with limb-threatening ischemia experienced the same benefits associated with attempted limb salvage.[4] Optimizing the risk stratification schema may help to identify which patients benefit most from multidisciplinary care and warrant appropriate allocation of these critical, though scarce resources. Similarly, the risk stratification schema will be critical to identifying those patients where multidisciplinary care represents overuse.

Appropriately powered prospective data collection comparing multidisciplinary care with standard care regimens will be required to validate our results externally. This will also aid in the clarification in the role of diabetes management upon outcomes. Future identification of other covariates that improve amputation-free survival will also require larger, likely multicenter cohorts. In spite of its limitations, the paper shows some of the earliest and best evidence to date that multidisciplinary care teams result in durable, superior amputation-free survival relative to the previous standard of sequential referrals to specialists as needed. The improved amputation-free survival was driven by improvements in limb salvage, as the major amputation rate was 50% lower in the multidisciplinary care arm.

REFERENCES

1. Chung J, Modrall JG, Ahn C et al. Multidisciplinary care improves amputation-free survival in patients with chronic critical limb ischemia. *J Vasc Surg*. 2015;61(1):162–9.
2. Sumpio BE, Armstrong DG, DPM, PhD, Lavery LA, DPM, MPH, Andros G. The role of interdisciplinary team approach in the management of the diabetic foot: A Joint statement from the Society for Vascular Surgery and the American Podiatric Medical Association. *J Vasc Surg*. 2010;51:1504–6.
3. Gerhard-Herman MD, Gornik HL, Barrett C et al. 2016 AHA/ACC Guideline on the Management of Patients With Lower Extremity Peripheral Artery Disease: Executive Summary: A Report of the American College of Cardiology/American Heart Association Task Force on Clinical Practice Guidelines. *J Am Coll Cardiol*. 2017;69(11):e71–e126.
4. Mayor J, Chung J, Zhang Q, Montero-Baker M, Schanzer A, Conte MS, Mills JL Sr. Using the Society for Vascular Surgery Wound, Ischemia, and foot Infection classification to identify patients most likely to benefit from revascularization. *J Vasc Surg*. 2019 Sep;70(3):776–85.

Chapter 42

Pediatric Renovascular Hypertension: 132 Primary and 30 Secondary Operations in 97 Children

Stanley JC, Criado E, Upchurch GR, Brophy PD, Cho KJ, Rectenwald JE, Michigan Pediatric Renovascular Group et al. J Vasc Surg. 2006 Dec;44(6):1219–28; discussion 1228–9. Epub 2006 Oct 20

ABSTRACT

Purpose This study was undertaken to characterize the contemporary surgical treatment of pediatric renovascular hypertension.

Methods A retrospective analysis was conducted of the clinical data of 97 consecutive pediatric patients (39 girls, 58 boys), aged from 3 months to 17 years, who underwent operation at the University of Michigan from 1963 to 2006. All but one patient had refractory hypertension not responsive to contemporary medical therapy. Developmental renal artery stenoses accounted for 80% of the renal artery disease, with inflammatory and other ill-defined stenoses encountered less frequently. Splanchnic arterial occlusive lesions affected 24% and abdominal aortic coarctations, 33%.

Results Primary renal artery operations were undertaken 132 times. Procedures included resection beyond the stenosis and implantation into the aorta in 49, renal artery in 7, or superior mesenteric artery in 3; aortorenal and iliorenal bypasses with vein or iliac artery grafts in 40; focal arterioplasty in 10; resection with re-anastomosis in 4; operative dilation in 4; splenorenal bypass in 2; and primary nephrectomy in 13 when arterial reconstructions proved impossible. Bilateral renal operations were done in 34 children, and 17 underwent celiac or superior mesenteric arterial reconstructions, including 15 at the time of the renal operation. Thirty patients underwent abdominal aortic reconstructions with patch aortoplasty (n = 19) or thoracoabdominal bypass (n = 11). Twenty-five of the aortic procedures were performed coincidently with the renal operations. Thirty secondary renal artery procedures were done in 19 patients, including nine nephrectomies. Hypertension was cured in 68 children (70%), improved in 26 (27%), and was unchanged in three (3%). Follow-up averaged 4.2 years. No patients required dialysis, and there were no operative deaths.

Conclusion Contemporary surgical treatment of pediatric renovascular hypertension emphasizes direct aortic implantation of the normal renal artery beyond its stenosis and single-staged concomitant splanchnic and aortic reconstructions when necessary. Benefits accompany carefully executed operative procedures in 97% of these children.

EXPERT COMMENTARY BY DAWN MARIE COLEMAN

Research Question/Objective This study was undertaken to characterize the contemporary surgical treatment of pediatric renovascular hypertension.

Study Design Single institution retrospective study.

Sample Size 97 children.

Follow-Up Follow-up averaged 4.2 years (range 3 months to 42 years).

Inclusion/Exclusion Criteria All consecutively pediatric patients presenting from 1994–2006 with sustained hypertension caused by renal artery occlusive disease treated surgically. Patients age 18 years or older were excluded.

Intervention or Treatment Received Open surgical renal artery revascularization, with or without concurrent aortic and splanchnic operation.

Results Primary renal artery operations were undertaken 132 times. Procedures included resection beyond the stenosis and implantation into the aorta in 49, renal artery in 7, or superior mesenteric artery in 3; aortorenal and iliorenal bypasses with vein or iliac artery grafts in 40; focal arterioplasty in 10; resection with re-anastomosis in 4; operative dilation in 4; splenorenal bypass in 2; and primary nephrectomy in 13 when arterial reconstructions proved impossible. Bilateral renal operations were done in 34 children, and 17 underwent celiac or superior mesenteric arterial reconstructions, including 15 at the time of the renal operation. Thirty patients underwent abdominal aortic reconstructions with patch aortoplasty (n = 19) or thoracoabdominal bypass (n = 11). Twenty-five of the aortic procedures were performed coincidently with the renal operations. Thirty secondary renal artery procedures were done in 19 patients, including nine nephrectomies. Hypertension was cured in 68 children (70%), improved in 26 (27%), and was unchanged in three (3%). Follow-up averaged 4.2 years. No patients required dialysis, and there were no operative deaths.

Conclusions Contemporary surgical treatment of pediatric renovascular hypertension emphasizes direct aortic implantation of the normal renal artery beyond its stenosis and single-staged concomitant splanchnic and aortic reconstructions when necessary. Benefits accompany carefully executed operative procedures in 97% of these children.

Study Limitations Limitations to this single-center retrospective study are intrinsic to the study design. Moreover, while the average length of follow-up was 4.2 years, some children had only short follow-up (i.e., 3 months) introducing the potential for type II error and limited longitudinal follow-up of hypertension and renal function (including hypertension "cure").

Relevant Studies The actual prevalence of clinical hypertension in children and adolescents is approximately 3.5%.[1,2] Renal disease followed by renovascular disease are among the most common secondary causes of hypertension in children, following primary hypertension is the predominant diagnosis.[3] The most recent clinical practice guidelines for screening and management of high blood pressure in children and adolescents from the American Academy of Pediatrics acknowledge no evidence-based criteria for the identification of children and adolescents who may be more likely to have renal artery stenosis, and that some experts perform an evaluation for such in those pediatric patients with stage 2 hypertension, those with significant diastolic dysfunction, those with hypertension and hypokalemia, and those with renal size discrepancy by standard renal ultrasound.[4] Hypertension treatment goals in this population aim to reduce the risk for target organ damage in childhood and reduce the risk for hypertension and related cardiovascular disease into adulthood with a treatment target goal in children to be a reduction in SBP and DBP to the <90th percentile and <130/80 mmHg in adolescents ≥13 years old (*Grade C, moderate recommendation*).[4]

Large surgical experiences with pediatric renovascular hypertension are uncommon. Although outcomes for blood pressure control in this series, of 70% cure and 27% improvement, are in line with important historic series from the Cleveland Clinic (N 56) and a combined experience from Vanderbilt University and the Children's Hospital of Philadelphia (N 50), a more contemporary report of 37 children from Great Ormond Street Hospital for Children in London reported a cure rate of only 46%.[5–7] Moreover, endovascular interventions are increasingly reported as a means of treating pediatric renovascular disease. While technically feasible, the blood pressure benefits appear inferior to open revascularizations with benefit in many series ranging from 54% to 69%.[8–10] Endovascular restenosis has been well described following pediatric renal artery angioplasty, ranging from 7% to 44% interventions, being more frequent following treatment of renal stenoses in children having defined syndromes like NF1. Additionally, the benefits from secondary open operations in these latter children may have limited benefits.[8,10–13]

More recent unpublished data from the same institution report on 169 children, noting hypertension cure rates of 44%, hypertension improvement rates of 46%, and re-intervention rates of 13% during a mean follow-up of 49 months. These authors report age at operation and abdominal aortic coarctation as independent predictors for re-operation, and that the 1/3 of children studied undergoing remedial operations are less likely to be cured of hypertension. They further conclude that established criteria for the diagnosis and management of pediatric RVH must consider specific patient phenotypes to define the most appropriate interventions and identify best practices, especially when balancing the risks of open operative and endovascular interventions.

Study Impact This contemporary report serves as the largest single institution experience with the surgical management of secondary renovascular hypertension in children, encompassing 132 primary operations and 30 secondary operations in nearly 100 pediatric patients. The authors carefully qualify refractory hypertension and identify themes in age- and gender-related disease patterns. Specifically, gender differences were most notable in the 21 boys and 11 girls with coexisting aortic disease. Vascular anatomy is similarly carefully qualified with the authors reporting ostial stenoses affected all 35 patients with concurrent abdominal aortic narrowings, often with a "gross hourglass appearance," while extraparenchymal segmental renal artery stenosis affected only 13 children as isolated lesions and five children with existing main renal artery disease. Histopathology reported consistent complex medial and perimedial dysplastic disease complicated with secondary intimal fibroplasia accounting for all but a few of the renal artery stenoses in this series. Concurrent aortic and splanchnic disease was common.

Within the manuscript, the authors review their careful and esoteric practice of renal revascularization that considers several tenets: (1) the use of a supra-umbilical transverse abdominal incision and medial visceral reflection; (2) intra-operative pharmacologic considerations including systemic anticoagulation, antiplatelet therapy and osmotic diuresis; (3) the importance of in situ reconstructions to avoid disruption of pre-existing collaterals; (4) single-staged operations that consider concurrent aorto-mesenteric vasculopathy; (5) the technique of renal artery reimplantation that employs intentional anterior/posterior spatulation and interrupted monofilament suture lines; (6) the use of internal iliac artery for autogenous conduit; and (7) aortic reconstruction that considers the use of ePTFE and patient size. The most common renal intervention was renal artery reimplantation onto the aorta (N 49), and primary nephrectomy was employed for 12 cases of irreparable renal disease. Patch aortoplasty was the preferred means of treating abdominal aortic coarctation over thoracoabdominal bypass when anatomy permitted, with patches made sufficiency large enough so as not to be constrictive as the child grows into adulthood.

With excellent surgical outcomes that include a 97% incidence of hypertension benefit, no cases or renal failure requiring dialysis, and no mortality, the study supports the role for open surgical reconstruction in carefully selected children with renovascular hypertension at centers of excellence with a multidisciplinary care team.

REFERENCES

1. Hansen ML, Gunn PW, and Kaelber DC. Underdiagnosis of hypertension in children and adolescents. *JAMA*. 2007;298(8):874–9.

2. McNiece KL, Poffenbarger TS, Turner JL, Franco KD, Sorof JM, and Portman RJ. Prevalence of hypertension and pre-hypertension among adolescents. *J Pediatr.* 2007;150(6):640–4, 4 e1.
3. Flynn JT, Alderman MH. Characteristics of children with primary hypertension seen at a referral center. *Pediatr Nephrol.* 2005;20(7):961–6.
4. Flynn JT, Kaelber DC, Baker-Smith CM et al. Clinical practice guideline for screening and management of high blood pressure in children and adolescents. *Pediatrics.* 2017;140(3).
5. Martinez A, Novick AC, Cunningham R, and Goormastic M. Improved results of vascular reconstruction in pediatric and young adult patients with renovascular hypertension. *J Urol.* 1990;144(3):717–20.
6. O'Neill JA, Jr. Long-term outcome with surgical treatment of renovascular hypertension. *J Pediatr Surg.* 1998;33(1):106–11.
7. Stadermann MB, Montini G, Hamilton G et al. Results of surgical treatment for renovascular hypertension in children: 30 year single centre experience. *Nephrol Dial Transplant.* 2010;25(3):807–13.
8. Shroff R, Roebuck DJ, Gordon I et al. Angioplasty for renovascular hypertension in children: 20-year experience. *Pediatrics.* 2006;118(1):268–75.
9. Courtel JV, Soto B, Niaudet P et al. Percutaneous transluminal angioplasty of renal artery stenosis in children. *Pediatr Radiol.* 1998;28(1):59–63.
10. Srinivasan A, Krishnamurthy G, Fontalvo-Herazo L et al. Angioplasty for renal artery stenosis in pediatric patients: An 11-year retrospective experience. *J Vasc Interv Radiol.* 2010;21(11):1672–80.
11. Rumman RK, Matsuda-Abedini M, Langlois V et al. Management and outcomes of childhood renal artery stenosis and middle aortic syndrome. *Am J Hypertens.* 2018;31(6):687–95.
12. Sharma S, Thatai D, Saxena A, Kothari SS, Guleria S, and Rajani M. Renovascular hypertension resulting from nonspecific aortoarteritis in children: Midterm results of percutaneous transluminal renal angioplasty and predictors of restenosis. *AJR Am J Roentgenol.* 1996;166(1):157–62.
13. Tyagi S, Kaul UA, Satsangi DK, and Arora R. Percutaneous transluminal angioplasty for renovascular hypertension in children: Initial and long-term results. *Pediatrics.* 1997;99(1):44–9.

CHAPTER 43

Late Results Following Operative Repair for Celiac Artery Compression Syndrome

Reilly LM, Ammar AD, Stoney RJ, Ehrenfeld WK. J Vasc Surg. 1985 Jan;2(1):79–91

ABSTRACT

The clinical significance of celiac artery compression by the median arcuate ligament of the diaphragm remains unsettled. The controversy stems from an undefined pathophysiologic mechanism and the existence of celiac compression in asymptomatic patients. This study was therefore conducted to evaluate the late results of operative therapy among our patients and possibly to identify parameters that might correlate with sustained symptom relief. Among 51 patients (12 men and 39 women) (mean age 47 years) who underwent operative treatment for symptomatic celiac artery compression, 44 (86%) were available for late follow-up. Their clinical status was determined between 1 and 18 years postoperatively (mean 9.0 years) by patient interview (36) or chart review (7). Operative treatment consisted of celiac axis decompression only (16 patients), celiac decompression and dilatation (17 patients), or celiac decompression and reconstruction by primary re-anastomosis or interposition grafting (18 patients). Sustained symptom relief occurred more often with a postprandial pain pattern (81% cure), age between 40 and 60 years (77%), and weight loss of 20 pounds or more (67%). A negative correlation with clinical improvement was demonstrated for an atypical pain pattern with periods of remission (43% cure), a history of psychiatric disorder or alcohol abuse (40%), age greater than 60 years (40%), and weight loss of less than 20 pounds (53%). Eight of 15 patients (53%) treated by celiac decompression alone remained asymptomatic at late follow-up in contrast to 22 of 29 patients (76%) treated by celiac decompression plus some form of celiac revascularization. Late follow-up arteriograms (18 studies) showed a widely patent celiac artery in 70% of asymptomatic patients but a stenosed or occluded celiac axis in 75% of symptomatic patients. These findings suggest that persistent clinical improvement in patients with symptomatic celiac axis compression can be achieved by an operative technique that ensures celiac axis patency. Although some clinical features are identified that correlate with long-term benefit, reliable diagnosis of the symptomatic patient awaits definition of the pathophysiologic mechanisms involved in this syndrome.

EXPERT COMMENTARY BY JUAN CARLOS JIMENEZ

Research Question/Objective What is the optimal treatment for patients with symptomatic celiac artery compression?

Study Design Nonrandomized, single-center retrospective review.

Sample Size 51 patients (12 men and 39 women).

Follow-Up Mean follow-up interval was 9 years. Seventy-seven percent of patients had 5-year follow-up and 47% had longer than 10-year follow-up.

Intervention or Treatment Received

1. Surgical exposure of the celiac artery through midline, thoracoabdominal or thoracoretroperitoneal incision
2. Release of the median arcuate ligament and resection of periarterial neural tissue only (n = 16)
3. Release of the median arcuate ligament and graduated celiac dilation (n = 17)
4. Release of the median arcuate ligament and celiac artery reconstruction (n = 18)
   a. Resection and primary anastomosis (n = 7)
   b. Use of a graft (saphenous, arterial autograft, or Dacron) (n = 18)

Results

1. No perioperative deaths
2. Eighty-six percent of patients available for late follow-up
3. At late evaluation:
   a. Asymptomatic: 68%
   b. Persistently symptomatic: 32%
4. Patient group who underwent celiac decompression alone: 53% asymptomatic
5. Patient group who underwent celiac decompression with either dilation of reconstruction: 76% asymptomatic
6. Persistent celiac artery stenosis or occlusion on late angiogram predicted persistent refractory symptoms
7. Predictors for sustained symptom relief included:
   a. Patients with a postprandial pain pattern
   b. Age between 40–60 years
   c. Weight loss of 20 lbs or more
8. Predictors for negative clinical improvement
   a. An atypical pain pattern with periods of remission
   b. A history of psychiatric disorder or alcohol abuse
   c. Age greater than 60
   d. Weight loss of less than 20 lbs

Study Impact

Dr. Reilly and colleagues' landmark 1985 study validated a surgical treatment protocol for patients with Median Arcuate Ligament Syndrome (MALS) for the first time in the vascular surgery literature. They demonstrated improved outcomes with MAL release, celiac ganglionectomy and more extensive arterial reconstruction compared with MAL release, and ganglionectomy alone. Their excellent outcomes were impressive despite the absence of routine use of CT angiography, endovascular techniques and devices, and laparoscopic or robotic surgery. The 32% failure (to alleviate symptoms) rate in Dr. Reilly's entire patient cohort supports similar outcomes in recent studies in the current literature including our own experience with treating these patients.[1,2] This is not an operation where certain complete symptomatic relief should be advertised to patients, and MAL release, either open or minimally invasive, should only be a last resort for patients who have failed all medical treatments.

This milestone paper also characterized the patient population with MALS and attempted to delineate optimal patient selection for surgery. Inclusion in the study required an extensive gastrointestinal workup, preoperative angiograms, and even a psychiatric and substance abuse history. Decades later, patient selection and predicting which patients will improve with surgery remains our biggest challenge in treating MALS. Accurate diagnosis of this disorder is difficult due to our lack of understanding of the pathophysiologic mechanism of the disease. We continue to further characterize and choose appropriate surgical candidates. At our institution, we have instituted the use of noninvasive mesenteric duplex with both full inspiration and expiration to assess real-time compression of the celiac artery. Celiac artery compression by the MAL is associated with full expiration.[3] Patients are tested in a fasting state to reduce artifact from bowel gas. In our experience, this has served to make us more selective for our surgical patients because individuals with normal duplex scans are not offered surgery despite axial imaging findings.

As the authors discuss, there are two proposed mechanisms for development of symptoms in MALS. The first is arterial insufficiency from the MAL compressing the celiac artery leading to end-organ ischemia and pain. The other is physical compression of the celiac ganglion by the MAL leading to subsequent somatic pain. Dr. Reilly's paper's evidence suggests that arterial patency is the main determinant of late symptom relief. The finding that most asymptomatic patients had patent celiac arteries postoperatively and that most symptomatic patients had persistent stenosis or occlusion suggests a mechanism of pain caused by ischemia. Conflicting evidence toward an ischemic etiology involves the abundant collateral beds between the celiac and superior mesenteric arteries (in mostly young patients free from significant atherosclerosis) and overall good results reported following conservative treatment of celiac artery dissection and thrombosis.[4,5]

In the more recent minimally invasive era, we are using laparoscopic and robotic techniques to release the MAL. The well-described natural history of in-stent restenosis with bare metal mesenteric stents has limited their role at our institution where intra-luminal interventions are rarely performed in these patients. In our recent published series, we demonstrated overall early and intermediate clinical improvement rates using robotic and laparoscopic decompression of the MAL alone similar to Dr. Reilly's outcomes with open surgical reconstruction.[6] Complete surgical dissection of the celiac ganglion is our primary focus with minimally invasive techniques and has led to excellent symptom relief postoperatively. One possible reason that surgical reconstruction resulted in better long-term outcomes in Dr. Reilly's paper is that a more complete celiac ganglionectomy and exposure of the artery is required for reconstruction or bypass.

This groundbreaking study by Dr. Reilly and colleagues was the first to characterize a complex disease process which is not completely understood decades later. The meticulous design study and long-term follow-up (up to 18 years) raises the importance of this paper above all other published series on MALS. It is an honor to include this pioneering work in our collection.

REFERENCES

1. Tulloch AW, Jimenez JC, Lawrence PF et al. Laparoscopic versus open celiac ganglionectomy in patients with median arcuate ligament syndrome. *J Vasc Surg*. 2010;52:1283–9.
2. Khrucharoen U, Juo YY, Chen Y, Jimenez JC, and Dutson EP. Robotic-assisted laparoscopic median arcuate ligament release: 7-year experience from a single tertiary care center. *Surg Endosc* 2018;32:4029–35.
3. Reuter, S.R. and Bernstein, E.F. The anatomic basis for respiratory variation in median arcuate ligament compression of the celiac artery. *Surgery*. 1973;73:381–5
4. Kueht ML, West CA, Mills JL, and Gilani R. Visceral collateralization with symptomatic occlusion of the celiomesenteric trunk. *J Vasc Surg* 2017;66:910
5. Hosaka A, Nemoto M, and Miyata T. Outcomes of conservative management of spontaneous celiac artery dissection. *J Vasc Surg* 2017;65:760–5.
6. Khrucharoen U, Juo YY, Chen Y, Jimenez JC, and Dutson EP. Short- and intermediate-term clinical outcome comparison between laparoscopic and robotic-assisted median arcuate ligament release. *J Robot Surg* 2020. Feb;14(1):123–9. doi: 10.1007/s11701-019-00945-y.

Chapter 44

Repair of Type IV Thoracoabdominal Aneurysm with a Combined Endovascular and Surgical Approach

Quiñones-Baldrich WJ, Panetta TF, Vescera CL, Kashyap VS.
J Vasc Surg. 1999 Sep;30(3):555–60

ABSTRACT

We report an unusual case of type IV thoracoabdominal aneurysm (TAA) with superior mesenteric artery (SMA), celiac artery, and bilateral renal artery aneurysms in a patient who underwent repair of two infrarenal abdominal aortic aneurysm (AAA) ruptures. Due to the presence of four visceral artery aneurysms and earlier transabdominal and retroperitoneal operations, surgical treatment through either approach using an inclusion grafting technique was considered difficult. A combined surgical approach achieving retrograde perfusion of all four visceral vessels and endovascular grafting allowing exclusion of the TAA was recommended. The procedure was performed in 1998 and the patient has been followed for 23 years. Complete exclusion of the aneurysm and normal perfusion of the patient's viscera were initially documented by CT imaging at 3 and 6 months and every year thereafter. The repair of a type IV TAA with a combined endovascular and surgical approach (CESA) allowed us to manage both the aortic and visceral aneurysms without thoracotomy or re-do retroperitoneal exposure while minimizing visceral ischemia time. The durability of this approach is now confirmed and represents an alternative in patients with complex aortic pathology.

AUTHOR COMMENTARY BY WILLIAM J. QUINONES-BALDRICH AND MEENA ARCHIE

This case report was inspired by what I believed at the time to be the future of vascular surgery. The patient was a 61-year-old gentleman with a longstanding history of smoking who was being evaluated for back pain with an MRI. The imaging demonstrated a contained rupture, and he was urgently repaired at an outside institution with an infrarenal tube graft through a midline transperitoneal incision. After surviving this, he experienced severe abdominal pain several months later at his son's wedding in Boston and was diagnosed with rupture below the previous infrarenal AAA repair. This was treated with a bifurcated graft reconstruction through a retroperitoneal approach. Notably, he also had an open repair of a left popliteal artery aneurysm. When I met the patient in December of 1997, his aorta had degenerated into a 5.5 cm type IV thoracoabdominal aneurysm (TAAA) that involved the origins of the celiac, superior mesenteric, and bilateral renal arteries.

I was inclined to agree with the referring surgeon that there were no good surgical options. After all, his aneurysms were quite extensive, suggestive of aorto-megaly. After considering the alternatives and having experience with endovascular repairs since 1994, a hybrid approach consisting of an endovascular thoracoabdominal aneurysm repair with open abdominal debranching was recommended. At the time, endograft options were limited, and the only endograft large enough to obtain a proximal and distal seal was the Corvita endograft. I contacted my friend and colleague, Dr. Thomas Panetta, who was the principal investigator of the Corvita device national trial.[1] With determination and a dash of luck, we were able to obtain surgical privileges for Dr. Panetta at UCLA, institutional approval for using the device, and FDA approval for "compassionate use"—a feat that I do not believe I could accomplish today. The patient even offered to pay for all additional expenses including travel!

The operation performed was a retrograde graft limb-ilio-birenal bypass, ilio-SMA, ilio-celiac bypass, and placement of two 27 mm × 14 cm Corvita stent endografts. This was performed in a single stage. Due to the tortuosity of the aorta, the endovascular portion required both antegrade and retrograde access through the right axillary and iliac arteries, respectively, with a single, very stiff wire that was flossed through the patient (aortic endografts were not known for their conformability at the time). Suffice it to say that a significant amount of wire straining was necessary to advance and deploy the endografts in a very tortuous descending thoracic aorta. The patient tolerated the surgery well and was discharged after 1 week.

This case demonstrates the versatility of hybrid vascular surgery. As a community, we have been vigilant to embrace technology with all its advantages and disadvantages. Vascular surgeons are now able to treat a broad spectrum of vascular disease, recognizing when one modality is preferred to the other. We have repeatedly shown that there is no "one size that fits all" any longer. This is true in all of vascular surgery, from aortic reconstruction to dialysis access. In this example, we appreciate that both initial open repairs were necessary to save the patient's life. In addition, they were quite durable two decades later. However, an entire open repair of his TAAA would have required distal visceral and renal bypasses due to origin aneurysms in

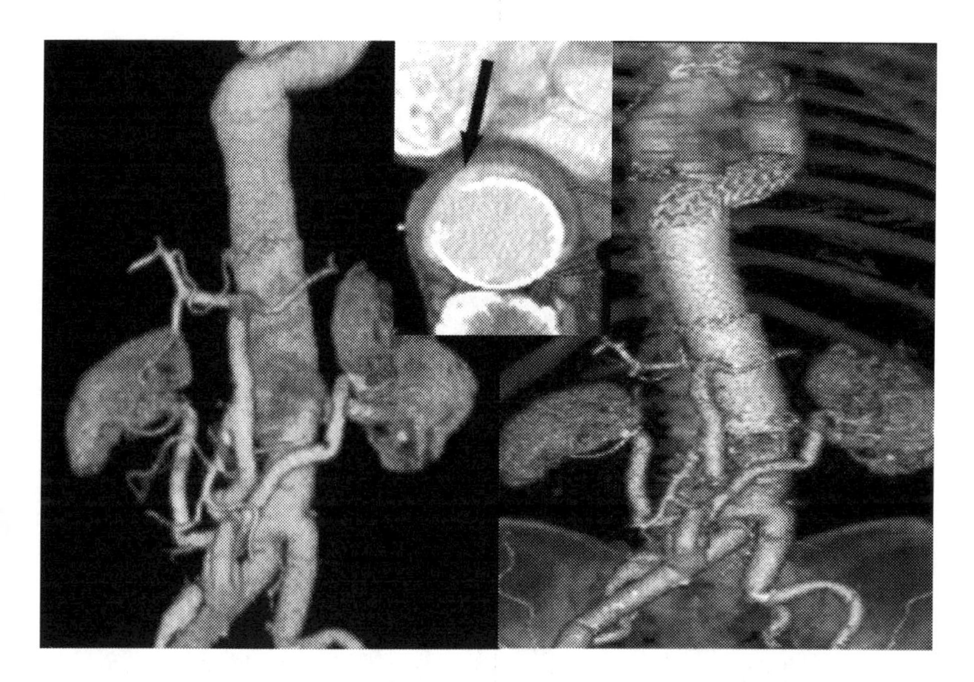

Figure 44.1 Type 1A endoleak developed 13 years after initial debranching and was successfully treated with a Gore C-TAG device.

these arteries. While this is feasible, it would certainly have increased morbidity and perhaps mortality. On the contrary, some may argue that today this could be treated entirely by endovascular techniques. It is unlikely that a fenestrated repair would provide a durable outcome given the extent of his visceral and renal aneurysms. From cases like this, we appreciate that the modern vascular surgeon needs to understand the benefits (and pitfalls) of utilizing both open and endovascular surgery. Combining the old with newer technologies allows treatment of complex pathology in patients with lower overall risk.

To complete the narrative, we followed the patient for 23 years after the combined endovascular and surgical repair. He developed a type 1a endoleak after 13 years, which was treated successfully with a Gore C-TAG device (Figure 44.1). After 22 years, he developed a type 3 endoleak from substantial aortic remodeling, and this was also sealed with a Gore C-TAG (Figure 44.2). Both open repaired segments were stable. It is notable that it has been the endovascular portion of the repair that has led to additional interventions underscoring the need for lifelong follow-up. He was seen a few months ago, and his imaging demonstrated a stable aneurysm sac with no evidence of endoleak. He is now 83 years old.

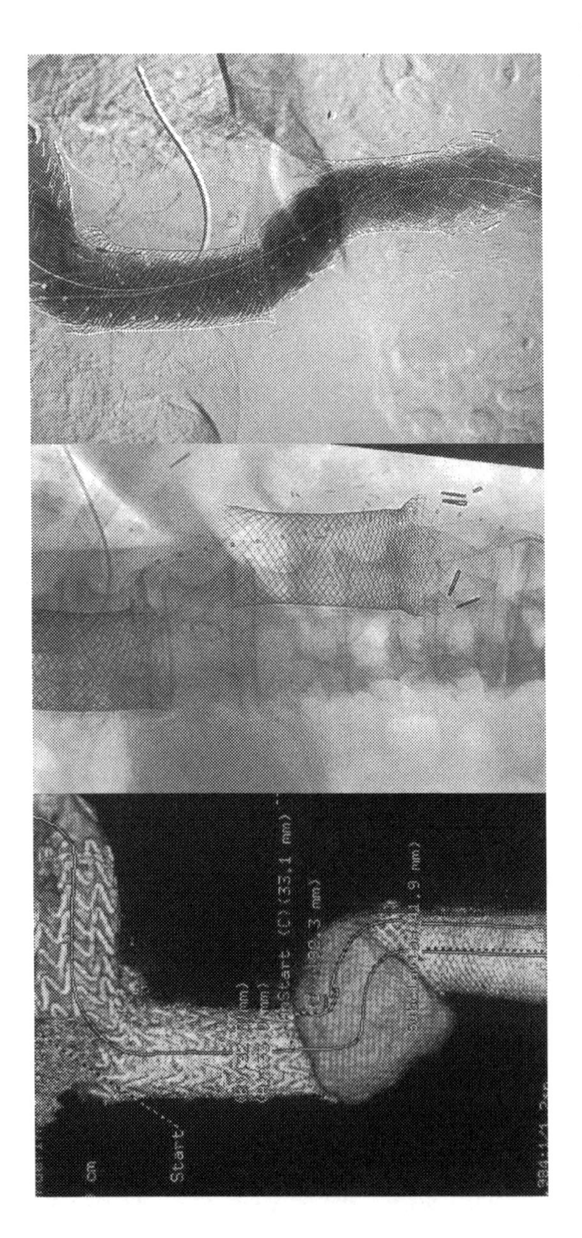

Figure 44.2 (Left) 3D reconstruction of complete abdominal debranching with retrograde graft limb-ilio-birenal bypass, ilio-SMA, ilio-celiac bypass. (Center) Type 3 endoleak due to component separation of the Corvita graft. (Right) Completion 3D reconstruction following retrograde graft limb-ilio-birenal bypass, ilio-SMA, ilio-celiac bypass, and endovascular repair of type 4 thoracoabdominal aortic aneurysm.

REFERENCE

1. Dereume JPE, and Ferreira J. *The Corvita System. Endovascular Surgery for Aortic Aneurysms*. Philadelphia, WB Saunders; 1997:122–39.

CHAPTER 45

The Contemporary Management of Renal Artery Aneurysms

Vascular Low-Frequency Disease Consortium, Klausner JQ, Lawrence PF, Harlander-Locke MP, Coleman DM, Stanley JC, Fujimura N. J Vasc Surg. 2015 Apr;61(4):978–84. doi: 10.1016/j.jvs.2014.10.107. Epub 2014 Dec 20

ABSTRACT

Background Renal artery aneurysms (RAAs) are rare, with little known about their natural history and growth rate or their optimal management. The specific objectives of this study were to (1) define the clinical features of RAAs, including the precise growth rate and risk of rupture, (2) examine the current management and outcomes of RAA treatment using existing guidelines, and (3) examine the appropriateness of current criteria for repair of asymptomatic RAAs.

Methods A standardized, multi-institutional approach was used to evaluate patients with RAAs at institutions from all regions of the United States. Patient demographics, aneurysm characteristics, aneurysm imaging, conservative and operative management, postoperative complications, and follow-up data were collected.

Results A total of 865 RAAs in 760 patients were identified at 16 institutions. Of these, 75% were asymptomatic; symptomatic patients had difficult-to-control hypertension (10%), flank pain (6%), hematuria (4%), and abdominal pain (2%). The RAAs had a mean maximum diameter of 1.5 ± 0.1 cm. Most were unilateral (96%), on the right side (61%), saccular (87%), and calcified (56%). Elective repair was performed in 213 patients with 241 RAAs, usually for symptoms or size >2 cm; the remaining 547 patients with 624 RAAs were observed. Major operative complications occurred in 10%, including multisystem organ failure, myocardial infarction, and renal failure requiring dialysis. RAA repair for difficult-to-control hypertension cured 32% of patients and improved it in 26%. Three patients had ruptured RAA; all were transferred from other hospitals and underwent emergency repair, with no deaths. Conservatively treated patients were monitored for a mean of 49 months, with no acute complications. Aneurysm growth rate was 0.086 cm/y, with no difference between calcified and noncalcified aneurysms.

Conclusions This large, contemporary, multi-institutional study demonstrated that asymptomatic RAAs rarely rupture (even when >2 cm), growth rate is

0.086 ± 0.08 cm/y, and calcification does not protect against enlargement. RAA open repair is associated with significant minor morbidity, but rarely a major morbidity or mortality. Aneurysm repair cured or improved hypertension in >50% of patients whose RAA was identified during the workup for difficult-to-control hypertension.

AUTHOR COMMENTARY BY PETER F. LAWRENCE AND DAWN MARIE COLEMAN

Research Question/Objective To define the clinical features natural history of renal artery aneurysms (RAAS), including growth rate and risk of rupture; to examine the current management and outcomes of RAA treatment using existing guidelines; to examine the appropriateness of current criteria for the repair of asymptomatic RAAs.

Study Design Multi-institutional retrospective study.

Sample Size 865 RAAs in 760 patients.

Follow-Up Conservatively managed patients were observed for a mean of 49 ± 5 months.

Inclusion/Exclusion Criteria All patients with RAAs defined as RAAs as focal, isolated dilatation of all three layers of the arterial wall that measured >1.5 times the diameter of the disease-free proximal adjacent arterial segment. Patients with pararenal or juxtarenal aortic aneurysms and proximal RAAs that originated from an aortic aneurysm were excluded.

Intervention or Treatment Received Open surgical repair, endovascular treatment, or conservative surveillance.

Results A total of 865 RAAs in 760 patients were identified at 16 institutions. Of these, 75% were asymptomatic; symptomatic patients had difficult-to-control hypertension (10%), flank pain (6%), hematuria (4%), and abdominal pain (2%). The RAAs had a mean maximum diameter of 1.5 ± 0.1 cm. Most were unilateral (96%), on the right side (61%), saccular (87%), and calcified (56%). The majority were located at the renal artery bifurcations. Elective repair was performed in 213 patients with 241 RAAs, usually for symptoms or size >2 cm; the remaining 547 patients with 624 RAAs were observed. Endovascular stent graft repair was performed when the RAA was located in the main renal artery. Major operative complications occurred in 10%, including multisystem organ failure, myocardial infarction, and renal failure requiring dialysis. RAA repair for difficult-to-control hypertension cured 32% of patients and improved it in 26%. Three patients had ruptured RAA; all were transferred from other hospitals and underwent emergency repair, with no deaths. Conservatively treated patients were monitored for a mean of 49 months, with no acute complications.

Aneurysm growth rate was 0.086 cm/y, with no difference between calcified and noncalcified aneurysms.

Conclusions This large, contemporary, multi-institutional study demonstrated that asymptomatic RAAs rarely rupture (even when >2 cm), growth rate is 0.086 ± 0.08 cm/y, and calcification does not protect against enlargement. RAA open repair is associated with significant minor morbidity, but rarely a major morbidity or mortality. Aneurysm repair cured or improved hypertension in >50% of patients whose RAA was identified during the workup for difficult-to-control hypertension.

Study Limitations Retrospective study design precluded the capture of all RAAs, so the true natural history of RAAs remains unknown because only outcomes of patients who did undergo aneurysm repair could be analyzed. Although most patients had an imaging study to evaluate their aneurysm, the modality used was not standardized, so recommendations about optimal imaging are limited to the observation that measurement of aneurysm growth can be obtained with CT angiogram or MR angiogram and that serial growth rates and aneurysm size can be determined and may be used as criteria for repair.

Relevant Studies RAAs are rare, with an estimated incidence of approximately 0.1% in the general population. Although infrequent, incidental diagnosis is increasingly common as RAAs are identified during cross-sectional imaging performed to evaluate other pathology. Previously accepted indications for elective repair included symptoms, size >2 cm, and aneurysms in women of childbearing age. These criteria were based on studies conducted before the widespread use of cross sectional imaging, during a time of higher reported rates of rupture with increased associated rupture-related mortality. Importantly, contemporary reports do not uphold historic data describing rupture rates approaching 30% and rather current rupture rates are estimated at 3%–5%. Moreover, most ruptures are diagnosed at the time of rupture presentation, in contrast to during surveillance of a known aneurysm, and most authors report no ruptures during surveillance.[1–5] Nongestational rupture-related mortality has similarly improved from historic rates approximating 80% to modern-day rates of <10%. As such, there has remained significant controversy surrounding RAA treatment criteria because the incidence, risk of rupture, and growth rate have not been determined.

Study Impact This contemporary study reports a very large, multi-institutional series of RAAs encountered during a time when cross-sectional abdominal imaging was routinely employed for the diagnosis of many nonarterial abdominal diseases and when both open surgical and endovascular techniques were available for treatment. The authors conclude that rupture of asymptomatic RAAs is exceedingly rare, the growth rate of RAAs is very slow, and open surgical repair, while associated with significant minor morbidity, is rarely complicated by major morbidity or mortality.

The study follows a single institution experience with RAA that questions whether the current size threshold for elective repair may be too aggressive.[6] To that end, a total of 88 RAAs >2.0 cm in maximum diameter (mean diameter 2.7 ± 0.1 cm) at 13 different institutions were not surgically repaired. During a mean follow-up of 29 ± 5 months, no acute complications were reported, suggesting that conservative management of some asymptomatic RAAs between 2 and 3 cm may be safe. Moreover, with only 3 ruptures in 865 aneurysms, including 88 aneurysms >2 cm and 7 aneurysms >3 cm, this study further confirms that RAA rupture is an exceedingly rare event (0.03%). All ruptured RAAs were measured >3 cm (mean diameter, 3.7 ± 0.2 cm) and among RAAs >3 cm, the rate of rupture was 18% (3 of 17 RAA).

Finally, the current study used 454 aneurysms from 16 different institutions to calculate a growth rate of 0.086 cm/yr. On the basis of this calculated growth rate, the authors propose that 46% of the asymptomatic aneurysms in this study would in theory not require surgical repair during the next 10 years if the size threshold for asymptomatic repair were increased to 3 cm. It was demonstrated that following young patients with serial imaging is safe because most RAA's do not increase significantly in size.

The authors question the current size criteria for repair of asymptomatic RAAs at 2 cm, supporting the development of updated practice guidelines as current guidelines recommending repair to prevent rupture for asymptomatic RAAs measuring >2 cm may be too aggressive. In fact, the Society for Vascular Surgery Clinical Practice Guidelines for the Management of Visceral Artery Aneurysms are currently drafted to support that patients with noncomplicated RAA of acceptable risk be considered for treatment for aneurysm size >3 cm (Grade 2C). As treatment guidelines remain limited by the absence of prospective and/or randomized data, as expected with a rare disease, ongoing study is essential to optimize patient selection for surgery by clinical phenotype and direct best practices for repair (i.e., open vs. endovascular treatment). This study nicely lays the foundation for such.

REFERENCES

1. Wayne EJ, Edwards MS, Stafford JM et al. Anatomic characteristics and natural history of renal artery aneurysms during longitudinal imaging surveillance. *J Vasc Surg*. 2014;60(2):448–52.
2. Henke PK, Cardneau JD, Welling TH et al. Renal artery aneurysms: A 35-year clinical experience with 252 aneurysms in 168 patients. *Ann Surg*. 2001;234:454–62.
3. Robinson WP 3rd, Bafford R, Belkin M et al. Favorable outcomes with *in situ* techniques for surgical repair of complex renal artery aneurysms. *J Vasc Surg*. 2011;53:684–91.
4. Tsilimparis N, Reeves JG, Dayama A et al. Endovascular vs open repair of renal artery aneurysms: Outcomes of repair and long-term renal function. *J Am Coll Surg*. 2013;217:263–9.
5. Klausner JQ, Harlander-Locke MP, Plotnik AN, Lehrman E, DeRubertis BG, and Lawrence PF. Current treatment of renal artery aneurysms may be too aggressive. *J Vasc Surg*. 2014;59:1356–61.
6. Tham G, Ekelund L, Herrlin K, Lindstedt EL, Olin T, and Bergentz SE. Renal artery aneurysms: Natural history and prognosis. *Ann Surg*. 1983;197:348–52.

CHAPTER 46

The Society for Vascular Surgery Lower Extremity Threatened Limb Classification System: Risk Stratification Based on Wound, Ischemia, and Foot Infection (WIfI)

Mills JL Sr, Conte MS, Armstrong DG, Pomposelli FB, Schanzer A, Sidawy AN, Andros G; Society for Vascular Surgery Lower Extremity Guidelines Committee. J Vasc Surg. 2014 Jan;59(1):220–34.e1-2

ABSTRACT

Critical limb ischemia, first defined in 1982, was intended to delineate a subgroup of patients with a threatened lower extremity primarily because of chronic ischemia. It was the intent of the original authors that patients with diabetes be excluded or analyzed separately. The Fontaine and Rutherford Systems have been used to classify risk of amputation and likelihood of benefit from revascularization by subcategorizing patients into two groups: ischemic rest pain and tissue loss. Due to demographic shifts over the last 40 years, especially a dramatic rise in the incidence of diabetes mellitus and rapidly expanding techniques of revascularization, it has become increasingly difficult to perform meaningful outcomes analysis for patients with threatened limbs using these existing classification systems. Particularly in patients with diabetes, limb threat is part of a broad disease spectrum. Perfusion is only one determinant of outcome; wound extent and the presence and severity of infection also greatly impact the threat to a limb. Therefore, the Society for Vascular Surgery Lower Extremity Guidelines Committee undertook the task of creating a new classification of the threatened lower extremity that reflects these important considerations. We term this new framework, the Society for Vascular Surgery Lower Extremity Threatened Limb Classification System. Risk stratification is based on three major factors that impact amputation risk and clinical management: Wound, Ischemia, and foot Infection (WIfI). The implementation of this classification system is intended to permit more meaningful analysis of outcomes for various forms of therapy in this challenging, but heterogeneous population.

AUTHOR COMMENTARY BY JOSEPH L. MILLS

Background The global epidemic of diabetes, a prime example of a noncommunicable disease, dramatically changed the landscape of healthcare delivery over the last decade. Diabetes is increasing in prevalence in virtually every country for which statistics are available and currently affects nearly 400 million people in the world. The most common manifestation of diabetes is the seemingly mundane diabetic foot ulcer (DFU). Approximately one in four people with diabetes will develop a foot ulcer during their lifetime and 80% of amputations in people with diabetes are heralded by a DFU. DFUs are most commonly caused by neuropathy, but are often complicated by peripheral artery disease (PAD). Even though PAD is detectable in 1/2–2/3 of patients with DFU, in many modern healthcare systems, patients presenting with DFU do not see a vascular specialist and in fact are not even referred for basic vascular noninvasive testing to diagnose and grade the severity of PAD, if present.[1] The diabetic foot literature was replete with DFU classification systems and algorithms of care, many of which either lacked routine assessment for PAD or simply graded PAD as a binary variable (present or absent). Neither approach was satisfactory from the standpoint of a vascular surgeon or specialist. The vascular surgical literature had long been satisfied with the concept of "critical limb ischemia" or CLI, a dated concept that originated in 1982 and was never intended to include patients with diabetes.[2] Similarly, both the widely utilized Fontaine[3] and Rutherford[4] classification systems failed to address numerous issues of critical importance to the assessment, management, and selection for revascularization of patients with DFU. DFUs are almost always initiated by a combination of motor, sensory, and autonomic neuropathy, but are frequently complicated by infection. In addition, wounds in those with diabetes are frequently more complex than a shallow, simple ischemic ulcer or a dry, gangrenous toe resulting from pure ischemia such as occurs in a smoker with PAD but without diabetes. Perfusion requirements for healing are likely greater in patients with diabetes, yet the vascular literature seemed stagnated by the concept of CLI and insistent that there was a specific hemodynamic cutoff for healing. None of these issues was adequately addressed by the concept of CLI or by the two most prevalent vascular classification systems, both of which were insufficiently granular.

Premises and Application of the WIfI Classification for Chronic Limb-Threatening Ischemia (CLTI) With these issues as a backdrop, the Society for Vascular Surgery (SVS) created and published a new classification system in 2014 intended to be applicable to both patients with and without diabetes. This system is based on grades of wound, ischemia, and foot infection, and has been termed WIfI.[1] A free "SVS IPG" app is available to help individuals and limb-salvage units calculate the WIfI grades and clinical stages. There were several important premises underlying WIfI. First, limb threat is a broad disease spectrum, especially in people with diabetes. Thus, the change to the term chronic limb-threatening ischemia or CLTI was recommended, to recognize the broader spectrum of PAD which may contribute to limb threat. Second, although important, perfusion is only one determinant of outcome (healing or amputation); wound extent and the presence and severity of concomitant infection also exert major impacts on outcomes. WIfI was intended to be a limb staging system, analogous to the TNM (tumor, nodes, and metastases) system used to stage cancer. The purpose of a limb staging system was to accurately provide risk stratification (1-year amputation and wound healing) and to help determine which patients would most likely benefit from revascularization. Eventually, it could be used to compare outcomes of various forms of treatments for limbs at comparable risk.

WIfI mandates grading of each of its three components (wound, ischemia, and foot infection) on a scale from 0 to 3. Thus, every patient presenting with possible CLTI, including those with the manifestations of ischemic rest pain, foot ulcer, or gangrene requires assessment of each of these factors, and importantly, hemodynamic assessment is mandated. Based on the combination of grades, using a Delphi consensus process, the limb was placed into one of four clinical stages intended to correlate with progressively increased amputation risk and delayed wound healing (Figure 46.1). WIfI has been adopted and validated globally (United States, Asia, Europe, and

	Ischemia – 0				Ischemia – 1				Ischemia – 2				Ischemia – 3			
W-0	1	1	2	3	1	2	3	4	2	2	3	4	2	3	3	4
W-1	1	1	2	3	1	2	3	4	2	3	4	4	3	3	4	4
W-2	2	2	3	4	3	3	4	4	3	4	4	4	4	4	4	4
W-3	3	3	4	4	4	4	4	4	4	4	4	4	4	4	4	4
	fI-0	fI-1	fI-2	fI-3	fI-0	fI-1	fI-2	fI-3	fI-0	fI-1	fI-2	fI-3	fI-0	fI-1	fI-2	fI-3

KEY: **I = Ischemia** **W = Wound** **fI = foot Infection**

Clinical Stage 1 or Very low risk
Clinical Stage 2 or Low risk
Clinical Stage 3 or Moderate risk
Clinical Stage 4 or High Risk
Clinical Stage 5 = Unsalvageable limb

Premises:

a. Increase in wound class increases risk of amputation (based on WIfI, PEDIS, UT and other wound classification systems)
b. PAD and infection are synergistic (Eurodiale); infected wound + PAD increases likelihood revascularization will be needed to heal wound
c. Infection 3 category (systemic/metabolic instability): moderate to high-risk of amputation regardless of other factors (validated IDSA infection guidelines)

Figure 46.1 SVS WIfI clinical limb stage based on estimated risk of amputation at one year.

South America). WIfI has been endorsed by many societies including the SVS, the APMA (American Podiatric Medical Association), the ESVS (European Society of Vascular and Endovascular Surgery), the ESC (European Society of Cardiology), the Japanese Society for Vascular Surgery, the Japanese Circulation Society, the IWGDF (International Working Group on the Diabetic Foot), and, most recently, by the Global Guidelines Committee on CLTI.[5]

Impact of WIfI Classification for CLTI The initial WIfI clinical limb stage strongly correlates with intermediate- and long-term prognosis. WIfI has been shown to predict the 1-year risk of amputation in patients with CLTI as well as those with diabetic foot ulcer. There is a striking contrast between the 1-year amputation rates for WIfI clinical stage 1 (<3%) versus clinical stage 4 limbs (>20%), even with revascularization.[6] A recent meta-analysis by Van Reijen of 12 studies comprising 2,669 patients with CLTI demonstrated that the likelihood of amputation at 1 year increased progressively with increasing WIfI stage, 0%, 8% (95% CI 3–21%), 11% (95% CI 6–18%), and 38% (95% CI 21–58%) for WIfI stages I–IV, respectively.[7] Other analyses have yielded similar findings (Table 46.1).[5,6] WIfI stages have also been shown to correlate with other important clinical endpoints such as wound healing time, wound healing rate, major adverse limb events after revascularization, hospital length of stay, and hospital cost.[6] WIfI may also be used to predict the likelihood of benefit of revascularization, although the data supporting this particular utility of WIfI are less robust.[8,9]

Routine WIfI baseline assessment of the patient and after the period of initial therapy,[8] analogous to restaging patients after receiving a course of therapy for cancer, is a major step forward in the treatment of patients with CLTI and DFU. It should be

Table 46.1 One-Year Major Limb Amputation Rate by the Society for Vascular Surgery (SVS) Wound, Ischemia, and foot Infection (WIfI) Clinical Stage

Study (Year): No. of Limbs at Risk	Stage 1	Stage 2	Stage 3	Stage 4
Cull (2014): 151	37 (3)	63 (10)	43 (23)	8 (40)
Zhan (2015): 201	39 (0)	50 (0)	53 (8)	59 (64)[a]
Darling (2016): 551	5 (0)	110 (10)	222 (11)	213 (24)
Causey (2016): 160	21 (0)	48 (8)	42 (5)	49 (20)
Beropoulis (2016): 126	29 (13)	42 (19)	29 (19)	26 (38)
Ward (2017): 98	5 (0)	21 (14)	14 (21)	58 (34)
Darling (2017): 992	12 (0)	293 (4)	249 (4)	438 (21)
Robinson (2017): 280	48 (2.1)	67 (7.5)	64 (7.8)	83 (17)
Mathioudakis (2017): 217	95 (4)	33 (3)	87 (5)	64 (6)
Tokuda1 (2018): 163	16 (0)	30 (10)	56 (10.7)	61 (34.4)
N = 2982 (weighted mean)	307 (3.2)	757 (7.0)	859 (8.7)	1059 (23.3)
Median (1-year major limb amputation)	0%	9%	9.4%	29%

Note: The number of limbs at risk in each WIfI stage is given, with percentage of a amputations at 1 year in parentheses. Mean in totals (in parentheses) are weighted.

[a] Falsely elevated because of inadvertent inclusion of stage 5 (unsalvageable) limbs.

noted that WIfI is a limb staging system. It incorporates aspects of the wound, modified from the International Working Group and the UT classifications. The infection component is based on the IDSA classification. The ischemia component is graded objectively; in patients with diabetes, toe pressures and waveforms are preferred due to falsely elevated ABIs, but alternative measures of perfusion are also useful when available, including skin perfusion pressure, transcutaneous oxygen pressure, and indocyanine green angiography.

It would potentially be a major step forward to mandate an assessment of all three of these major limb factors whenever evaluating patients with DFU and limb threat for the potential benefit of revascularization. Recent data compiled from 10 centers across the globe shows that specific WIfI stage subsets benefit greatly from revascularization.[9] WIfI is a clinical impactful tool to be utilized by limb-salvage centers as it allows stratification of amputation risk, predicts the need for revascularization, and allows comparison of outcomes between centers and after alternative modes of treatment. When incorporated into algorithms that include overall patient risk assessment and the Global Limb Anatomic Staging System (GLASS) described in the recent Global Guidelines on CLTI,[5] it should be possible to treat and evaluate outcomes of a broad spectrum of patients with CLTI and select the best evidence-based methods of treatment.

REFERENCES

1. Mills JL, Conte MS, Armstrong DG, Pomposelli F, Schanzer A, Sidawy AN, Andros G. The Society for Vascular Surgery Lower Extremity Threatened Limb Classification System: Risk stratification based on Wound, Ischemia and foot Infection (WIfI). *J Vasc Surg*. January 2014;59:220–34.
2. Bell PRF, Charlesworth D, DePalma RG, Eastcott HHG, Eklöf B, Jamieson CW et al. The definition of critical ischemia of a limb. Working Party of the International Vascular Symposium. *Br J Surg*. 1982;69(Suppl):S2.
3. Fontaine R, Kim M, Kieny R. [Surgical treatment of peripheral circulation disorders.]. *Helv Chir Acta*. 1954;21:499–533.
4. Rutherford RB, Baker JD, Ernst C, Johnston KW, Porter JM, Ahn S et al. Recommended standards for reports dealing with lower extremity ischemia: Revised version. *J Vasc Surg*. 1997;26:517–38.
5. Conte MS, Bradbury AW, Kolh P, White JV, Dick F, Fitridge R, Mills JL, Ricco JB, Suresh KR, Murad MH. Global vascular guidelines on the management of chronic limb-threatening ischemia. *J Vasc Surg*. 2019;69:3S–125S.
6. Mayor JM, Mills JL. The correlation of the Society for Vascular Surgery Wound, Ischemia, and foot Infection threatened limb classification with amputation risk and major clinical outcomes. *Indian J Vasc Endovasc Surg*. May 2018;5(2):83–6.
7. Van Reijen NS, Ponchant K, Ubbink DT, Koelelmay MJW. The prognostic value of the WIfI classification in patients with chronic limb threatening ischemia: A systematic review and meta-analysis. *Eur J Vasc Endovasc Surg*. 2019;58:362–71.
8. Leithead C, Novak Z, Spangler E, Passman MA, Witcher A, Patterson MA et al. Importance of postprocedural Wound, Ischemia, and foot Infection (WIfI) restaging in predicting limb salvage. *J Vasc Surg*. 2018;67:498–505.

9. Mayor J, Chung J, Zhang Q, Montero-Baker M, Schanzer A, Conte MS, Mills JL. Using the Society for Vascular Surgery (SVS) Wound, Ischemia and foot Infection (WIfI) classification to identify patients most likely to benefit from revascularization. *J Vasc Surg*. September 2019;70:776–85.

CHAPTER 47

Long-Term Results in Patients Treated with Thrombolysis, Thoracic Inlet Decompression, and Subclavian Vein Stenting for Paget-Schroetter Syndrome

Kreienberg PB, Chang BB, Darling RC 3rd, Roddy SP, Paty PS, Lloyd WE, Cohen D, Stainken B, Shah DM. *J Vasc Surg. 2001 Feb;33(2 Suppl):S100–5*

ABSTRACT

Purpose In an effort to minimize long-term disability related to effort thrombosis of the subclavian vein, selected patients were treated with thrombolysis, thoracic inlet decompression, percutaneous transluminal angioplasty (PTA), and subclavian vein stenting. We evaluated the long-term outcomes of patients treated with this algorithm.

Methods Between 1994 and 2000, 23 patients were evaluated with effort thrombosis of the subclavian vein. Thrombolysis was instituted on an average of 9.4 days (range, 1–30 days) after initial onset of symptoms. Average time to clot lysis was 34 hours (range, 12–72 hours). After immediate supraclavicular thoracic inlet decompression, all patients underwent PTA. Fourteen patients with residual vein stenosis (>50%) after PTA underwent stenting of the subclavian vein. Complications in this series included three wound hematomas that required drainage in two patients and one subpleural hematoma that required thoracotomy for decompression.

Results All patients who underwent PTA are patent, with a mean follow-up of 4 years (range, 2–6 years). In the veins treated with stents, 9 of 14 veins are patent, with a mean follow-up of 3.5 years (range, 1–6 years). Two veins had early occlusions (2 days); two veins occluded at 1 year; and seven veins occluded at 3 years. Three of the patients (including those patients who experienced the early failed procedures) were later identified with factor V Leiden. Early failures also had clot extending into the brachial vein.

Conclusion Patients with short-segment venous strictures after successful lysis and thoracic outlet decompression may safely be treated with subclavian venous stents and can expect long-term patency.

AUTHOR COMMENTARY BY R. CLEMENT DARLING III AND PAUL B. KREIENBERG

Research Question/Objective This study was designed to ascertain the outcomes of subclavian vein thrombolysis, thoracic inlet decompression, percutaneous transluminal angioplasty, and subclavian vein stenting in patients presenting with axilla subclavian vein thrombosis. In addition, we evaluated the long-term outcomes of these patients treated with this algorithm via questionnaire.

Study Design Between 1994 and 2000, 23 patients were evaluated with effort thrombosis of the subclavian vein. Thrombolysis commenced on an average of 9.4 days after initial onset of symptoms. After successful lysis, immediate supraclavicular thoracic inlet decompression was performed in all patients who underwent percutaneous transluminal angioplasty. Additionally, 14 patients required stent placement for residual stenosis greater than 50%.

Follow-Up Routine follow-up was 4 years with a range of 2–6 years.

Results In the veins treated with stents, 14 veins remained patent with a mean follow-up of 3–1/2 years. Two veins had early occlusions at 2 days; two veins occluded at 1 year; and seven veins occluded at 3 years. Of note, three of the patients including those who experienced early failures had factor V Leiden. Early failure was also demonstrated when clot extended into the brachial vein.

Study Limitations Limitations of this study are due to the small sample size. Because of the rarity of the condition, large numbers are not obtainable. In addition, this is retrospective analysis of our treatment algorithm.

Relevant Studies Subclavian vein effort thrombosis typically affects young healthy active people. The treatment of this syndrome has evolved over time with initial treatments being conservative, including resting the extremity, elevation, and anticoagulation. However, this treatment algorithm left as many as 75% of those treated with significant residual symptoms at follow-up.[1] To improve the outcomes, several other approaches have been adapted including a staged approach that uses anticoagulation, then thoracic inlet decompression, thrombectomy, first rib resection, and venous bypass procedures.[1–5] At the time of publication of this paper, more recent therapeutic approaches had demonstrated lytic therapy being effective in reestablishing the patency in the thrombosed subclavian vein. This did not obviate the need for thoracic inlet decompression that produces better long-term results.[5–8] Investigators championed a staged approach that delayed thoracic inlet decompression for 3 to 4 months. However, given the high incidence of persistent stenosis in the vein, thrombosis was a common finding. Therefore, our treatment protocol of both lytic therapy, thoracic and inlet decompression, and angioplasty or vein stenting all in single admission to the hospital was designed to prevent that and allow more rapid resolution of the syndrome.

Study Impacts This paper was born out of the need to see the long-term results of a treatment algorithm for subclavian vein thrombosis. At the time the study was undertaken, several treatment paradigms existed. These included involving lytic therapy and first rib resection, venous reconstruction, or angioplasty. The approach to these patients is three-fold: first to open the occluded vein, second to perform first rib resection to open the thoracic inlet, and third to treat the chronically scarred vein with either surgical or percutaneous reconstruction. We put forth the algorithm that we could perform lytic therapy, rib resection, angioplasty plus or minus stenting all in the same hospital admission. In addition, we reserved stenting for patients who had residual greater than 50% stenosis. Our intent was to look at the long-term outcomes of these patients treated with this algorithm.

Our follow-up survey demonstrated that no patient had experienced a development of symptoms in the contralateral limb. All patients treated with angioplasty were able to continue the same recreational and occupational activities that they participated in prior to the procedure. Three of the 14 patients of the stented group have made major changes in their recreational activities. In the three, this is mainly secondary to their anticoagulation.

Several important observations can be drawn from this study. First, patients who present with long segments of occluded vein do not respond well to this treatment algorithm. It was our observation that those patients who had long segments of vein that required stenting sustained early thrombosis. In addition, a significant proportion of patients in the study who had early occlusions also had a hypercoagulable state and tested positive for factor V Leiden. It therefore becomes important in the treatment algorithm to assess patients for this hypercoagulable state. Currently, because of these factors, all patients presenting with axillo-subclavian vein thrombosis undergo a hypercoagulable workup, which includes evaluation for factor V Leiden.

Publications that are more recent include the use of mechanical thrombectomy devices to clear the thrombosed subclavian vein. These include both the ANGIOJET™[9] and Penumbra Indigo System™[10] mechanical aspiration system. These devices may decrease the amount of lytic agent that needs to be used and shorten the lysis time. By using these devices it may decrease the possibilities for bleeding complications related to the lytic treatment.

Current trends we see in our practice of venous thoracic outlet referrals demonstrate an increased volume of patients presenting. In addition, patients for the most part tend to be younger and more active than we have seen in the past. The increased number of patients seen may be due to a keener awareness of the syndrome among the referring primary care physicians in our area.

We now have begun to adopt the use of the Indigo system thrombectomy device to hopefully shorten the treatment times for these patients and decrease their bleeding risk secondary to TPA administration.

We have also begun doing the rib removal by an infraclavicular approach which allows removal of the key segment of rib and reduce the risk of brachial plexopathy.

In summary, the findings of the study support existing data that early operative intervention is safe and effective after catheter directed thrombolysis for effort thrombosis of the subclavian vein. Angioplasty performed after first rib resection produces excellent long-term patency and symptomatic relief. Patients with short segment venous structures that persist after angioplasty may be safely treated with stents and can expect long-term patency.

REFERENCES

1. Tilney ML, Griffiths HJG, and Edwards EE. Natural history of major venous thrombosis of the upper extremity. *Arch Surg*. 1970;101:792–6.
2. Paget J. Clinical lectures and essays. In: Howard M (ed.) *Anonymous*. London: Longmens green; 1875.
3. Aziz S, Straehley CJ, and Whelan TJ. Effort -related axillosubclavian thrombosis. *Am J Surg*. 1986;152:57–61.
4. Kunkel JM, and Machleder HI. Treatment of Paget Schroetter syndrome: A staged, multi-disciplinary approach. *Arch Surg*. 1989; 124:1153–8.
5. Molina JE. Need for emergency treatment in subclavian vein effort thrombosis. *J Am Coll Surg*. 1995;181:414–20.
6. Taylor LM, McAllister WR, Dennis DL, and Porter JM. Thrombolytic therapy followed by first rib resection for spontaneous ("effort") subclavian vein thrombosis. *Am J Surg*. 1989;124:1153–8.
7. Machleder HI. Evaluation of a new treatment strategy for Paget Schroetter syndrome, spontaneous thrombosis of the axillary subclavian vein. *J Vasc Surg*. 1993;17:305–17.
8. Porter JM, Bergan JJ, Goldstone J, and Greenfield LJ. Axillary subclavian vein thrombosis. *Perspect Vasc Surg*. 1991;4:85–98.
9. Shah AD, Bajakian DR, Olin JW, and Lookstein RA. Power pulse spray thrombectomy for treatment of Paget Schroetter syndrome. *AJR*. 2007;188:1215– 7.
10. Maldonado TS. Early multicenter experience using Indigo system for upper extremity DVT secondary to venous TOS. *Presented at the Veith symposium* 2017.

CHAPTER 48

Age Stratified, Perioperative, and One-Year Mortality after Abdominal Aortic Aneurysm Repair: A Statewide Experience

Rigberg DA, Zingmond DS, McGory ML, Maggard MA, Agustin M, Lawrence PF, Ko CY. *J Vasc Surg. 2006 Feb;43(2):224–9*

ABSTRACT

Objective The purpose of this study was to determine the in-hospital, 30-day, and 365-day mortality for the open repair of abdominal aortic aneurysms (AAAs), when stratified by age, in the general population. Age stratification could provide clinicians with information more applicable to an individual patient than overall mortality figures.

Methods In a retrospective analysis, data were obtained from the California Office of Statewide Health Planning and Development (OSHPD) for the years 1995 to 1999. Out-of-hospital mortality was determined via linkage to the state death registry. All patients undergoing AAA repair as coded by International Classification of Diseases, 9th Revision (ICD-9) procedure code 38.44 and diagnosis codes 441.4 (intact) and 441.3/441.5 (ruptured) in California were identified. Patients <50 years of age were excluded. We determined in-hospital, 30-day, and 365-day mortality, and stratified our findings by patient age. Multivariate logistic regression was used to determine predictors of mortality in the intact and ruptured AAA cohorts.

Results We identified 12,406 patients (9,778 intact, 2,628 ruptured). Mean patient age was 72.4 ± 7.2 years (intact) and 73.9 ± 8.2 (ruptured). Men comprised 80.9% of patients, and 90.8% of patients were white. Overall, intact AAA patient mortality was 3.8% in-hospital, 4% at 30 days, and 8.5% at 365 days. There was a steep increase in mortality with increasing age, such that 365-day mortality increased from 2.9% for patients 51 to 60 years old to 15% for patients 81 to 90 years old. Mortality from day 31 to 365 was greater than both in-hospital and 30-day mortality for all but the youngest intact AAA patients. Perioperative (in-hospital and 30-day) mortality for ruptured cases was 45%, and mortality at 1 year was 54%.

Conclusions There is continued mortality after the open repair of AAAs during postoperative days 31 to 365 that, for many patients, is greater than the perioperative death rate. This mortality increases dramatically with age for both intact and ruptured AAA repair.

AUTHOR COMMENTARY BY DAVID RIGBERG AND MARK AJALAT

Research Question Given that the goal of AAA repair is to prolong life and prevent eventual aneurysm rupture and death, what is the age stratified perioperative and 1-year mortality associated with open AAA repair?

Study Design This was a retrospective review of data obtained from the California Office of Statewide Health Planning and Development (OSHPD). From 1995–1999, all California residents at nonfederal institutions undergoing AAA repair for ruptured or intact aneurysms were identified and mortality was determined by review of the state death registry. Demographic data, Charlson Comorbidity Index, and annual hospital volume were recorded for both ruptured and intact aneurysms undergoing repair. Mortality rates at 0–30 days, 31–365 days, and 0–365 days after surgery were stratified by patient age and intact versus ruptured diagnosis, and this data was compared to age-matched data from the general population. Multivariate logistic regression analysis was used to determine predictors of mortality at each of the time periods.

Sample Size The study population consisted of all California residents aged 51–100 years who underwent open AAA repair for intact or ruptured aneurysms in nonfederal state institutions. Non-California residents were identified by ZIP code and excluded due to inability to track after discharge. A total of 12,406 patients who underwent repair were analyzed in this study. Only patients who underwent elective repair (planned admission >24 hours) or emergency rupture repair were included. Demographic review demonstrated that the majority of the patients were white (90.8%) and male (81%).

Follow-Up The OSHPD data is linked to the state death certificate to allow for determination of mortality rates at 30 and 365 days. Mortality rates were stratified by age and ruptured versus intact status, and results were compared to age-matched data from the general population obtained from the National Vital Statistics report.

Exclusion Criteria (1) Patients who were not California residents, (2) intact aneurysms but unscheduled admissions (846 patients), and (3) patient age <50 years.

Intervention or Treatment Received Patients with either intact or ruptured AAA all received open AAA repair.

Results In this study, the patient's average age was 73 years, 78.8% of repairs were for intact aneurysms, 90.8% of patients were white, and 81% males. For patients who underwent repair for intact AAAs, overall mortality was 3.8% in-hospital, 4% at 30 days, and 8.5% at 1 year. These results were stratified by age and demonstrated increasing mortality with increase in age as well as a 31–365-day mortality higher

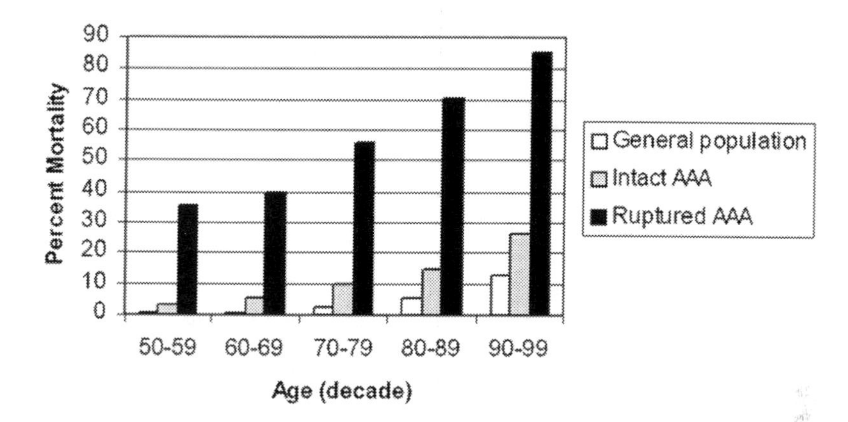

Figure 48.1 Overall 365-day mortality is displayed for both elective and nonelective abdominal aortic aneurysm (AAA) repair vs mortality of age-matched population controls for a 1-year period.

than that for age-matched population data (Figure 48.1). For all patients >59 years old who underwent repair for intact AAA, mortality at the balance of postoperative year was greater than the perioperative period. For patients who underwent repair for ruptured AAAs, overall mortality was 45.7% in-hospital, 45.1% at 30 days, and 53.5% at 1 year. Stratification of this data by age similarly demonstrated the general trend of increasing mortality with increasing age at all three time points (i.e., a 1-year mortality for 51–60 years is 35.4% and for >80 years is >70%). Multivariate logistic analysis demonstrated advancing age and Charlson Comorbidity Index were independent risk factors for mortality at all time points. Annual hospital volume analysis demonstrated mortality association with low volume hospitals for patients with intact and ruptured AAAs at the 30-day and 1-year time periods.

Study Limitations (1) The OSHPD data does not have any data regarding aneurysm size and how it relates to mortality. (2) ICD codes used in this study included the less technically demanding cases. (3) This study also solely focuses on open repair of AAA but the majority of AAA repair today is performed via EVAR. (4) The great majority of subjects in this study were white males and results may have limited applicability to patients of differing backgrounds. (5) Open repair of AAA may have significant associated morbidity and this data was not included.

Relevant Studies Included in reference list.

Study Impact The overall goal of aortic aneurysm repair is to prolong life by preventing eventual aneurysm rupture. With this in mind, perioperative and long-term mortality should be a vital part of the discussion during the preoperative evaluation. The findings of this study allow for the discussion to be tailored toward individual patients rather than a generalized population. Not only is it evident that mortality at all time points increases with age, but there is continued mortality beyond the perioperative period which is higher than that anticipated in the general population. Age stratified mortality rates during the perioperative period as well as overall 1-year mortality can be included in the preoperative discussion so that the patient can make an informed decision.

Mortality rates in this study are similar to other large scale studies which have investigated perioperative mortality in different populations. Schermerhorn et al. conducted a large retrospective study of the U.S. Medicare population using propensity score modeling and found in-hospital, 30-day, and 90-day mortality after open repair of intact AAA to be 4.6%, 4.8%, and 7%, respectively.[1] Additionally, they found that the excess surgical risk associated with open surgery does not return to the baseline until about 3 months postoperatively.[1] This parallels the numbers quoted in the aforementioned study of 3.8% in-hospital, 4% at 30 days, and 8.5% at 1 year. There is a paucity of studies which have addressed the 1-year mortality, with mortality rates ranging between 6%–10% for intact aneurysms and 45%–53% for ruptured AAA.[2] Findings from the aforementioned study are also similar in value.

This study was one of the first to stratify perioperative and long-term mortality rates by age group in those undergoing open repair of intact and ruptured AAA. Subsequent studies have also determined advancing age to be a risk factor for increased mortality. A large retrospective database analysis performed by Hicks et al. demonstrated significantly greater perioperative and 1-year mortality for open aortic repair in octogenarians when compared to nonoctogenarians (20.1% vs. 7.1% and 26% vs. 9.7%, respectively).[3] Additional studies have found up to a five-fold increase in mortality associated with open repair of intact AAA as compared to EVAR in patients aged >70 years.[4] Hence, open repair of AAA in the elderly population should be approached with caution. According to the CDC, the average life expectancy of the U.S. population is 78.6 years and the risk of death in patients without AAA is substantial.[5] Therefore, AAA repair may have a limited survival benefit in elderly patients with short life expectancy and an individualized patient risk assessment is crucial for determining the appropriateness for elective AAA repair.[3]

Selecting the right patient to undergo a major elective vascular operation such as open AAA repair involves a thorough preoperative evaluation and integration of multiple clinical factors. Several models and indices have been developed to help guide the clinician and patient during the preoperative discussion to determine those who may be at higher risk of adverse outcomes with an elective operation. Recently, there has been a focus on the association of patient frailty with adverse outcomes of vascular surgical procedures. The modified frailty index (mFI) is one model which has been found to be applicable to the vascular surgery patient population and may be a better indicator for morbidity and mortality when compared to other risk calculators.[6] The clinical frailty score (CFS) is another rapid assessment tool which has shown to be useful in predicting postoperative morbidity and mortality for those undergoing elective open AAA repair.[7] Furthermore, the CFS may also be useful in predicting the likelihood of nonhome discharge with long-term institutionalization as well as loss of independence.[8] This may be an essential part of the preoperative conversation between the patient and physician and can help manage expectations before a major elective surgery.[8] Additionally, it may provide the opportunity to address and manage modifiable risk factors which may optimize late outcomes after open aortic repair.[9] A systematic review conducted by Khashram et al. found that the use of statins, beta-blockers, and aspirin prior to elective AAA repair offers a distinct long-term survival advantage.[9] Last, there is a multitude of other determinants of long-term outcomes including operative technique, gender, ethnicity, and specific aneurysm pathophysiology and anatomy which are being investigated today.[10]

Overall, this landmark study has provided valuable information regarding age stratified mortality during the perioperative and 1-year time points which is helpful in guiding clinical decision-making. This targeted data allows for a meaningful patient-physician discussion whether in an elective or emergent setting. In addition to the increase in mortality rate with age after open repair of intact and ruptured AAA, it is important to also recognize the continued mortality which occurs beyond the initial perioperative period. Further studies will need to be conducted to investigate the etiology of this long-term mortality to allow for risk reduction in the postoperative period.

REFERENCES

1. Schermerhorn ML, Giles KA, Sachs T et al. Defining perioperative mortality after open and endovascular aortic aneurysm repair in the US Medicare population. *J Vasc Surg*. 2012;55(6):1834.
2. Dueck AD, Kucey DS, Johnston KW et al. Long-term survival and temporal trends in patient and surgeon factors after elective and ruptured abdominal aortic aneurysm surgery. *J Vasc Surg*. 2004;39(6):1261–1267.
3. Hicks CW, Obeid T, Arhuidese I et al. Abdominal aortic aneurysm repair in octogenarians is associated with higher mortality compared with nonoctogenarians. *J Vasc Surg*. 2016;64(4): doi:10.1016/j.jvs.2016.03.440.
4. Locham S, Lee R, Nejim B et al. Mortality after endovascular versus open repair of abdominal aortic aneurysm in the elderly. *J Surg Res*. 2017;215:153–159.
5. FastStats - Life Expectancy. *Centers for Disease Control and Prevention*, Centers for Disease Control and Prevention, 17 Mar. 2017, www.cdc.gov/nchs/fastats/life-expectancy.htm.
6. Ehlert BA, Najafian A, Orion KC et al. Validation of a modified frailty index to predict mortality in vascular surgery patients. *J Vasc Surg*. 2016;63(6): doi:10.1016/j.jvs.2015.12.023.
7. Al Shakarchi J, Fairhead J, Rajagopalan S et al. Impact of frailty on outcomes in patients undergoing open abdominal aortic aneurysm repair. *Ann Vasc Surg*. 2019; doi:10.1016/j.avsg.2019.11.017.
8. Donald GW, Ghaffarian AA, Isaac F et al. Preoperative frailty assessment predicts loss of independence after vascular surgery. *J Vasc Surg*. 2018;68(5):1382–1389.
9. Khashram M, Williman JA, Hider PN et al. Management of modifiable vascular risk factors improves late survival following abdominal aortic aneurysm repair: A systematic review and meta-analysis. *Ann Vasc Surg*. 2017;39:301–311.
10. Chandra V, Trang K, Virgin-Downey W et al. Long-term outcomes after repair of symptomatic abdominal aortic aneurysms. *J Vasc Surg*. 2018;68(5):360–1366.

CHAPTER 49

Transaxillary Decompression of Thoracic Outlet Syndrome Patients Presenting with Cervical Ribs

Gelabert HA, Rigberg DA, O'Connell JB, Jabori S, Jimenez JC, Farley S. J Vasc Surg. 2018 Oct;68(4):1143–9. doi: 10.1016/j.jvs.2018.01.057. Epub 2018 Apr 25

ABSTRACT

Objective The transaxillary approach to thoracic outlet decompression in the presence of cervical ribs offers the advantage of less manipulation of the brachial plexus and associated nerves. This may result in reduced incidence of perioperative complications, such as nerve injuries. Our objective was to report contemporary data for a series of patients with thoracic outlet syndrome (TOS) and cervical ribs managed through a transaxillary approach.

Methods We reviewed a prospectively maintained database for all consecutive patients who underwent surgery for TOS and who had a cervical rib. Symptoms, pre-operative evaluation, surgical details, complications, and postoperative outcomes form the basis of this report.

Results Between 1997 and 2016, there were 818 patients who underwent 1,154 procedures for TOS, including 873 rib resections. Of these, 56 patients underwent 70 resections for first and cervical ribs. Cervical ribs were classified according to the Society for Vascular Surgery reporting standards: 25 class 1, 17 class 2, 5 class 3, and 23 class 4. Presentations included neurogenic TOS in 49 patients and arterial TOS in 7. Operative time averaged 141 minutes, blood loss was 47 mL, and hospital stay averaged 2 days. No injuries to the brachial plexus, long thoracic, or thoracodorsal nerves were identified. One patient had partial phrenic nerve dysfunction that resolved. No hematomas, lymph leak, or early rehospitalizations occurred. Average follow-up was 591 days. Complete resolution or minimal symptoms were noted in 52 (92.8%) patients postoperatively. Significant residual symptoms requiring ongoing evaluation or pain management were noted in four (7.1%) at last follow-up. Somatic pain scores were reduced from 6.9 (pre-operatively) to 1.3 (at last visit). Standardized evaluation using shortened Disabilities of the Arm, Shoulder, and Hand scores indicated improvement from 60.4 (pre-operatively) to 31.3 (at last visit).

Conclusions This series of transaxillary cervical and first rib resections demonstrates excellent clinical outcomes with minimal morbidity. The presence of cervical ribs, a positive response to scalene muscle block, and abnormalities on electrodiagnostic testing are reliable indicators for surgery. A cervical rib in a patient with TOS suggests that there is excellent potential for improvement after first and cervical rib excision.

AUTHOR COMMENTARY BY HUGH GELABERT

The cervical rib is central to our understanding of thoracic outlet syndrome. In 1818, A.P. Cooper described the association of cervical ribs with the development of neurovascular symptoms in the same extremity.[1] This was called the cervical rib syndrome. This was a seminal observation which has informed our understanding of compressive syndromes of nerves and blood vessels. Thus, when H. Coote resected a cervical rib (1861) via a transcervical approach,[2] it was predicated on Cooper's observations. Since then, the resection of cervical ribs has most often been accomplished via the same approach used by Coote in 1861.

Roos first described the transaxillary resection of first ribs[3] and the transaxillary resection of cervical ribs.[4] He promoted the advantages of this approach: more direct visualization of the rib and reduced potential for injury to blood vessels and nerves. Despite these benefits, custom, familiarity, and bias have directed surgical preferences toward supraclavicular resection of the cervical rib. When "Transaxillary decompression of thoracic outlet syndrome patients presenting with cervical ribs" was published, there was no prior manuscript which described the exclusive use of primary transaxillary cervical rib resection in a similar sized group.

At the time of publication, the largest series in literature was that of Sanders and Hammond[5] with 39 cervical rib resections done via a supraclavicular approach. More recently, Chang et al.[6] published a series of 20 patients who underwent 23 cervical rib resections via a combination of supraclavicular and transaxillary approaches. With 70 cervical rib resections, "Transaxillary decompression of thoracic outlet syndrome patients presenting with cervical ribs" is the largest series of transaxillary cervical rib operations in the literature.[8] It is a retrospective analysis of a prospectively accumulated cohort. The patient assessment was protocol driven, the surgical approach for cervical rib resection was standardized, and the follow-up protocols used standardized outcomes measures.

A total of 105 cervical ribs were identified (56 index and 49 contralateral) and a total of 70 symptomatic cervical rib operations were performed. No neurological or hemorrhagic complications were observed. Arterial cases required more time, incurring slighter more blood loss, yet having equal hospital stay. The overall follow-up period averaged 591 days. The outcomes were excellent with improvement in almost all. The large number of rib resections (70) allowed for a meaningful use of comparative statistical analysis of different cervical rib classes, operations, presentations, and genders. The data set provided the most granular description of a cervical rib patient population.

In keeping with the recently published Society for Vascular Surgery Reporting Guidelines,[7] the project made use of standardized outcomes measures such as QUICK DASH scores and Somatic Pain Scores to provide a more intelligible description of results. Analysis of the data indicated that the type of operation, the type cervical rib (class 1, 2, 3, or 4), and the gender made no difference as to outcomes. Arterial presentations were notable for having less pain and disability at the end of follow-up. About 27% of patients had prior surgical procedures and 62% had co-existing medical conditions which would adversely affect their outcomes. Despite this, the presence of a cervical rib was predictive of excellent outcomes: At the end of the study, 92% improved. Residual symptoms were noted only in neurogenic cases.

Impact This project allowed the most detailed description of the largest cohort of cervical rib patients—detailing the presentation, evaluation, management, and surgical outcomes. It has defined transaxillary surgical approach to cervical ribs. By using standardized measures, it has provided an unambiguous benchmark for comparison with future endeavors.

REFERENCES

1. Cooper A, and Travers B (Eds.). *An Exostosis. Surgical Essays*. London: Longman; 1821: p. 128.
2. Coote H. Exostosis of the left transverse process of the seventh cervical vertebra surrounded by blood vessels and nerves: successful removal. *Lancet*. 1951:i:360.
3. Roos DB. Transaxillary approach to first rib resection to relieve thoracic outlet syndrome. *Ann Surg*. 1966;163:354–358.
4. Roos DB. Experience with first rib resection for thoracic outlet syndrome. *Ann Surg*. 1971 Mar;173(3):429–42.
5. Sanders RJ, and Hammond SL. Management of cervical ribs and anomalous first ribs causing neurogenic thoracic outlet syndrome. *J Vasc Surg*. 2002 Jul;36(1):51–6.
6. Chang KZ, Likes K, Davis K, Demos J, and Freischlag JA. The significance of cervical ribs in thoracic outlet syndrome. *J Vasc Surg*. 2013 Mar;57(3):771–5.
7. Illig KA, Donahue D, Duncan A et al. Reporting standards of the Society for Vascular Surgery for thoracic outlet syndrome. *J Vasc Surg*. 2016 Sep;64(3):e23–35.
8. Gelabert HA, Rigberg DA, O'Connell JB, Jabori S, Jimenez JC, and Farley S. Transaxillary decompression of thoracic outlet syndrome patients presenting with cervical ribs. *J Vasc Surg*. 2018 Oct;68(4):1143–9.

CHAPTER 50

Stenting and Medical Therapy for Atherosclerotic Renal-Artery Stenosis

Cooper CJ, Murphy TP, Cutlip DE, Jamerson K, Henrich W, Reid DM, Cohen DJ, Matsumoto AH, Steffes M, Jaff MR et al. N Engl J Med. 2014 Jan 2;370(1):13–22. doi: 10.1056/NEJMoa1310753. Epub 2013 Nov 18

ABSTRACT

Background Atherosclerotic renal-artery stenosis is a common problem in the elderly. Despite two randomized trials that did not show a benefit of renal-artery stenting with respect to kidney function, the usefulness of stenting for the prevention of major adverse renal and cardiovascular events is uncertain.

Methods We randomly assigned 947 participants who had atherosclerotic renal-artery stenosis and either systolic hypertension while taking two or more antihypertensive drugs or chronic kidney disease to medical therapy plus renal-artery stenting or medical therapy alone. Participants were followed for the occurrence of adverse cardiovascular and renal events (a composite endpoint of death from cardiovascular or renal causes, myocardial infarction, stroke, hospitalization for congestive heart failure, progressive renal insufficiency, or the need for renal-replacement therapy).

Results Over a median follow-up period of 43 months (interquartile range, 31 to 55), the rate of the primary composite endpoint did not differ significantly between participants who underwent stenting in addition to receiving medical therapy and those who received medical therapy alone (35.1% and 35.8%, respectively; hazard ratio with stenting, 0.94; 95% confidence interval [CI], 0.76–1.17; P = 0.58). There were also no significant differences between the treatment groups in the rates of the individual components of the primary endpoint or in all-cause mortality. During follow-up, there was a consistent modest difference in systolic blood pressure favoring the stent group (–2.3 mmHg; 95% CI, –4.4 to –0.2; P = 0.03).

Conclusions Renal-artery stenting did not confer a significant benefit with respect to the prevention of clinical events when added to comprehensive, multifactorial medical therapy in people with atherosclerotic renal-artery stenosis and hypertension or chronic kidney disease (funded by the National Heart, Lung and Blood Institute and others; ClinicalTrials.gov number, NCT00081731).

EXPERT COMMENTARY BY TRISTEN T. CHUN AND STEVEN M. FARLEY

Research Question/Objective The Cardiovascular Outcomes in Renal Atherosclerotic Lesions (CORAL) study aimed to investigate the clinical outcomes of stenting in atherosclerotic renal artery disease. Specifically, this study was performed to assess the effects of renal-artery stenting on major cardiovascular and renal outcomes in patients with hypertension, chronic kidney disease, or both as a result of atherosclerotic renal artery stenosis.

Study Design This was a prospective, multicenter, unblinded and open-label, two-arm, randomized control trial which assigned study participants to either medical therapy plus stenting or medical therapy alone for renal artery stenosis.

Sample Size A total of 5,322 potential participants were initially screened for this study, and 947 underwent randomization. Of these, 459 participants were included in the medical therapy plus stenting group and 472 in the medical therapy alone group. The baseline characteristics of the participants were well-matched between the two groups. A total of 19 crossovers from the medical therapy alone group to the stent group occurred, and seven were ultimately approved by a designated crossover committee.

Follow-Up Study participants were followed for a median of 43 months with interquartile ranges from 31 to 55.

Inclusion/Exclusion Criteria Adult participants aged 18 years or older with severe renal artery stenosis as defined by the following criteria were enrolled into this study: angiography showing stenosis of at least 80% but less than 100% of the diameter or stenosis of at least 60% but less than 80% with a systolic pressure gradient of at least 20 mmHg. Severe renal artery stenosis could also be identified using duplex ultrasonography (systolic velocity >300 cm/sec), magnetic resonance angiography (stenosis greater than 80% or stenosis greater than 70% with certain features) or computed tomography angiography (stenosis greater than 80% or stenosis greater than 70% with certain features). Participants with documented history of hypertension on two or more antihypertensive medications or those who did not have hypertension but had renal artery stenosis in the setting of chronic kidney disease stage 3 or greater (estimated GFR less than 60 ml/min/1.73 m^2 of body-surface area) could be enrolled into this study.

Exclusion criteria included renal artery stenosis due to fibromuscular dysplasia, chronic kidney disease from causes other than ischemic nephropathy or chronic kidney disease with serum creatinine level greater than 4.0 mg per deciliter (354 μmol/L), length of the kidney less than 7 cm, renal artery stenosis not amenable for treatment with a stent, and renal artery size less than 3.5 mm or greater than 8.0 mm. Allergies to intravenous contrast and medications including aspirin, clopidogrel, and ticlopidine were also used as exclusion criteria.

Intervention or Treatment Received All randomized participants received antiplatelet therapy and antihypertensive medical therapies using the angiotensin II type-1 receptor blocker candesartan (Atacand, AstraZeneca), with or without hydrochlorothiazide and the combination agent amlodipine-atorvastatin (Caduet, Pfizer). These medications were provided free of charge to the study participants and were titrated to desired target blood pressure levels (140/90 mmHg or 130/80 mmHg depending on coexisting conditions) and lipid levels as per study guidelines. The participants in the medical therapy plus stenting group had a Palmaz Genesis stent (Cordis) placed with or without pre-dilation of the artery. For those who had more than one stenosis, stenting was performed either as a single procedure or multiple procedures at 2–4-week intervals.

Results The primary endpoint of this study was a composite of death from cardiovascular or renal causes, myocardial infarction, stroke, hospitalization for congestive heart failure, progressive renal insufficiency, or the need for permanent renal-replacement therapy. The secondary endpoints included all-cause mortality.

Stenting resulted in a significant reduction in renal artery stenosis. However, no significant difference was observed in the occurrence of the primary composite endpoint between the medial therapy plus stent group and the medical therapy alone group (35.1% vs. 35.8%; HR 0.94, 95% CI 0.76–1.17; P = 0.58). In addition, no significant differences were observed in the individual components of the primary endpoint or in all-cause mortality. A reduction in systolic blood pressure was observed in both treatment groups. Participants in the stent group had significantly lower systolic blood pressure than those in medical therapy only group (−2.3 mmHg; 95% CI −4.4–0.2 mmHg; P = 0.03) and this difference persisted throughout the follow-up period.

Study Limitations There were several limitations identified by the study authors. First, participants with mild renal artery stenosis (60% or more) could be enrolled into the study, and these participants may not benefit from intervention as there is an ongoing debate about the degree of stenosis that would necessitate intervention. The authors did, however, report that a subgroup analysis of participants with 80% or more stenosis still failed to show the benefit of intervention. Second, participants with fibromuscular dysplasia were excluded from this study, while there is evidence to suggest that percutaneous intervention could improve hypertension in this population. Third, not every eligible participant was enrolled into this study, and a significant number of participants were withdrawn at the discretion of treating physicians as they were believed to benefit from stenting due to their severity of disease.

Other issues raised by the study authors include whether the results of medical therapy can be replicated in routine clinical practice. A combination of an angiotensin II type-1 receptor blocker, with or without a thiazide-type diuretic, a calcium channel blocker, with the addition of a statin, and an antiplatelet agent was used in this study. Participants who were treated with these medications alone for their renal artery stenosis achieved remarkable results in terms of cardiovascular and renal outcomes, despite advanced age and other comorbidities including hypertension, diabetes, and chronic kidney disease.

Relevant Studies Several early studies from the 1990s suggested that renal-artery stent placement was technically feasible without major complications, and significant reduction in systolic blood pressure or stabilization of renal function could be achieved with renal artery angioplasty and stenting in patients with atherosclerotic renovascular disease.[1–4] However, randomized trials that followed, including the Angioplasty and Stenting for Renal Artery Lesions (ASTRAL) trial and the Stent Placement and Blood Pressure and Lipid-Lowering for the Prevention of Progression of Renal Dysfunction Caused by Atherosclerotic Ostial Stenosis of the Renal Artery (STAR) trial, failed to show the benefit of renal artery angioplasty and stent placement with regard to hypertension and renal function.[5–8]

This CORAL study was designed to address some of the criticisms that arose in these trials and to specifically detect a clinical benefit with respect to major cardiovascular and renal outcomes. The results of this study were described in a subsequent Cochrane systematic review, which reported that there were insufficient data to conclude that revascularization with renal artery balloon angioplasty with or without stenting is superior to medical therapy alone for the treatment of atherosclerotic renal artery stenosis.[9]

Study Impact The results of the CORAL trial have improved our understanding of how to treat atherosclerotic renal artery stenosis. Early, uncontrolled trials suggested that angioplasty and stenting for renal artery stenosis may result in clinical benefits including a reduction in blood pressure or stabilization of renal function. The result was an observed rapid increase in the volume of percutaneous renal artery interventions among Medicare beneficiaries in the United States. Renal artery angioplasty and stenting was poised to be a potential paradigm shift in the management of renovascular hypertension and chronic kidney disease. However, subsequent randomized trials were not able to replicate the findings of the early trials and failed to show a benefit of intervention with regard to blood pressure and kidney function. As a result, concerns about the efficacy and potential cost implications of renal artery stenting emerged.

The CORAL study was designed to elucidate the effects of renal artery stenting on major cardiovascular and renal outcomes and showed that when added to comprehensive medical therapy, stenting did not confer a significant clinical benefit, in accordance with the prior renal artery stenting randomized trials.

REFERENCES

1. Blum U, Krumme B, Flugel P et al. Treatment of ostial renal-artery stenoses with vascular endoprostheses after unsuccessful balloon angioplasty. *N Engl J Med.* 1997;336(7):459–65.
2. Burket MW, Cooper CJ, Kennedy DJ et al. Renal artery angioplasty and stent placement: Predictors of a favorable outcome. *Am Heart J.* 2000;139(1 Pt 1):64–71.
3. Harden PN, MacLeod MJ, Rodger RS et al. Effect of renal-artery stenting on progression of renovascular renal failure. *Lancet.* 1997;349(9059):1133–6.
4. Watson PS, Hadjipetrou P, Cox SV et al. Effect of renal artery stenting on renal function and size in patients with atherosclerotic renovascular disease. *Circulation.* 2000;102(14):1671–7.
5. Plouin PF, Chatellier G, Darne B et al. Blood pressure outcome of angioplasty in atherosclerotic renal artery stenosis: A randomized trial. *Hypertension.* 1998;31(3):823–9.
6. Webster J, Marshall, F, Abdalla M et al. Randomized comparison of percutaneous angioplasty vs continued medical therapy for hypertensive patients with atheromatous renal artery stenosis. *J Hum Hypertens.* 1998;12(5):329–35.
7. The ASTRAL Investigators. Revascularization versus medical therapy for renal-artery stenosis. *N Engl J Med.* 2009;361(20):1953–62.
8. Bax L, Woittiez AJ, Kouwenberg HJ et al. Stent placement in patients with atherosclerotic renal artery stenosis and impaired renal function: A randomized trial. *Ann Intern Med.* 2009;150(12):840–8.
9. Jenks S, Yeoh SE, Conway BR. Balloon angioplasty, with and without stenting, versus medical therapy for hypertensive patients with renal artery stenosis. *Cochrane Database syst Rev.* 2014;(12):CD002944.

Index

A

D

E

J

L

M

N

O

P

Q

R

S

T

Printed in the United States
by Baker & Taylor Publisher Services